Nature's Secrets
for
Health and Beauty

Minoo Golnazar

Copyright 1998 by Minoo Golnazar

This book demonstrates
various methods of preparation and application of herbal remedies. The
information provided is not for individuals with serious health problems, and
should not take place of one's doctor appropriate treatment.

ISBN # 0-9664814-0-2
Published by Minoo's Skin Care Co.
800-726-6466

Editor:Behzad Pirazizi
Copy Editor: Pamela Durham Bollanol

Book design & Illustrations : Sepehr Partnership

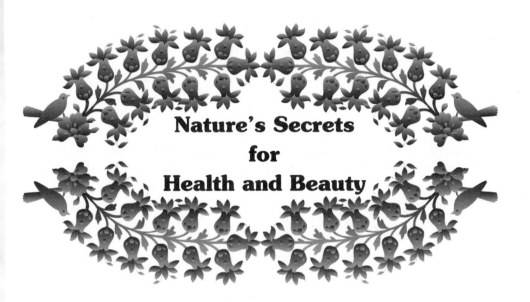

Nature's Secrets
for
Health and Beauty

Minoo Golnazar

MINOO
Natural
Skin Care

About the Author

Born and raised in Iran, Minoo's early interest in skin care came about when she was thirteen years old. At that time, her skin began undergoing a change in pigmentation. The dermatologist she consulted instructed her to keep out of the sun and gave her two products to use on her skin. After using his medications, which were primarily herbal, Minoo noticed that her skin responded positively. This made her curious to learn more about herbs, so she began reading herbal books and making her own extracts.

Soon she was collecting herbs and flowers that were therapeutic for the skin and body. After learning to dry them, cook them, and extract their oils and essences, she began making her own skin products, such as cleansers, toners, fresh fruit masks, and moisturizers. She also began experimenting with herbs in her food, creating numerous recipes for soups and salads.

By the time Minoo was eighteen, she had a little laboratory in her room that contained all kinds of herbal oils and essences. It was at this point in her life that she decided that the science of herbs would be her life's work.

True to her earlier decision, Minoo attended college and obtained a degree in botany. With the knowledge of biochemical interactions between plants and the human body, she was able to create preparations that were natural and beneficial, especially for the skin, the body's largest and most visible organ.

Today Minoo continues to study plants that benefit the skin and enable it to retain its suppleness throughout life. She also continues her research on new herbs that fight the primary foes of the skin — sun, dehydration, aging, and acne.

The herbs and essences Minoo uses in her completely natural products are gathered from all over the world. Each product has been tested under clinically controlled conditions in her American laboratory to assure purity and effectiveness.

Acknowledgments

I would like to acknowledge my inner voice, the inspiration that has always guided me in life and provided me with great hope, strength, and a positive attitude.

This book represents a strong belief in nature's energy and power and in my ability to use it for foods and natural medicines.

The preparation and foundation of this book would not have been possible without the encouragement of friends. I would like to thank all the students who participated in my classes and seminars.

I have been inspired by many people throughout my life to be a better human as well as better healer and educator. My desire is that this book will be a reward for all those people who have given care and encouragement to me.

I am grateful for the precious treasures in my life, especially my son, Parsa, whose friendliness and support throughout the work cannot be expressed by words and gestures.

My gratitude is especially due to my father who has truly inspired and supported me.

How to Use This Book

Nature's Secrets for Health and Beauty is a comprehensive guide to alternative medicines, health and beauty. It is designed for both professionals and individuals who desire a practical guide for the use and application of herbs. Practicing herbs is fun and safer than modern drugs for the mind and body. However, herbs can be powerful, so it is not possible to predict each individual's reaction to a given herb.

In addition to offering a general introduction and brief history of herbal medicine, this book also demonstrates various methods of preparation and application of herbal remedies. All nutritional, medicinal, and health information presented in this book is based on the personal research, training, and experience of the author and is correct to the best of her knowledge. Your response to any herbal remedy may differ from the author's experience. For this reason, Natures' Secrets for Health and Beauty shares both the beneficial as well as the undesirable effects associated with each herb, with the understanding that you will accept responsibility for your own health.

The result of a given treatment cannot be guaranteed, nor can the author or publisher be held responsible for any adverse conditions resulting from the use of remedies offered in this book. Please consult your professional healer as well as your own inner guidance as you make use of the information provided. May Natures' Secrets for Health and Beauty contribute a great deal of pleasure and health information.

Contents

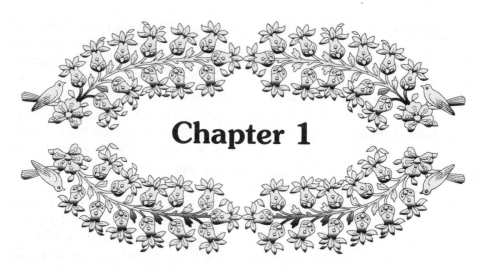

Chapter 1

Introduction

Knowledge of nature's beauty in general, and its plant types specifically, has interested many people who have partaken of it, either as a profession or hobby. In any case, the interest in plants and flowers dates back to my childhood in Iran. My mother and grandmother used to tend herbs and flowers in our backyard. Collecting, drying, and preserving those herbs and flowers triggered my interest and fascination. As I started helping them tend and collect the herbs, an emotional bond was set in me. At times, I could imagine that I could talk to plants, encouraging them to reach the best of their health and beauty.

At the age of thirteen, changes in the form of pigmentation appeared on my skin. Having consulted a dermatologist, I was given some skin care medication and was told to protect my skin from the sun. The result was positive. This event triggered my curiosity. Further investigations proved that the basic constituents of this medication were herbs. I started reading books about herbs and their beneficial uses, and as a hobby, I began collecting and preserving herbs, flowers and other types of plants. Gradually, I learned the ways of processing herbs in order to derive oils. Later my hobby became more methodical, and I started recording my experiences.

In Iran, herbs and wild flowers grow in the mountains. I often walked on wilderness trails looking for plants and herbs. Their various colors and methods of growing intrigued me, and I wanted to learn everything I could about those beauties of nature. Then I bought a large notebook, and on every excursion, I brought back herbs and wild flowers. After drying them, I glued them in my recording book, and with the help of my mother, I identified and described each of them in terms of their uses and medicinal values.

My formal training in science was another step forward. By then, I had learned the fine art of collecting certain herbs, the timing and methods of their harvesting, levels of energy, and uses.

In Iran, we were taught that each part of a plant has a different energy level which varies according to the season. For instance, in the spring, leaves and flowers contain high energy; in the summer, fruits obtain their energy level; and roots and seeds, in the winter. Thus, the herbs are classified according to these energies such as warm, cool, and neutral.

In Middle Eastern countries, everyone is raised with some knowledge of how and when to use herbs. They use plants for food, healing, and to treat different illnesses according to their energy level, taste, fragrances, and geographical location.

I still remember that when my grandmother suffered from a cold, cough, flu, or fever she would use herbs with a cool energy level. She would use flax or quince seeds, soaking them in hot water until the mucilage was attained to soothe her throat and suppress coughing. At times marshmallow root also helped as an alternative. When she was out of marshmallow root, she would use rice starch, stirring one tablespoon in a glass of hot water until it was thick, then drinking it. The rice starch would cool her throat because of its cool energy. Moreover, rice starch contains vitamin B complex which relaxes the throat tension.

I also learned from my grandmother that the taste of each plant provides information about its energy level and nutritional properties. For example, sweet plants are nutritional, sour plants aid digestion, bitter plants purify the blood, and salty plants balance the body's water and potassium levels.

Herbal Classification According to the Energy Level in Iran

The first step in classifying herbs and plants in Iran is to recognize their energy level. Each plants is believed to have varying amounts of energy and biochemical properties.

In Iran, even preparation of food is according to this energy classification. They believe in mixing foods of both cool and warm energy levels to maintain the physical, emotional and chemical balance of the body. They include fresh and dried herbs in salads or main meals everyday. A basket of fresh herbs such as tarragon, basil, mint, chives, marjoram, radish, green onion, watercress, and parsley is a prominent part of the Iranian food habit.

In Iran, lunch is heavier than the evening meal. The summer afternoon snacks made of fresh herbs, feta cheese, fresh bread, cucumbers, and tomatoes are widely welcome. A winter snack would consist of ground walnuts, chopped feta cheese, herbs, and breads served with a cup of fresh herbal, cardamom, or cinnamon tea.

During month of September, most Iranian housewives prepare jams from fresh organic fruits, pickle foods, and dry herbs as the supply of fresh fruits and herbs is scarce during the winter. Almost every family has a large store room for its winter food supplies such as organic fruit jams, jellies, tomato paste, dried herbs, onion, garlic, pickles and spices. During the winter in Iran, foods with warm energy are used to keep the body warm and protect it against colds and flu.

In ancient Middle Eastern culture, illnesses were thought to have different energy levels. Thus, every illness was treated with foods of the appropriate energy level. A person who suffered from a warm energy disease such as a fever, flu, or a sore throat would be treated with foods of cool energy such as sweet lime, cloves, rose hips and citrus fruits to cool the body temperature and soothe the pain. People suffering from cool energy illnesses such as low blood pressure or diarrhea, were treated with foods of warm energy such as dates, ginger, cinnamon, peppermint, honey and yarrow to balance their blood pressure and cure their

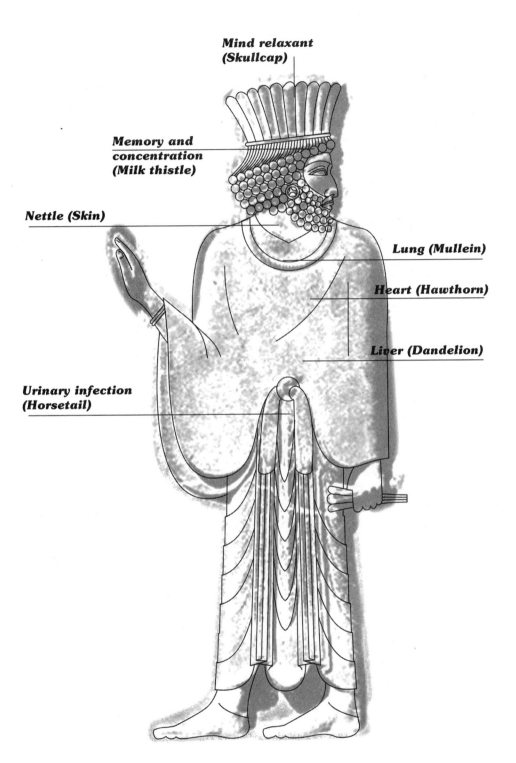

Mind relaxant
(Skullcap)

Memory and
concentration
(Milk thistle)

Nettle (Skin)

Lung (Mullein)

Heart (Hawthorn)

Liver (Dandelion)

Urinary infection
(Horsetail)

diarrhea.

Like herbs and foods, people have different energy levels too. In Middle Eastern foods, energies are coordinated with each person's natural energy level. People who have a cooler energy level eat foods with warm energy levels to avoid losing energy, whereas people who have a warm energy levels eat foods with cool energy level to stay balanced. For example, people with fair skin are believed to have cooler energy level than people with darker complexions. Therefore, fair skinned people should avoid eating a lot of foods with cool energy, as they may lose their energy, feel tired, and get a heavy muscle feeling and watery mouth. To heal this, they should eat dates, ginger, figs, and cinnamon which are foods of warm energy. If people with fair skin become constipated or get burning sensations with urination, they should take cooling foods, such as sweet lime, lemon, watermelon, and cool energy vegetables, and drink a lot of water to reduce the burning sensation. People with darker complexions should not eat too much of foods with warm energy, foods like dates, ginger, cinnamon, and other spices, because their mouths may get dry, their energy level may drop, and they may become constipated. These people feel better after eating foods with cool energy, such as cucumbers, yogurt, spinach, and lettuce.

Physicians in the Middle East believe that foods should be taken in equal quantity according to their energy levels. For example, to promote healthy liver function, a meal should consist of both cool and warm energy levels. Moreover, the liver has a tendency to store excesses of warm energy, which can be problematic. For instance, if too much food with warm energy such as cinnamon and chilies are taken, the energy that is stored in the liver may cause acne, liver spots, dry mouth, or other disorders. In this case, the liver must be detoxified with cool energy herbs such as dandelion, gentian, and bilberry juice. In Iran, cool energy herbs like gentian, dandelion, bilberry and flax are used to detoxify the liver and purify the blood.

Ancient Iranians used the energy and power of plants containing essential oils to treat emotional, mental, and physical pain and tension. Sometimes the aroma of flowers, such as roses and orange blossoms, and orange was used during delivery to ease pain and decrease the anxiety. They also massaged essential oils of rose and orange on the temples and shoulders to ease body tension during delivery . This technique helps essential oils to penetrate into the body through the pores of the skin and infiltrate to the bloodstream in order to ease anxiety, tension, and pain. Another remedy in cases of delivery consisted of a mixture of lemon balm, orange blossom, and blackberry tea. Steamed roses and sandalwood were also used to alleviate emotional pain during delivery.

Plants used in aromatherapy soothe the body when used in steam, massage, and baths. The herbs containing essential oils are separated during harvest. Sometimes, in order to relieve depression and other emotional disorders, herbal pillows are made to be used in bathing or during sleep. Such treatments also facilitate dreaming and psychological processes.

Warm energy herbs containing vola-tile oils such as garlic, rosemary, sage, and turnip can be mixed with cool energy herbs for liver detoxification. Volatile oils kill harmful bacteria and are found in garlic, onion, and sage, which all have warm energy and are also highly anti-septic and antibacterial. They are ideal for liver and gallbladder detoxification, as well as for antibiotic treatment of such internal disorders as infections of the bladder, kidneys, liver, or blood.

Classification of Common Herbs and Foods According to Their Energetic					
Warm	**Cool**	**Neutral**	**Warm**	**Cool**	**Neutral**
bell pepper	apricot	alfalfa	kiwi fruit	orange	
black pepper	beans	almond	lamb	peach	
bok choy	beef	apple	mango	plum	
broccoli	beef liver	calf liver	marjoram	potato	
cabbage	beer	carrot	onion	rhubarb	
cantaloupe	beets	corn	papaya	rice	
cauliflower	blackberry	kidney beans	parsley	root beer	
cheese	blueberry	pear	peanut,cashew	sour cherry	
chicken	celery	persimmon	pineapple	spinach	
chicken liver	cherry	rabbit	pistachio	strawberry	
chocolate	cilantro	salmon	pumpkin	sweet lemon	
cinnamon	cow's milk	squash	pumpkin seeds	tea	
clams	cranberry	turkey	quince	tobacco	
cocoa	cucumber	veal	radish	tomato	
coffee	dandelion	zucchini	raisin	watermelon	
date	duck		red cabbage	yogurt	
egg	egg plant		seeds		
garbanzo beans	fava beans		sesame		
fig	fish		shrimp		
garlic	grapefruit		sunflower seeds		
ginger	green beans		tarragon		
goat's milk	lemon, lime		urnip		
grape	lentil		walnut		
honeydew	nectarine		wheat		
horseradish	oats		wine		

This chart shows the types of energy existing in our daily foods. The chart can help balance our daily diet for better digestion.

Planting and Collecting Herbs

How to Collect and Dry Herbs and Plants

My strong interest in drying and collecting plants began during my teenage years, and the idea of collecting and preserving the beauty of nature throughout the year was quite fascinating. Later on because of my scientific training and experiences, I learned when to collect certain herbs and specific methods of drying them in order to preserve their special properties.

For instance, as mentioned earlier, the medicinal value and energy levels of certain plants is in their root system, thus they must be collected during winter before any fresh growth interferes with its energy level. If energy levels of buds and barks of certain plants are of interest, then spring is the best season for harvesting. This is the time of active growing and greatest energy in these parts.

By observing, comparing, and experimenting with plants over time, I learned to sort them according to their medicinal properties and energy values. Plants and flowers are sensitive and have certain energy levels. Thus, working with plants requires special care and knowledge.

Most medicinal herbs can be grown in your backyard or patio pots, but gathering, growing, and harvesting other plants should follow special rules. Plants need to grow in their own natural environment in order to obtain their active properties. Remember that plants should not be collected along highways, hiking paths, or areas with a possibility of pesticide pollution. Since it is difficult to know whether the plants you purchase are free from contamination, it is safe to find a reputable supplier who grows plants in the country under optimal conditions. Make sure that your supplier dries and preserves them correctly. When you cultivate your own herbs, you can be certain of their quality.

Plants must be handled with utmost care. Before picking a plant, be sure of its identity. It is very easy, for example, to confuse dandelions with certain poisonous plants that grow beside the roads or highways. Learn to identify plants by their color and aroma.

The exact reason for gathering a plant is also very important. Choose only healthy plants, and be aware of decay and insects. Separate the chosen plants from any surrounding leaves or grass, and wash the roots.

How to Plant Seeds

If you decide to grow herbs indoors, you can use either a glass container or clay pot. Mix equal parts of sand and peat with topsoil. Keep the temperature between 70 and 75 degrees Fahrenheit to speed germination of the seeds and growth of small saplings. Small soil heating cables are available in several sizes to keep the temperature stable. Pour the seeds as sparingly and as evenly as possible because seedlings growing very close to each other may have poor air circulation and succumb to damping-off disease. In case of crowding, saplings can be transplanted. Sprinkle one-fourth inch of top soil over the seeds, then press them with the palm of your hand.

Label each container and check daily. Never allow the soil to dry. If signs of dryness appear, add water. When the seeds sprout, move them to brighter light. From planting the seeds to harvesting, growing of herbs takes between six to ten weeks depending on type.

What Makes Plants Grow ?

Plant survival depends on the processes of photosynthesis and respiration. Photosynthesis is the process by which plants manufacture food by taking energy from the sun or any source of light, carbon dioxide from the air, and water from the soil. In the process, saccharine is created which is a versatile food and can supply immediate energy to plants, be stored as food for later use, or be used as building material within the plant body.

Nutrients added to the soil help in the production of saccharine and growth of plants. During photosynthesis, respiration also takes place. In respiration, carbon dioxide is consumed and oxygen is produced. Fertilizing is also a way to help plant growth. A proper fertilizer consist of liquid organic matter.

How to Dry Plants

If you are collecting and drying herbs for medicinal and healing uses, it is better to categorize and separate them according to their healing properties. Next, provide a thin muslin cover for shade. You will also need a box with a wire-screened bottom to permit full air circulation. Carefully spread herbs on the screen in a well-ventilated, partially shaded place. Turn them once a day so that they dry thoroughly and evenly, without decay or browning of their leaves.

To obtain the best color and flavor or herbal potency, store them in a glass jar or proper packaging. Remember to package in such a way that the stems and roots remain dry for long periods of time.

The Tradition of Herbs

Using herbs and plants as medicine has a long tradition in the Far and Middle East. Essentially every culture has learned about the variety of natural energy levels and therapeutic values of plants to be used as medicine or daily diet.

Traditional methods of the Chinese and Iranian cultures have changed little over the centuries. Traditional healers have always been weighing a series of herbs, giving them to the patient, and directing the use and duration. They usually prescribe herbs in standard formulas which may be slightly adjusted for present uses depending on the patient and specific conditions. The formula could include as many as four to twenty herbs with biochemical interaction between them that is as significant as their individual properties.

Thus, the energy and therapeutic value of herbs has played a vital role in medicinal traditions of many cultures since ancient times. Herbs have always been used at home for minor illnesses or supplemented for more potential remedies prescribed by professional heal-ers. However, herbs can be taken as beverages, quite simply as tea. Another way to enjoy herbs at home is to experience the pleasure of preparing real homemade herbal remedies. Although consumption of most of the herbs is quite safe, one should not always attempt self-prescription or exceed recommended doses.

In this chapter, various topics that include the making of extracts, herbal teas, beverages, tinctures, and decoctions for the treatment of pains and disorders, as well as daily use, are presented.

Mind and Nerve Relaxation

Daily life with its pressures, challenges, and tensions of ten leaves us no time to relax. A healthy diet, including fresh herbs and herbal drinks, plus regular exercise can increase our power over emotional stresses and release many physical tensions.

If the suffering from exhaustion or stress persists for longer periods, particularly mental stress, try herbal teas to relax the nervous system. Using the recipes for herbal teas at the end of this book is beneficial for the nervous system. Good health depends on a balanced nervous system as it is directly linked to the immune system. The immune system controls the ability of the body to resist infections and recover rapidly from injuries or diseases. Maintenance of health is the result of harmonious functioning of the nervous and immune systems. If your life is challenging and tense, it is best to block further negativity from your mind, drink herbal tea, lie down, and relax. Tea made from herbs such as ginseng, chamomile, vervain, passionflower, cowslip, and skullcap, either singular or in combination, can ease physical and emotional tensions. A healthy body has an infinitely greater capacity to adjust to external pressures and to adapt to the external world when the body's internal functioning remains normal.

Many herbs can act on the immune and nervous systems to help the body adapt more effectively to stress of all kinds, whether physical, mental, or emotional. Certain plants and their essential oils are considered adaptogenic, i.e., they are able to change the power of adaptability. These plants support the nervous system and ease emotional tension by acting directly with the body's physiological processes. Ginseng root, for example, is a fine remedy for mental and physical stresses. Herbal aromatherapy can also have a powerful calming effect on the mind, body, and nerves. There are two easy ways to use herbs for relaxation... boiling them for their aroma or soaking them in a bath. The essential oils of herbs are released by the hot water and absorbed through the skin into the bloodstream. Many herbs, such as sandalwood, rose, orange, and lavender, when used in aromatherapy are also excellent stress reducers. The oils or perfumes of these plants can be used for steaming and bathing (see section on aromatherapy for more details).

Alternatively, fill your bathtub with hot water, take a muslin pillow and fill it with lavender, rose, melissa, and orange peel, and then leave the pillow in the bathtub for ten to fifteen minutes to release the aroma. Lay in the tub for at least twenty minutes. Keep the window closed so that the steam of the herbs lingers in the bathroom, allowing for better results from the biochemical contents. Repeat at least two to four times a week. Tension reduction massages with the essential oils of lavender or rosemary can enhance the effect as these herbs are simultaneously soothing and stimulating.

Try to eat more carbohydrates because, in the case of mental stress, the brain uses more energy. Carbohydrates change into sugar and feed the brain, especially during mental stress. Steamed rice with yogurt is recommended for dinner. Rice contains Vitamin B complex and carbohydrates, both of which are beneficial for reducing mental depression.

Making Herbal Remedies

How to Make Herbal Extracts

If you intend to make your own extracts, please remember that one part of dry herbs is equivalent to three parts of fresh herbs. Herbal or plant extracts can be obtained from fresh or cooked plants as follows:

Fresh herbs

If you wish to make an extract from fresh or dry herbs, first combine the herbs containing the same healing properties, such as parsley, burdock, and yellow dock which are used for detoxification and blood purification. Wash, chop, add a cup of water, and place them in a heavy-duty food processor. Blend for approximately four to five minutes until all the extract and juice is removed. Then strain all the liquid. Finally, pour the extract in a clean jar and store it in your refrigerator for not more than a few days in order to have fresh extract.

Cooked herbs

Fresh or dried herbs can be cooked to obtain extracts. First, sort and wash the herbs. Place three ounces of fresh herb in a pot with two cups of water. Boil for twenty minutes. Beat the cooked herbs in a blender for two minutes. Strain the extract, and store it in the refrigerator. The same method applies for dried herbs, but use three parts of water to one part of dried herbs. Beat for five minutes in the blender, then strain. Store as above.

The importance of mixing several herbs

When using herbs, try to mix several types as a single herb may prove too strong and direct. Besides, you may desire several effects that cannot be obtained from a single herb. Such combinations are essential in treating chronic ailments where many organs have been affected. For example, in the case of a simple headache, select the proper herb (processing the primary healing property), then add a small amount of secondary herbs as a stimulant to promote the action of the primary herb. Add a small amount of an antispasmodic herb to reduce muscle tension, and finally, add a pinch of soothing herbs to relax the body and protect the system.

The best methods of obtaining the flavor and scent of an herb are: a) chopping and grinding, b) pounding (mostly for scents), and c) soaking in hot water and placing them in a warm oven for a few hours.

How to make herbal infusions, decoctions, tinctures, and ointments.

Infusion:

Making an infusion is like making tea, and it is perhaps the most common method of using fresh or dried herbs. Leaves, flowers, or green stems are the proper plant parts for infusions, as the desired substances become easily accessible.

To make an infusion rich in aromatic oil, first chop or grind the herbs into smaller pieces, especially when using leaves. Then measure the required amount of herbs into a glass. For each tablespoon of dried herbs, use sixteen ounces of boiled water (divide this figure by three if using fresh herbs). Cover the herbs with boiling water, and simmer for fifteen minutes. Strain and store.

Herbs with high volatile oil contents and possible disintegration of their biochemistry are known as herbs sensitive to heat. When using herbs sensitive to heat, cold infusion is recommended. The ratio of herbs to water is the same as for herbs less sensitive to heat, but in this case, the infusion should be left for six to twelve hours in a well-sealed pot. Make sure to strain the liquid before use.

Decoction:

Decoction is made from the hard and woody parts of plants, such as bark, root, or nut. It can be prepared in the same manner as an infusion. Add one large tablespoon of chopped and dried root or bark to sixteen ounces of boiled water and simmer for fifteen to twenty minutes. Strain while hot, and store in a glass jar.

When preparing a mixture of soft and woody herbs, it is best to prepare an infusion and decoction separately to ensure the correct treatment of herbs sensitive to heat. First, decoct the roots or barks, using one large tablespoon of mixture to sixteen ounces of boiling water. Simmer it, then pour the whole decoction over the soft parts of the plant such as flowers, aerials, and leaves, then infuse for fifteen minutes. Strain, and store in a glass jar.

Tincture:

A tincture is made with an alcohol base, as alcohol is generally a better solvent for plants' biochemical components than water. There are several ways to make a tincture. You can use straight spirits, mixing the liquor with a little cold or hot water. When hot water is used some of the alcohol evaporates.

To make a tincture, place two ounces of finely chopped or ground dried herbs in a glass container which can be closed tightly. Pour sixteen ounces of 35 percent vodka over the herbs, and close the container tightly. If you are using fresh herbs, measure twice as much herbs as alcohol. Keep the container in a warm place, and try to shake it twice a day. After two weeks, pour the mixture into a cheesecloth and squeeze it over a bowl to wring out all the liquid. Then pour the liquid into a tinted glass container, and use as recommended. As tinctures are more concentrated than infusions, one should be cautious about the amount to be used.

Ointment:

In ancient times, Iranians made herbal ointments with a lard base. Yet today, you can replace the lard with pure unsalted butter, beeswax, or petroleum jelly. Personally, I recommend beeswax or pure organic butter. The oil enables the herb's active penetration to the skin for a longer period, thus promoting the healing process.

Ointments are especially effective for injuries such as burns and wounds. For example, while making ointments to soothe a burn or heal a wound, herbs such as comfrey, marigold, and lavender should be selected. Mix one ounce of each fresh herb with thirty two ounces of boiling water. In a separate dish, melt ten ounces of beeswax, and mix it with the herbs. Bring this mixture to a boil, stirring constantly. Press the mixture through a cheesecloth to remove all the liquid, then cool and store in a tightly closed glass jar.

Making Herbal Beverages

Using herbs can be referred to as the domestic interaction between humans and green nature. Herbs can make a delicious addition to everyday life and open up a whole world of joy and pleasure. They can be used as foods, beverages, medicines, and even aromatherapy.

Though preparation of herbs at home appears complicated, the pleasure of using homemade herbal products is worthwhile. If one learns to use herbs correctly, one can discover the magic of herbal power for physical and spiritual healing.

Although most of the herbs are safe for use, always remember to consult an expert and to not exceed recommended dosages. In dealing with herbs, one should note that interactive properties of herbs are as important as their individual properties. Thus, many times a primary herb is used to treat a problem, and a secondary herb is added to promote the former action.

Everyone has a favorite herb to be used in foods or beverages. Many herbs are not only delicious, but also promote health, especially when combined in special ways. Herbs such as rose hips, chamomile, rosemary, sage, lavender, and lemon verbena are used for their flavors as well as their healing powers.

Making herbal tea is just like making an infusion, i.e., activation of herbal properties. When selecting your herbs, remember that one part dried herbs equals three parts fresh herbs. In the case of fresh herbs, make sure the herbs are chopped or minced so it will be easier to measure with a spoon. In later chapters you will be offered some recipes for making herbal beverages.

Aromatherapy

Aromatherapy is using the aroma of herbs through their essential oils. These oils are effective in treating anxiety, depression, and physical and emotional stresses. Essencial oils can be massaged into the skin, or inhaled as vapors. They have small molecules which penetrate quickly into the body through the pores of the skin and indirectly to blood stream. Then it simulates the nerve in central nervous system, which in turn stimulate the part of the brain that controls emotions.

From the beginning of human history, plants have been used to cure diseases. Ancient Egyptians perfected the study of the medicinal power of plants to cure diseases as well as control the emotions. Like the Egyptians, the Greeks also developed medicines from different parts of plants, as well as aromatherapy. Since the essential oil's absorption by the skin is for a short period of time, its application must be scheduled. For example, after exercise or during anxiety. the essential oils can be applied to the face, backs of hands, soles of feet, chest, and back. In cases of rheumatic pain, the oil may be applied to the painful area.

Essential oils cannot be taken internally and must be used with great care, particularly in the cases of children and pregnant woman. When using oil for a child, remember to dilute the oil to half strength. Before using any essential oils, a skin test is a must.

Skin test

Everyone should conduct a skin test before using essential oils, especially if suffering from hay fever or asthma. Put one drop of the essential oil you wish to use on a cotton swab, and place it on the inside of your elbow. Cover the area with a small adhesive bandage, and leave it unwashed for twenty-four hours. If redness or any other reaction occurs, then you had better avoid using that oil.

Methods of Oil Extraction

For aromatherapy, it is very important to use the method which will yield the highest quality oil with greatest therapeutic value. Different methods of extraction yield different products as each process extracts different biochemical contents from the plant. No matter which method is chosen, extraction of essential oil is a difficult process because the amount of oil present in any plant is little. Large quantities of plants are needed to extract large amounts of oil. For example, 250 pounds of fresh lavender produces one pound of essential oil. That is why essential oils are expensive.

There are various methods for extracting essential oils. Some of these methods are elaborated below.

Using Oil

You will need eight ounces of fresh herbs or four ounces of dried herbs for every pint of grapeseed or soy oil. First wash and dry the fresh herbs; then carefully place fresh or dried herbs in a clear glass bottle. Cover the herbs completely with grapeseed or soy oil, seal the bottle, and leave it on a sunny windowsill for three weeks. Remove the oil and pour into a dark bottle. The oil is now ready for use.

Using Steam Distillation

This method was used by the ancient Egyptian thousands of years ago. They placed raw herbs in a large clay pot with hot water and heated them. The steam would pass through cotton or linen, trapping the oil. Then the oil would be squeezed. This method is in use even today.

The easiest way to use steam distillation at home is to place fresh organic herbs containing essential oil in a tea kettle. Then add hot water and heat it. Conduct the steam through a pipe and collect it in jar.

Using Volatile Solvent

Extraction with volatile solvents involves dissolving the plant oil in alcohol and then evaporating the solvents. In this method, the basic herbs are placed in a large tank similar to a pressure cooker. Volatile solvents are then heated and poured through the tank. The solvents ,saturated with the plants' essential oil, evaporate, leaving the residue. This process is used in the perfume industry and products extracted by this method are not pure essential oil. Thus, such oils are not used in aromatherapy.

Checking Quality

It is difficult to check the quality of essential oils. A simple way for checking is through smelling, unless you are allergic. If the smell is very strong or if it causes irritation in throat, then it has some impurities or is synthetic. Another way to ascertain the quality of oil is to extract it at home. Though homemade oils are not as strong as the purchased ones, they still are effective and safe to use.

Storing Essential Oils

Essential oil should always be stored in dark bottles of either glass or metal and kept in dark and cool places. An oil bottle must be properly sealed because air can affect and damage the oil.

Aromatherapeutic Massage Application

There are many ways to use essential oils. One the most effective ways is by massaging it on skin. The essential oil easily passes through the skin. Since the essential oils are absorbed by the skin for a short duration, its application must be scheduled. For massage application, the essential oil can be applied over the skin to reduce physical pain and emotional tension. Aromatherapeutic massage applications are as follows:

■ Place two drops of essential oil on your fingertips, then apply it with pressure at several points on the face and neck.

■ Working in parallel lines, press both thumbs between the brows and move upward towards the hairline applying pressure at several points along the way. This method is good for headaches and sinus pains.

■ Working from the inner corner of the nose out to the ears, use four fingers to apply pressure under the cheekbone near the sinus area.

■ Apply pressure over the upper lips with the thumbs. Then work with the pressure on the chin at intervals along the lines from the mouth to the nose.

■ Use all ten fingers to apply pressure at several points on the face along the jawbone.

■ Apply pressure to the forehead with the thumbs, moving toward the hairline. Then apply pressure with thumbs and index finger above the eyebrows. Pinch and lift the eyebrows, and then press. This method is good in the case

of sinus pain.

■ Apply pressure with the thumbs between the eyebrows. At the same time, using the middle and ring fingers, apply pressure at the temple and move thumbs toward the inner corners of the eyes.

■ Press the fingers gently against the ears. Massage the whole ear, then move to the back of the neck and massage the neck.

■ Using the thumbs and fingers together, massage the shoulders and spine, applying deep, but gentle, pressure.

In the case of reducing tension, a body massage by a massage therapist with essential oils is recommended.

Inhalation Aromatherapy

This method is very useful for congestive ailments such as catarrh, colds, stuffy nose, and flu. It involves inhalation of eucalyptus, wintergreen, or rosemary oil by putting a towel over the head and directly taking in the vapors.

Inhalers are also useful and are available in pharmacies. Otherwise, place a drop of the chosen oil on one palm and rub the palms together to warm the oil. Cup the palms over the nose, making sure the hands are firmly closed. Inhale deeply several times, and the curative properties of the oil will be absorbed quickly.

Facial Sauna Aromatherapy

Add two drops of oil to a pot of boiling water, put a towel over your head, and let the steam on your face for at least fifteen minutes. The essential oil in the steam will be absorbed in the skin. Otherwise, add a few drops of oil to hot water in the bathtub and lay in the water for at least ten minutes. Close the door so the aroma and vapor will linger in the room and be absorbed by the skin for a longer period of time.

Oils

There are a variety of oils and essences that can be used. Some of the essential oils to be used at home or office are as follows:

Oil of Bergamot

This oil is particularly good for relieving mental depression and physical tension. Bergamot oil is produced from the rind of a bitter orange. The oil is extracted by pressing the peel or grating it without touching the white inner

part. Its color is emerald green, and the oil has a spicy lemon scent.

The oil can be used as steam inhalation, or it can be massaged around the temples and forehead to reduce depression.

Oil of Chamomile

Chamomile oil is excellent for reducing tension. The essential oil of chamomile is made from fresh or dried flowers. The oil is sweet, and at first, the color is a bluish pastel, later turning greenish-yellow. The most important constituent is azulene, a fatty aromatic substance that is an anti-inflammatory and promotes rapid healing of eczema and boils.

Chamomile oil can be used as steam inhalation to reduce tension or it can be massaged around the temples and forehead to reduce muscular, as well as emotional, stress.

Oil of Eucalyptus

Essential oil of eucalyptus is highly antiseptic. It is an effective remedy for coughs, bronchitis, sinus pain and pressure, flu, colds, and catarrh. Eucalyptus essential oil is also beneficial for rheumatic conditions. The leaves of both young and mature trees are distilled for the oil. The color is pale yellow. Its aroma is fresh and clean.

Eucalyptus can be used as steam inhalation or massaged. In the case of steam inhalation, fresh eucalyptus leaves can be placed in hot water and brought to a boil a create steam that can kill the bacteria around the home and unblock the mucous membranes. In the case of massage, eucalyptus oil can be used to reduce muscle tension and sinus pressure.

Oil of Geranium

Geranium oil is the most important oil in aromatherapy. This oil is distilled from the freshly cut green parts before flowering. It is beneficial for treating fatigue and exhaustion. It can be used for children, but always remember to use half-strength. Essential oil of geranium is also good for skin disorders like eczema.

Geranium oil can be massaged over muscles or forehead to reduce tension and headache.

Oil of Lavender

The essential oil of lavender is very therapeutic and mostly used for tension and depression. The color varies from dark yellow to dark greenish-yellow, and it is highly scented. There are different kinds of lavenders. French lavender is considered to be better than the English one, as it is richer in linalyl acetates. The oil is distilled from the flowers.
Essential oil of lavender can be used directly over muscles or by steam in-

halation either in boiled water or in a bath to reduce tension and emotional stress.

Oil of Melissa (lemon balm)

The essential oil of lemon balm is known as melissa in aromatherapy. Its soothing properties disperse depression and negativity. The plant is harvested from May to June before the first flowers appear. The oil is steam-distilled from the leaves and tops. The color is pale yellow, and it has a warm, lemony aroma.

Essential oil of melissa can be used both as steam inhalation or direct massage around the temples and forehead to reduce anxiety and depression.

Oil of Neroli

Essential oil of neroli reduces tension and anxiety and induces calm and sleep. Neroli essential oil is extracted from the fragrant flowers of the bitter source orange tree. The flowers of the Seville orange are steam-distilled, and oil is obtained. The fresh oil is yellowish, but turns into a reddish-brown color as it is exposed to air or light.

Essential oil of neroli can be used as steam inhalation or massaged directly over muscles in order to reduce emotional stress and anxiety. It can also be used in a bath with other herbs, such as lavender and melissa.

Oil of Orange

This essential oil is antidepressant and soothing. The oil is extracted from the bark or fruit. The color is pale orange with an orange fragrance.

The oil can be used via steam inhalation or massage to relieve depression or stress. It can also be placed with other soothing herbs in a bath.

Oil of Rose

Essential oil of rose is very valuable for easing tension in women. The essential oil is steam-distilled from petals. It is a pale yellow-green and has a very strong aroma.

Essential oil of rose is best used as a massage around the forehead to reduce mental depression, especially during loss of a loved one or separation. Another way of using rose oil is by making a pillow with rose, lavender, orange, and melissa for use during the night to release mental and emotional depression.

Oil of Rosemary

Essential oil of rosemary is stimulating, and it alleviates physical and mental weariness and depression. It raises the energy level and is a powerful antiseptic that is also used to treat rheumatism and respiratory problems. It has yellowish-green color.

Essential oil of rosemary can be diluted and used as a massage oil to reduce muscle tension and headache, or it can be used as steam inhalation, either fresh or the bottled oil.

Oil of Sage

Essential oil of sage helps to cure general fatigue, irritability, and depression. It raises the energy level and helps in dispersing negativity. If you are negative, feel down, and have a low energy level, either burn or boil sage in your home. For those who are suffering from anxiety and swelling or puffiness due to menstrual tension or menopause, the oil can be massaged. The oil is steam-distilled from the leaves and has a pale yellowish color with a camphor-like aroma.

Oil of Sandalwood

Essential oil of sandalwood is useful for treating both tension and anxiety, and it acts as sexual stimulant. Sandalwood oil is used for chronic bronchitis, urinary problems, bladder infections, and inflammation and is very popular in Europe.

It is steam-distilled from the flowers. Once distilled, it is kept in the distillery for about six months so it can achieve the desired maturity and fragrance. It has a pale to brownish-yellow color and a sweet aroma.

Oil of sandalwood can be used as steam inhalation or can be used as a massage oil to reduce anxiety and emotional tension.

Oil of Ylang Ylang

Essential oil of ylang ylang is highly scented and very antidepressant. It has a relieving action on pain and can be used as a sedative. The essential oil is steam-distilled from the flowers of a tree known as the "Perfume Tree," which originated in the Philippines and spread throughout tropical Asia. In France, the oil is used for treating malaria, typhus, and other fever types, intestinal infections, diarrhea, and flatulence. Ylang ylang is also a sexual stimulant. Ylang ylang oil is yellowish and has a pleasant aroma.

Ylang ylang can be massaged over the forehead and around the temples to reduce tension and also it can be used as steam inhalation.

Herbs and Health (Mind And Body Cleansing)

ealth is the reflection of the balance between our body, mind, environment, and diet. If you are searching for perfect, everlasting health and happiness in life, the key to it is self-recognition, believing in yourself, learning and understanding your body and mind.

Knowledgeably understanding nutrients and what nature provides for us is fascinating and is the foundation of our physical, emotional, and spiritual health and behavior. One must understand the basic causes of illness at physical, emotional, and spiritual levels in order to discover a logical way for its cure.

Health is related to the idea of balance between the needs of the body and mind. So it is not far from reality to say, "you are what you eat," and believe that "you are what you think and do." This belief forms your mode of action in life. Knowledge gives one the power to think, eat, and behave in such a way that benefits you the most. The more you know about your body and how to keep it healthy, the better your chances are to live longer and well.

There are many factors to good health and keeping well. If you truly know your body, you would know that the food you eat is your medicine too. Illness by itself does not exist; every illness and disorder indicates a lacuna. Some believe bacteria in the body cause illness. You must remember that impediments in the immune system permit bacteria and free radicals' entrance into the body, hence the illness. If there is a lack of nutrients, the body weakens, and body's defense mechanisms weaken too. Thus, bacteria can conquer. Proper nutrition and a healthy diet strengthen the immune system.

Though drugs help in obtaining a faster recovery and are widely used, they have side effects which render them less desirable. In such cases, nature knows best. By using herbs, one takes nature's side in combating the disease. We all deserve healthy bodies and happiness in this life, and the key to it is in our hands.

For thousands of years, herbs and plants have been regarded as potential medicines. In the last century, synthetic pharmaceuticals have taken over, hindering individuals' use of herbs as remedies.

To my amazement, I found that herbalists worldwide are routinely discovering remarkable herbs for food and medicine. The chemical content of such herbs can prevent or cure diseases and disorders. I am also fascinated by the curative value of herbs. Herbs are used both as food in everyday diet for better health and energy and as medicine by means of their therapeutic power and biochemical content.

Instead of always worrying about what is bad for you, make a small change in your diet by deliberately eating more natural foods and herbs. This will bring positive effects. You may prevent both acute and chronic diseases; such as infections, heart disease, high blood pressure, diabetes, cancer, constipation, gastrointestinal diseases, ulcer, arthritis, skin disorders, headache, low energy, and insomnia.

Never before have scientists and herbalists around the world united in such an exciting investigation… the remarkable impact of the chemical content of herbs on human health.

Modern synthetic medicines may relieve quickly, but they often have side effects. Herbs, unlike the chemical drugs, promote the natural functions of the body and play an important role in the process of strengthening it from within. They are effective in removing health problems and stress, but if a proper diet is omitted, the natural herbal remedies may become ineffectual. Disease sometimes gives one an opportunity for a better understanding of one's body, and the process of healing is a reflection of a new awakening, which means learning to listen to one's body. Through using herbal remedies to heal diseases we learn not only the healing properties and therapeutic value of the herbs, but also how to listen to the body and understand its chemistry better.

Staying Healthy

We have to learn to listen to our bodies and learn their needs. They can tell us everything. For example, if sometimes one suddenly craves for certain foods, that is the time when the body lacks a particular nutrient, and one should satisfy that need. As another example, if one feels fairly healthy and rarely gets a headache, but suddenly a severe headache is experienced, then one should search for the cause. It may be that the person has not eaten the right food, may have had insufficient sleep, or might have experienced prolonged emotional trauma.

As most of us know, the key to staying healthy and in shape is eating a healthy and balanced diet, getting enough sleep, increasing the resistance of the immune system to free radicals, exercising, drinking plenty of fluids (especially water), and making sure that the daily diet is incorporated with some antioxidants. An antioxidant is a free radical scavenger. It also helps the body produce melatonin which plays a role in the body's defense and immune system.

What is Melatonin?

Melatonin is a hormone that appears to have important and positive effects upon almost every system of the human body. Melatonin seems to affect the body in several different ways. It is a powerful antioxidant and a key component of the immune system. According to current research, melatonin may be one of the body's most effective weapons against free radicals. As a hormone, melatonin influences the aging process, reproductive cycle, and sleep cycle. Melatonin helps to keep the body's natural defense system strong and, as an antioxidant, melatonin on a molecular level limits the damage to organs and tissues caused by free radicals.

What are Free Radicals?

Free radicals are molecules that contain one or more unpaired electrons. These unstable molecules, in an attempt to stabilize themselves, try to combine with healthy cells in the body. So they often damage cell membranes. There is growing evidence that the major killer diseases, especially cardiovascular disease and cancer, are influenced by the presence of an excess of free radicals and the biochemical reactions they cause in the body.

Free radicals are produced inside the

body. They also come into the body through the air. The damage that is done by free radicals goes beyond the first cell it attacks. Not only is that cell injured, but its ability to reproduce and metabolize is permanently impaired. This chain reaction may continue, deforming cell after cell. If it damages the immune system, the body becomes vulnerable to infection. Then free radicals disrupt enzyme production, which is vital for regulating biochemical reactions in the body, and the stage is set for premature aging of any number of organs in the system.

A free radical's damage is also linked to some of the cosmetic impacts of aging. Recent estimates by dermatologists show that as much as seventy percent of age-related skin damage comes from exposure to free radical-rich ultraviolet rays from the sun. To stabilize the immune system against free radicals, one should include antioxidants in the diet, drink purified water, exercise in fresh clean air, and avoid canned and frozen foods.

What are Antioxidants?

Antioxidants are molecules that prevent the reaction of oxygen with other substances that results in the creation of free radicals. They protect cells from being damaged. Major antioxidants are beta-carotene, vitamins A, E, and C , and selenium.

If you follow a balanced diet, there is no need to worry about cholesterol, saturated fats, vitamins, trace minerals, or most of today's other nutritional concerns. We must eat a variety of fresh foods in order to get a full variety of nutrients, knowing that different foods provide different elements. Therefore, the diet that emphasizes one group of foods or just one food should be discarded. We should let our body to cleanse itself. The human body has a wonderful, effective, and astonishingly complex mechanism for ridding itself of waste and toxins. Using simple and safe herbs will support this natural process. Herbs that are good for detoxification are dandelion, gentian, centaury, parsley, peppermint, fennel, peach leaves, and papaya leaves.

Herbal
Reference
Guide

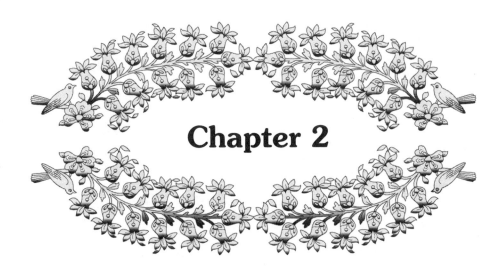

Chapter 2

Medicinal and Cosmetic Uses of Herbs

P lants are chemical factories. The medicinal value of plants resides in whatever principle property they have that makes them capable of producing a physiological effect on human body tissue. The interaction between plants and people dates back to centuries ago and has influenced human life, culture, and beliefs. People are interested in plants for their biochemical content as medicine, food, and drink, their essential oil properties for cosmetics and aromatherapy, and as fuel and shelter. When we use plants as medicine or food, they directly interact with our body chemistry and are absorbed by the body. Once reaching the bloodstream, they can influence the whole human system with their active biochemical contents. The purpose of using plants is to attain their effects in order to balance and strengthen the body's responses without harmful side effects.

Medical biologists in the USA believe that less than half of the beneficial active principles of plants have yet been isolated from herbs. Those most useful in medicine include essential oils, alkaloids, and glycosides. There are many plants for different uses and purposes. Plants are used as cosmetic products, flavors, or sources of perfume. They also have a wide range of other applications. A herb that is prized for cooking may also be of value against pests in the garden; one that is used in beauty care may also be used for preparing dyes, medicines, internal cleansers, and remedies. Therefore, each herb and plant has its own personality and benefits to human beings.

This next chapter shows how the magical biochemistry of herbs makes these diverse properties possible. The herbs and plants listed in this chapter have been in use traditionally from the beginning of the history. Also listed are plants that have been used extensively in medicine, aromatherapy, and food. This chapter also is a summary of the main uses of the various herbs, the research findings on their effects, specific applications, and their chemical effects on the body.

Agrimony (agrimonia)

Parts used: Aerial parts.

Biochemical contents: Tannins, silica, essential oils, bitter glycosides, vitamins B and K, and iron.

Energy: Warm.

Country of origin: United Kingdom

Harvest time: Agrimony should be gathered during the spring when the flowers are blooming.

Properties: Agrimony has astringent, tonic, and diuretic properties.

Cosmetic uses: Agrimony can be used in most skin creams especially for those who have sensitive and inflamed skin, owing to its tannins. This plant has healing properties, and as an ointment, it will help the healing of wounds and bruises.

Medicinal uses: Agrimony has been well known for centuries and has been used for its medicinal values in many countries, especially in Egypt and Greece. Bitter glycoside content and tonic properties make it particularly valuable for the digestive system, regulation of liver function, and gallbladder secretion. Ancient Iranians used agrimony to treat the urinary tract and stones. The silica content in the plant makes it helpful for active bone and cartilage

Alfalfa (Medicago Sativa)

Parts used: Aerial portion and sprouting seeds.

Biochemical contents: Alkaloid, flavonoids, vitamins A, E, K, and C, minerals, and enzymes, leaves contain 20% protein.

Energy: Cool.

Country of origin: Iran, about 700 B.C., taken to Greece about 500 B.C., 100 B.C. migrated to Italy and later to other European countries.

Harvest time: Alfalfa is harvested mostly in the summer.

Properties: Alfalfa has cleansing, estrogenic, and anti-inflammatory properties.

Main uses: For centuries, alfalfa has been harvested for its nutritional and medicinal properties. It is used more therapeutically as a food than as a medicine. Alfalfa helps in the penetration of nutrients and is best used fresh in a daily salad. Alfalfa has estrogenic properties and can be used for the treatment of menopausal and menstrual problems. It is good for bones and cartilage. Its infusion with honey is beneficial for children. In China, it is used in salads with spinach and beet root. As alfalfa can cause stomach gas, it would be favorable to take it with peppermint. In Iran, it is a favorite summer time afternoon snack.

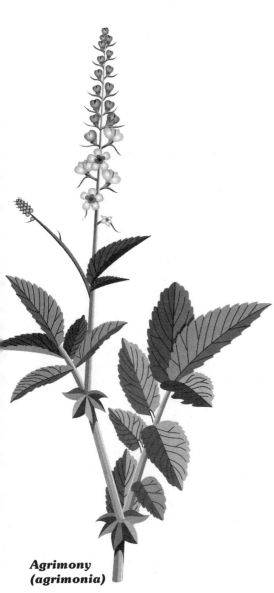

Agrimony (agrimonia)

formation. The French drink it as a tea once a week for liver detoxification.

Algae:

Parts used: Seaweed extract (algae).

Biochemical contents: Up to 90% mucilaginous; polysaccharides, amino acids, and most of the minerals.

Energy: Warm.

Country of origin: Asian countries.

Harvest time: Algae grows in deep sea at a depth of 100 feet below the surface. Algae plants are harvested from rocks at the seaside. Clean seaweed, after it has been boiled with sulfuric acid, sets a jelly named agar.

Properties: Agar has anti-inflammatory, antispasmodic, stimulating, and purgative properties.

Medicinal uses: Agar contains large amounts of mucilage that makes it very useful for soothing the intestinal tract, stimulating bowel activity, and increasing metabolism. In most scientific research laboratories, agar is used as a culture for growing microorganisms. Agar is also used as a thickening agent for food, such as ice cream.

Allspice (Pimenta Officinalis)

Parts used: Berries and essential oil.

Biochemical contents: Volatile oil, vitamins A, C, B1, B2, protein, fat, and many minerals.

Energy: Warm.

Country of origin: Central and South America.

Harvest time: The berries are harvested before they are ripe, since the volatile oil content decreases as they ripen.

Properties: Allspice has stimulating, antispasmodic, aromatic, and antiseptic properties.

Main uses: Allspice has been used by Africans, Indians, and South and Central Americans to reduce flatulence. It is highly effective in increasing the appetite and has a slight cathartic effect. The volatile oil in this plant makes it quite antiseptic and qualifies it as an appetite stimulant. The essential oil in allspice cannot be taken internally, however.

Caution: Do not take allspice during pregnancy

Aloe Vera (Syn. A. Barbadensis)

Parts used: Gel and juice.

Biochemical contents: Saponin, lignin, tannin, mucilage, glycosides, antibiotics, vitamins, minerals, amino acids, mucopolysaccharides, and mucoprotein.

Energy: Cold

Country of origin: South Africa, Iran, India.

Harvest time: Aloe vera mostly grows in warm climates. The leaves are collected all year round to obtain the gel and bitter liquid. Aloe vera can tolerate a scarcity of water for a long period of time. Its vital energy and vitamins are in the leaves.

Properties: Aloe vera has cleansing, penetrative, soothing, anti-inflammatory, healing, antiseptic, antibacterial, antihistamine, antipyretic and antibiotic properties. Saponin contained in aloe vera acts as a natural cleanser used in the cosmetic and skin care industry. It is excellent for skin cleansers and shampoos. The Indians applied the fresh gel of aloe vera leaves to their hair with water and noticed some lathering effects. Lignin is able to penetrate the skin if used topically, and if used internally, it is able to permeate nutrients in the body.

Cosmetic Use: Aloe is a cleanser for all skin types, and it can be used for skin irritation and inflammation. It soothes and heals sensitive skins. Its emollient properties moisturize dry skin. It is used for some skin disorders. Aloe maintains beauty, minimizes wrinkles, and penetrates the tissues.

Medicinal Uses: Aloe vera gel is one of the most healing substances known.

Aloe heals cuts, burns, and wounds and is an antiseptic, antibiotic, local anesthetic, bactericide, antipyretic, anti-inflammatory, and antihistamine. Aloe vera relieves pain both on the surface and deep in the tissues, including joint pain and muscle soreness. Aloe vera is bactericidal. If maintained in a high concentration for several hours in direct contact with bacteria, it acts as an antibiotic that may destroy bacteria even when highly diluted. It acts homeostatically, reducing both topical and below the surface bleeding. As an antipyretic, it reduces fever and the heat of sores. It is an anti-inflammatory and antipruritic, stopping itching. This last property is especially beneficial for athlete's foot, plant rashes, and insect bites.

Aloe provides a wide range of vitamins, minerals amino acids, mucopolysaccharides, and mucoproteins. Muccopolysaccharides are very important in protecting the body against invasions by organisms such as bacteria, fungi and viruses. The body slows its production of these compounds or completely eliminates it at puberty, therefore, we must obtain mucopolysaccharides from foods. Foods that contain substantial amounts of mucopolysaccharides and mucoproteins are crustaceans and deep sea cold water fish. They dilate the capillaries, increasing the blood supply in the areas to which they are applied. They are natural moisturizers both at the surface and throughout the tissue. They apply a protective barrier, which slows evaporation of natural moisture in the skin. It has healing and soothing properties for cuts and burns. Aloe Vera can be taken internally to cleanse the system and also helps the absorption of vitamins and minerals in the body.

Iranians use aloe vera for both external and internal treatment. They apply aloe vera in the form of a jelly, ointment, or massage cream to release tension and muscle exhaustion. It is also used to reduce inflammation and burning sensation after sunburn and cut. Indians use extract of aloe vera for vision improvement.

Angelica (Angelica)

Parts used: Leaves, stem.

Biochemical contents: Tannins, silica, lignin, angelica acid, and bitter glycoside.

Energy: Warm.

Country of origin: Iran, India

Harvest time: Angelica root is collected in the fall of its first year, and the leaves should be collected in the summer.

Properties: Angelica has diuretic, stimulant, and tonic properties.

Cosmetic uses: It is great for healing and reducing skin inflammation and

irritation. It soothes and relaxes irritated skin.

Medicinal uses: Angelica resembles celery. It has purplish stems. Angelica's dried leaves have an odd, strong, but not unpleasant odor. Angelica has stimulating and aromatic properties. Its lignin content helps to stimulate the appetite, promote digestive secretions, and help with the absorption of nutrients. In Iran, they use angelica for coughs and colds, as well as to reduce chest inflammations. They also use angelica leaves in a variety of soups and steamed vegetables, especially in winter.

Anise (Pimpinella Anisum)

Parts used: Seeds and leaves.

Biochemical contents: Volatile oil, glycosides, and fatty oil.

Energy: Warm.

Country of origin: European countries, Iran

Harvest time: Anise seeds should be collected as dry fruit between midsummer and early fall.

Properties: Anise has antispasmodic, anti-microbial, and tonic properties.

Cosmetic uses: It can be used as a toner and conditioner for all types of skin.

Medicinal uses: The volatile oil in anise serves as a remedy for intestinal colic and flatulence, and it has an anti-spasmodic properties that can be helpful for coughs, colds, and bronchitis. Anise tea eases indigestion. Anise leaves can be used in a variety of soups and salads.

Arnica (Arnica Montana)

Parts used: Flower, flower head, and extract for ointment.

Biochemical contents: Volatile oil, carotenoids, flavonoids, tannin, bitter glycosides, alkaloid, unstable fatty essential oil.

Energy: Warm.

Country of origin: France, Iran.

Harvest time: Arnica is collected or harvested between the early and late summer.

Properties: Arnica has antiseptic, anti-inflammatory, and soothing properties.

Cosmetic uses: Arnica can be used in most skin cleansers and creams. Arnica ointment is helpful on irritated and sensitive skins. It is an excellent remedy for bruises and reduces inflammation.

Medicinal uses: Arnica is a popular plant in Iran. Iranians make ointment with arnica to heal wounds and skin bruises. They also massage the muscles

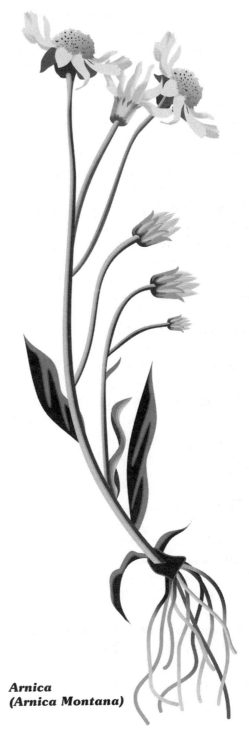

**Arnica
(Arnica Montana)**

and joints to relieve rheumatic or other pains and inflammation of the muscles. especially after accidents. Iranians also use arnica to treat coughs, whooping cough, and to reduce fever. Arnica is homeostatic, reducing both topical and below the surface bleeding.

Caution: External use of this herb may cause skin rash in some people.

Barberry (Berberis Vulgaris)

Parts used: Berries.

Biochemical contents: Alkaloid, tannin, resin, fruit acid, vitamin C, pectin, wax, alkaloid berberine.

Energy: Cool.

Country of origin: Iran, India.

Harvest time: Gather ripe berries in summer and dry in either sun or shade. Use fresh berries for juice.

Properties: Barberry has purgative, antispasmodic, and soothing properties.

Medicinal uses: Ancient Egyptians used fresh barberry for colds, sore throat, and better digestion. Barberry fruit is very sour and rich in vitamin C. The fruit not only has medicinal properties, but the leaves and bark also have medicinal value. Barberry fruit promotes the secretion of bile and helps lower high blood pressure, blood cho-

lesterol, and blood sugar. Barberry can help to cleanse and purify the blood. Barberry produces an edible wax that can be used in the cosmetic industry as an emulsifier. Iranians make iced tea with barberry and peppermint to treat indigestion and for internal cleansing also.

Caution: Do not use barberry during pregnancy due to berberin content in this plant (berberin stimulates the uterus).

Basil (Ocimum Basilium)

Part used: Leaves, fresh and dried, seeds.

Biochemical contents: Essential oil, tannins, and camphor.

Energy: Warm.

Country of origin: Iran, Mediterranean countries

Harvest time: Basil can be harvested throughout the year, especially in summer and fall.

Properties: Basil has astringent and tonic properties.

Cosmetic uses: Basil has healing properties that reduce irritation and inflammation. It is an antiseptic and can be used to condition and balance oily skin, plus reduce irritation.

Medicinal uses: Basil has been used in many countries since ancient times, as food and medicine. It is used raw or cooked, mostly in Italians and Iranian foods.

In Iran, the extract of basil is used with sugar to treat coughs, asthma, chest pain, bladder, and kidney infection. They also make an ointment with essencial oil of basil and peppermint for arthritis and rheumatic pain.

In China, basil leaves are used to increase the appetite, tone stomach tissue, and to release flatulence.

In India, bacil has been used traditionally to treat bronchitis, bloody diarrhea, and fever. They smash its fresh leaves and use it for burns, and mosquitoes stings.

Chinese, and Indians smoke basil leaves to reduce arthritis, and joint pain. An infusion of basil's seeds can be used to treat tension headache, and nervousness.

In Philippine, they soak basil's seeds in boiling water for fifteen minutes to release sticky substance then they add honney, and give it to women after childbirth to increase menstrual flow.

In Indonesia, infusion of basil's seeds are made to treat constipation, and urinary infection.

There are a variety of herbs, like mar- joram, oregano, thyme, tarragon, mint, dill weed, and savory, that have the same properties of benefiting the skin and body, that could be mixed with basil to make soups or to be added to salads. These herbs belong to the same botanical family and have the same properties and effects. See the chapter on recipes for cold summer soup with basil.

Bayberry (Myrica Corifera)

Parts used: Dried roots and bark.

Biochemical contents: Tannin, alkaloid, flavonoid, glycoside ,resin, and wax.

Energy: Cool.

Country of origin: Iran.

Harvest time: Bayberry root is unearthed in the spring, and the bark is gathered in the fall. They are dried in shade.

Properties: Bayberry has antispasmodic, diuretic, and soothing properties.

Medicinal uses: Bayberry is used to treat inflammation and infection of the gastrointestinal tract. Iranians use bayberry to treat throat infections, colds, and fever, and to release excessive mucus in the sinuses. Bayberry produces an edible wax that is used for making candles and chewing gum, and it can also be used in the cosmetic industry as an emulsifier.

Caution: Excess use of bayberry may cause potassium excretion and sodium retention.

Bearberry (Arctastaphylos Uva-ursi)

Part used: Leaves.

Biochemical contents: Tannins, phenolic acid, allantoin, volatile oil, arbutin, glycosides, and flavonoids.

Energy: Cool.

Country of origin: Iran

Harvest time: Bearberry leaves are best picked and dried in late summer when there is more energy in the leaves and fruit.

Properties: Bearberry has antispasmodic, antiseptic, and soothing properties.

Cosmetic use: Volatile oil and phenolic acid make this plant very antiseptic, while the allantoin and tannins make bearberry very soothing and healing. Bearberry also reduces skin irritation and inflammation. It is great for all skin types, especially dry skin.

Medicinal uses: Iranians use bearberry for internal cleansing and urinary infections. They make an infusion with leaves to use as a douche for vaginal

infections. Dried bearberry leaves are useful as a diuretic, astringent, antiseptic, and mild disinfectant of the urinary tract. It soothes, tones, and strengthens the urinary system. It can be used with marshmallow root as an infusion for the urinary system, especially in cases of infection, kidney stones, and ulceration of kidneys and bladder.

Caution: The arbutin in the plant is converted to hydroqunione, therefore, long use of bearberry may produce toxic properties, since hydroqunione is poisonous.

Bentwood (English Ivy)

Parts used: Leaves, and fruits.

Biochemical contents: Saponin, glucose.

Energy: Warm.

Country of origin: Asia, Europe, and Iran.

Harvest time: Bentwood fruits and leaves are harvested during summer.

Cosmetic uses: Because of the saponin content in bentwood, this plant is an ideal ingredient for cleansers and conditioners for all skin types. It can also be used for acne, for problem skins, and in moisturizers.

Medicinal uses: It has antispasmodic, antiseptic and laxative properties. Chinese make tea with bentwood for tension headaches, coughs, and to regulate menstruation. Bentwood has tiny black fruits which are cathartic (dose should not exceed 10-12 pieces). Bentwood can be used externally as a compress to reduce skin inflammation. It is also wound healer. In Asia, they mix ground bentwood leaves with sugar, cinnamon, and charcoal to reduce pain and inflammation of skin wounds and burns. Soaked bentwood leaves are very useful for baldness if used repeatedly for few weeks.

Bergamot (Monarda Didyma)

Parts used: Leaves, flowers, and oil for aromatherapy.

Biochemical contents: Volatile oil and tannic acid, essential oil.

Energy: Warm.

Country of origin: European countries, Iran.

Harvest time: Bergamot leaves and flowers are collected during late spring to summer.

Properties: Bergamot has antidepressant, soothing, antiseptic, and aromatic properties.

Main uses: Bergamot has a pleasant aroma. Its oil is used in aromatherapy for depression, anxiety, and emotional stresses. It can be applied directly on the skin or by steam inhalation. It is also used in baths or pillows along with other soothing herbs like lavender, rose, and melissa (lemon balm). For the bath, the use of either dried flowers or oil is best. When using dried flowers, place them in a bath filled with hot water and let the perfume and aroma be released in the water for at least ten minutes before bathing. Soak your body in the bath.

Betel Nut (Piper Betel L.)

Parts used: Fruits, leaves, root, seeds.

Biochemical contents: Essential oil, phenol, antibiotics, and enzymes.

Energy: Neutral.

Country of origin: India, China, Malaysia, Philippines, and North Africa.

Harvest time: Betel nut leaves and fruits are collected from late summer to fall.

Properties: Betel nut has antiseptic, antibacterial, aromatic, and toning properties.

Cosmetic uses: Leaves are highly aromatic and their extract can be used in beauty creams as perfume. It can also be used in skin conditioners. Its extract is great for acne.

Medicinal uses: Indians make some

sort of chewing gum substance with betel nuts. While its leaves are popular, even its seeds and roots are also employed as remedies for bloody diarrhea, fever and to increase secretion of salvia. Chewing gums made from betel leaves are useful in stimulating nerves. Steamed dried leaves have extremely beneficial topical uses, especially for women after childbirth as they help relax muscles. Betel nut is also beneficial for coughs. Steamed dried leaves, mixed with olive oil and massaged, are good for stomach ailments, wounds, burns, acne, and boils. The antibacterial property of its essential oil is useful for stomach ulcer and upper respiratory inflammations. Chewing betel nut leaves strengthens gums and teeth, freshens mouths, and alleviates coughs and indigestion. When used for indigestion, combine it with cardamom seeds for best results. Steamed, chopped betel leaves can decrease liquid accumulation in the prostate, with the results appearing after three days. Warm betel nut leaves can be applied over the prostate to reduce the swelling. Eight leaves taken with salt may relieve constipation.

Bilberry (Vaccinium Myrtillus)

Parts used: Berries and leaves.

Biochemical contents: Tannin, pectin, organic acid (alpha hydroxy acid), vitamins C and B, arbutin.

Energy: Cold.

Country of origin: Iran.

Harvest time: Bilberry fruits are gathered in June and July and carefully dried in shade.

Properties: Bilberry has astringent, diuretic, and detoxifying properties.

Cosmetic uses: This is useful in skin softening, exfoliating, skin toning, and conditioning. Bilberry contains organic alpha hydroxy acid that increases skin exfoliation at the cellular layer and helps the skin gain tone and become soft and younger looking.

Medicinal uses: Bilberry is ideal for high blood pressure, blood cleansing, liver detoxifying, and skin disorders such as acne and boils. There are two different kinds of bilberry, red and black. Black bilberry juice is good for high blood pressure, diabetes, and high cholesterol levels. Bilberry juice has cool energy, and it is especially helpful for people suffering from skin disorders such as acne and boils. Taking one to two glasses a day helps cool down and purify the blood. It also soothes skin inflammation.

Bilberry juice is ideal during the holiday season after all those heavy, sweet, and greasy foods which stress the liver. It cleanses the liver and helps to promote the secretion of bile. Bilberry seeds contain a bitter glycoside that is cleansing and detoxifying to the liver.

Bilberry juice lowers blood pressure, blood sugar, and blood cholesterol. Bilberry leaves are diuretic and also control diarrhea. Bilberry is a popular in Iran; for blood purifying and internal cleansing, almost every family drinks bilberry juice during the holiday season.

Black Cohosh (Cimicifuga Racemosa)

Parts used: Root and rhizome dried.

Biochemical contents: Various glycosides, salicylic acid, tannin, and resin.

Energy: Warm.

Country of origin: Iran, India.

Harvest time: Black cohosh roots with rhizomes are collected in the fall after the fruits have ripened.

Properties: Black cohosh has sedative, tonic, and antispasmodic, and anti-inflammatory properties.

Medicinal uses: Black cohosh has an excellent reputation in treating arthritis, whooping cough and large intestine problems. Since it has a normalizing property on the balance of female sex hormonal activity, it may be used for delayed periods, ovarian cramps or pain in the uterus, menstrual pain, and the discomfort of menopause. Black cohosh also has a reputation for relieving labor pain. Indians make an infusion of black cohosh combined with borage and valerian during labor pain. They also combine black cohosh with skullcap and passion flower to reduce nervous tension during labor and after childbirth. Black cohosh is used to relieve all kinds of nervous conditions, such as insomnia and nerve pain. Because of its content of various bitter glycosides, this plant is an effective remedy for helping liver cleansing.

Black Haw (Viburnum Prunifoliuml)

Part used: Dried bark of root, stem or trunk.

Biochemical Content: Tannin, saponins, bitter principle.

Energy: Warm.

Country of origin: Iran, Asia.

Harvest time: The stem and the bark from the root are collected in the fall. Bark from the branches should be collected in the spring or summer.

Properties: Black haw has tonic, antispasmodic, and sedative properties.

Cosmetic uses: Black haw possesses cleansing and soothing properties that makes it very useful for cleansing and conditioning of all skin types and moisturizing properties for sensitive to normal skins.

Medicinal uses: The part used as medicine is the bark of the root or stem. It has a definite function as a uterine sedative in threatened abortion. Black haw is a powerful relaxant of the uterus and is used to stop false labor pains. It may also be used to prevent menstrual pain, labor pain and miscarriage. To prevent possible miscarriage, infusion of black haw should be taken everyday, four to five weeks before the expected birth. Blackhaw is a superior plant for easing the discomfort of menopause. It also prevents excessive flow of perspiration.

Black Peppermint (Mentha Piperita)

Parts used: Leaves dry or fresh, extract ,essential oil.

Biochemical contents: Volatile oil, menthol, azulenes, tannin, and rosmarinic acid.

Energy: Warm.

Country of origin: Iran, India, European countries.

Harvest time: Black peppermint can be gathered all year round.

Properties: Black peppermint has tonic, digestive, and antispasmodic properties.

Cosmetic uses: It is an excellent conditioner for oily and sensitive skin, reduces skin inflammation and irritation; azulene oil contained in peppermint soothes and heals the sensitive skin.

Medicinal uses: Black peppermint is highly antiseptic and antibacterial because of its volatile oil contents. It is excellent for the digestive system. It relieves colic and helps in removing excess water and cramp-causing gas from the stomach. It also soothes stomach ulcers. Iranians eat black peppermint with their meals and also make an infusion with black peppermint and marjoram for menstrual pain and indigestion.

Bladder wrack (Fucus Vesiculosus)

Parts used: Whole plant.

Biochemical contents: Mucilage, volatile oil, potassium, iodine, and other minerals.

Energy: Neutral.

Country of origin: Iran, Asian countries.

Harvest time: The entire bladderwrack plant is collected in early summer from rocks around the seashore and allowed to dry in the sun.

Properties: Bladderwrack has properties that oppose both hyperthyroidism and rheumatism.

Cosmetic uses: This plant is highly antiseptic, thus together with its astringent properties, it makes an effective toner and conditioner for all skin types. Its anti-inflammatory properties make it a superior lotion or ointment for acne in sensitive, irritated skin.

Medicinal uses: Bladderwrack supplies minerals to the body and is a fine source of iodine. Because of its effects on underactive thyroid glands, bladderwrack is an excellent remedy for rheumatic pain, arthritis, and joint inflammation and has a weight reduction reputation.

Iranians make soup with bladderwrack. They also add it in salads, especially during illnesses like flu, colds, and muscle spasm.

Blessed Thistle (Cnicus Benedictus)

Parts used: Root, aerial, and seeds.

Biochemical contents: Mucilage, tannin, alkaloid, essential oil, bitter glycoside, and flavonoids.

Energy: Cool.

Country of origin: Iran, India.

Harvest time: Blessed thistle's leaves and flowers should be collected when the plants are blooming from the early to late summer, and the seeds should be collected in the fall.

Properties: Blessed thistle has tonic, antibacterial, astringent, and anti-inflammatory properties.

Medicinal uses: Blessed thistle has an excellent reputation to increase the flow of breast milk. Because of its bitter glycoside content, it has a bitter taste and is, therefore, used as a digestive tonic. It stimulates the liver and increases the secretion of bile. Because of its alkaloid and tannin content, it is a superior remedy for fever and headache and may be used for diarrhea.

Iranians make a decoction with blessed thistle root, burdock root, and devil's claw to treat tension headache and also to treat arthritis and joint pain.

Caution: Do not use during pregnancy. Strong infusion may be emetic and cause diarrhea.

Bloodroot (Sanguinaria Canadensis)

Parts used: Root and rhizome.

Biochemical contents: Alkaloids, resin.

Energy: Hot.

Country of origin: India, Iran.

Harvest time: Bloodroot rhizome is unearthed in the early summer and can be dried in the fall in shade.

Properties: Bloodroot has antispasmodic, antiseptic and cardiac properties.

Cosmetic uses: It can be used in many skin toners and conditioners, especially those for sensitive and sunburned skin.

Medicinal uses: Bloodroot is primarily used for sinus congestion, chronic coughs, colds, laryngitis, sore throat, and asthma. Due to its stimulating properties, it may relax the bronchial muscles. Bloodroot can be combined with other herbs, such as licorice and eucalyptus oil, to massage the chest and neck and used externally on athlete's foot. Ancient Indians used bloodroot with clover to treat gum diseases and tooth pain.

Caution: Large doses can be poisonous. Bloodroot is classified by US Food and Drug Administration (FDA) as unsafe.

Blue Cohosh (Caulophyllum Thatictroides)

Parts used: Root and rhizomes.

Biochemical contents: Alkaloids, glycosides, saponin, starch, salt, phosphoric acid.

Energy: Warm.

Country of origin: Iran, Egypt, Asia.

Harvest time: Blue cohosh roots are collected in the fall after ripening of the fruits.

Properties: Blue cohosh has antispasmodic, sedative, and tonic properties.

Medicinal uses: Blue cohosh has a great reputation and power for relaxing and normalizing female reproductive systems as well as treating arthritis and is also useful in decreasing labor pains.

Ancient Egyptians used blue cohosh for menstrual irregularities and for easing the cramping pain of menstruation. Long ago, American Indian women drank the tea of blue cohosh a few weeks before childbirth to make the process swift and easy. Ancient Iranians used blue cohosh with peppermint and borage for treating muscle spasm and tension headache.

Caution: The seeds are poisonous. The herb should not be taken during pregnancy, high blood pressure, or heart diseases.

Blue Flag (Iris Versicolor)

Parts used: Rhizome.

Biochemical contents: Volatile oil, glycosides, salicylic acid, tannin, alkaloid, and starch.

Energy: Warm.

Country of origin: Iran, Asia.

Harvest time: The blue flag rhizome is best when collected in the fall.

Properties: Blue flag has diuretic, laxative, antiseptic, and anti-inflammatory properties.

Cosmetic uses: Being antiseptic and antibacterial due to its volatile oil content, it has anti-inflammatory properties to soothe and reduce the irritation of sensitive and inflamed acne skin. Blue flag has a reputation of being a blood purifier and effective neutralizer of toxins. It soothes and cools the blood and is superb for treatment of most skin diseases, especially eczema, psoriasis, and acne.

Medicinal uses: Salicylic acid and alkaloid content in blue flag makes it an excellent remedy for rheumatism, headache, and muscle pain. Blue flag is especially good for liver congestion and cleansing, because of its glycoside content. Ancient Iranians used blue flag to treat rheumatism, liver congestion, digestive problems, and heartburn. They made an infusion with burdock root, yellow dock root, blue flag, and bilberry to purify the blood and to treat acne. Recent studies have demonstrated that blue flag tends to reduce the craving for food, permitting control and reduction of the appetite.

Boldo (Peumus boldo)

Parts used: Leaves.

Biochemical contents: Flavonoid glycoside, alkaloids, tannins, resin, and volatile oil.

Energy: Cool.

Country of origin: Iran, Mediterranean countries.

Harvest time: Boldo is harvested from late spring to summer.

Properties: It has anti-inflammatory, antispasmodic, diuretic, and antibacterial properties.

Principle uses: Boldo contains large amounts of volatile oil from which this plant gains its antiseptic properties. Ancient Egyptians used boldo for treating urinary infections and discomfort. Boldo stimulates the liver and gallbladder and increases the flow of bile. Its alkaloid content makes this plant useful for killing pain and reducing fever. Iranians use an infusion of boldo with other herbs such as agrimony horsetail, and parsley to relieve urinary infection pain and crush kidney and bladder stones.

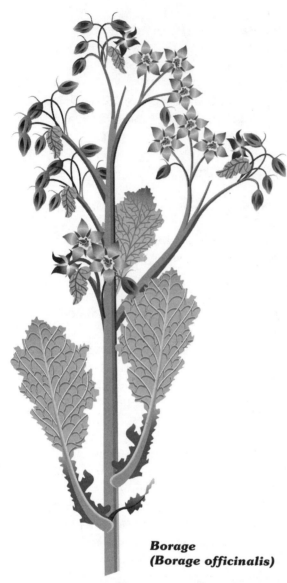

**Borage
(Borage officinalis)**

Borage (Borage officinalis)

Parts used: Leaves, flowers, mostly dried.

Biochemical contents: Mucilage, tannins, alkaloids, essential oil, calcium, and potassium.

Energy: Cool.

Country of origin: Iran, India.

Harvest time: Borage leaves can be collected when the plant is setting to flower in early summer. Borage should not be collected when wet with rain or dew.

Properties: Borage has diuretic, tonic, anti-inflammatory, and emollient properties.

Cosmetic uses: Borage has anti-inflammatory properties which soothe and relax irritated skin. It is moisturizing and healing. Borage helps in retaining moisture and absorbing nutrients in dry skin. It is highly emollient and used to regain moisture in the skin.

Medicinal use: Borage was originally introduced from Iran to Europe. It has a lovely lavender blue flower, but its leaves are the part which is dried when the plant is to be used as medicine. Iranians, use borage for menstrual pain, depression, and anxiety especially during the hormonal changes of menstruation. A high gamma linoleic acid level (GLA) makes it especially great for menstrual pain. GLA helps stimulate the production of progesterone It may also affect the sex hormones, progesteron is naturally produced by the body.

Ancient Iranian's used borage during depression, and they believed borage would bring courage and cheer. Iranians still use borage for menstrual pain, for depression during menopause and menstruation, and for regulating heartbeat. They combine borage with valerian and peppermint to make an infusion, then add rock candy and drink. Borage leaves may increase the milk supply of nursing mothers. In Europe, people use borage for coughs, colds, and flu.

Buchu (Barosma Betulina)

Parts used: Leaves.

Biochemical contents: Volatile oil, mucilage, flavonoids, resin, camphor, and essential oil.

Energy: Cool.

Country of origin: South Africa.

Harvest time: Buchu leaves are harvested in summer.

Properties: It has antispasmodic, antiseptic, aromatic, and diuretic properties.

Medicinal uses: Buchu has a strong aroma, and Africans use the leaves as body perfume. They also use the oil for aromatherapy to reduce physical and emotional stress. Early Europeans used buchu as a remedy for urinary infection. Iranians combine buchu with other herbs, such as juniper and goldenrod, to treat bladder infection

(cystitis). Buchu is a diuretic, and the oil is highly antiseptic. These qualities make it especially helpful for treating bladder and urinary infections.

Caution: Avoid using buchu if you have kidney infection.

Burdock (Arctium Lappa)

Parts used: Leaves, extract, roots.

Biochemical contents: Volatile acid, polyphonic acids, tannin, bitter glycoside, 45% inulin in root and leaves, unstable essential oil in root, 60 % linoleic acid, burdock seeds contain 16-20% fixed oil.

Energy: Cool.

Country of origin: Iran, Asia, and Europe.

Harvest time: The best time to harvest burdock is midsummer. Burdock takes two years to complete its cycle. Leaves develop in the first year. Burdock leaves and stalks are purplish-red, similar to rhubarb, and they are very bitter.

Properties: Burdock has anti-tumor, anti-pyretic, anti-rheumatic, antibiotic, astringent, tonic, and hypoglycemic properties.

Cosmetic uses: Burdock is prescribed for skin diseases, especially disorders such as acne, boils, eczema, and psoriasis. Burdock is very antiseptic and antimicrobial and is a super blood cooler for skin inflammation. Therefore, it is very useful for easing pains and healing inflamed, reddened, heated skin conditions, such as acne, chronic rashes, eczema, cysts, infected wounds, burns, itchy skin, and herpes.

Medicinal uses: Burdock root has strong medicinal power. Its energy goes into the root after the summer, at which time it is harvested for medicine. Chinese use burdock seeds for sore throats, colds, and flu. In Japan, people use burdock root, leaves, and stalks to increase their immune system and to increase secretion of sweat glands. Iranians use burdock for menstrual flow, inflammation, and infection. They also use burdock seeds with honey and vinegar for rheumatic pain. Iranians also use burdock to reduce blood sugar, treat skin diseases such as cold sores, and remedy baldness. They have been known to make infusion of burdock with licorice to treat stomach ulcers. Infusion of its root with brown sugar is used to treat both headache and measles, while burdock root with olive oil is used to treat wound and scratches. In India, people use burdock for blood purifying and detoxification. Burdock seed oil is used daily as a strengthening and nourishing tonic for hair follicles with thinning hair from stress. Rub a palm full of bur-

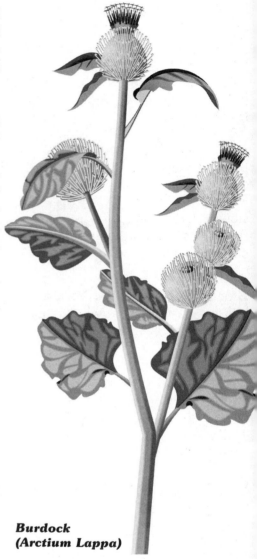

**Burdock
(Arctium Lappa)**

dock oil into the scalp, then cover the head with a wet towel or shower cap for at least an hour. Repeat this topical treatment once a week, in addition to internal use of burdock, for hair loss or hair thinning.

Burdock increases the flow of urine, reduces urinary inflammation and bladder irritation, and cures chronic urinary problems. Burdock purifies and cleanses the blood and tissues. It lowers blood sugar, thus making it suitable for treating diabetes. Burdock also has a reputation for curing rheumatic joints, back pains, and skin disorders such as acne and eczema. Burdock works throughly and slowly, individuals who are using Burdock should not be in hurry for cure, using Burdock takes 6 -12 weeks to get result.

Burweed (Xanthium spinosum L.)

Parts used: Fruits, leaves, and seeds.

Biochemical contents: Vitamin C, fat, linoleic acid, tannin.

Energy: Warm.

Country of origin: Asia, Iran, India, and European countries.

Harvest time: Burweed leaves and fruits are harvested in the summer and seeds in the fall.

Properties: Burweed has soothing and tonic actions.

Medicinal uses: Burweed is one the most famed plants in Korea for treating colds, flu, rheumatism, and skin disorders. In China, burweed has been used since ancient times for treating rheumatism and reducing fever. The part of this plant having the most powerful medicinal properties are the seeds and fruits. In China and India, they also use burweed externally to reduce inflammation and itching on the skin. They also get an extract from the leaves and apply it over wounds to kill bacteria and prevent infection. The fruits are also used for eye strength and ear pain. Burweed root contains bitter principle which make this plant very useful for liver cleansing and digestion. Scientific research shows that burweed may cure some cancers.

Cabbage: (Brassica oleracea "L." DC.)

Parts used: Leaves

Biochemical content: Glycosides, carbohydrate, protien, myrosin, Vitamins (A, B1, B2, B3, and C), minerals (potassium, iron, calcium, and phosphate).

Energy: Warm

Country of origin: Europe, Iran, Asia

Harvest time: Summer cabbage is planted in the fall and harvested late spring.

Properties: Cabbage has anti rheumatic, antibiotic, astringent and tonic action.

Medical uses: Ancient East Indins ate cabbage heaves to tone stomach and heart tissues, and applies smashed cabbage externally to treat theumatic pain. Steamed cabbage and cabbage roots relieve headaches, sharpen vision, and increase the flow off urine.

Iranians, apply extract of cabbage leaves and garlic externally to treat muscle tension and arthrities pain. They also make variety of dishes, and pickles with cabbage (see chapter 19 recipe on stuffed cabbage leaves or dolmeh cabbage).

Cabbage seed have a laxative effect, they kill bacterica and intestinal worms and they stimulate sexual desire.

Ancient Iranians used to mix chopped steamed cabbage with barley and apply it externally to reduce inflammation and treat measles, and skin cancer. They also mixed it with vinegar ang egg white to treat burns. Cabbage paste mixed with fenugreek, and vinegar is helpful for joint, and arthritis pain.

The French mix cabbage-leaf extract with honey and take in doses three to four tablespoon to relive coughs, soothe chest pain, kill intestinal worms, and increase sperm production.

Cabbage and its close relatives (broccoli, brussels, sprout, cauliflower and kale) are among the most powerful cancer-prevention plants. In the last 25 years, scientists have learned through experiments and long-term studies that certain foods contain natural chemicals with the power to fight cancer-causing free radicals. These foods are helpful both in preventing cancer and in slowing its effects. Certain foods have been shown to have power in combating particular types of cancer. Scientists hope that with further research they will discover foods that will specifically combat every type of cancer.

Dr. Lee Wattenberg professor at university of Minnesota has proven that diet centering on natural foods can destroy cacerous free radicals in the body. For 30 years, from 1960 until less than a decade ago, Dr. Wattenberg has extensively researched the effects of simple foods such as cabbage and its relatieves, delving into their biochemical effects in stopping cancerous cells.

In the mid-seventies, Dr. Saxon Graham and his staff studied 256 patients who had intestinal cancer. The diet of this group of patients proved deficient in the members of the cabbage family as well as in carrots, lettuce, and cucumber. Dr. Graham compared this group to another sample, who were oldder and did not have intestinal cancer, but had a diet rich in these vegetables. The finding published in 1979 in "Epidemiology" magazine, indicated that eating these vegetables daily may insure health and well-being. Other researches have revealed that diets rich in cabbage, apple, hot pepper, ginger, pumpkin, and carrot fight cancerous free radicals in the colon and thus prevent colon cancer.

Each 100 grams of raw cabbage contain:

Water	91	gm
Protein	2/7	gm
Fat	0/2	gm
Carbohydrate	4	gm
Calcium	25	mg
Phosphate	56	mg
Iron	1/1	mg
Sodium	13	mg
Potassium	295	mg
Vitamin A	60	IU
Thiamin A	0/11	mg
Riboflavin	1/10	mg
Niacin	0/7	mg
Vitamin C	87	mg

Twenty to thirty percents of above nutrition will deplete after cooking.

Calendula (Calendula Officinalis)

Parts used: Flowers and leaves.

Biochemical contents: Volatile oil, tannin, mucilage, saponin, flavonoid, bitter glycoside.

Energy: Neutral.

Country: of origin Iran, European countries.

Harvest time: Calendula flowers are gathered in early summer and early fall.

Properties: Calendula has anti-inflammatory, astringent, antimicrobial, and tonic properties.

Cosmetic uses: Calendula is qualified to be used for all skin types, especially sensitive and irritated skin. Because of its mucilage and tannin contents, calendula is an anti-inflammatory endowed with wound-healing properties. It relaxes and soothes irritated skin. Its astringent and antiseptic properties also reduce skin irritation and rashes.

Medicinal uses: Calendula is one of the most healing plants in Iran. Ancient Iranians used it for treating varicose veins and as a facial soothing mask. They combined calendula with cucumber, used as a mask, to soothe the skin after facial massage. Iranians also make an infusion with calendula and marshmallow for treating stomach pain.

Caraway (Carum carvi)

Parts used: Seeds.

Biochemical contents: Tannin, glycoside, volatile oil.

Energy: Neutral.

Country of origin: Iran.

Harvest time: Caraway should be

gathered in the summer when flowers are blooming.

Properties: Caraway has anti-microbial, antispasmodic, and astringent properties.

Medicinal uses: Caraway has the best reputation in Iran for flatulence and colic relief. In the case of nursing mothers, they use an infusion of caraway with fennel to help increase milk flow and also release stomach gas to prevent baby's colic. Caraway has an antispasmodic property; it can help to relieve period pain and muscle spasms.

Some Iranians use caraway with cardamom seeds and peppermint for arthritis pain and muscle tension.

Cardamom (Elettaria Cardomumum)

Parts used: Seeds.

Biochemical contents: Volatile oil, camphor, essential oil.

Energy: Warm.

Country of origin: Iran, India, Egypt.

Harvest time: Cardamom seeds are harvested in the fall and dried in the sun.

Properties: Cardamom seeds have antispasmodic, antiseptic and aromatic properties.

Medicinal uses: Cardamom has warm energy and is highly aromatic. One can steam the nasal passages with cardamom seeds and let the aroma linger in the home for a very soothing, calming atmosphere. Cardamom is used in most Iranian and Mediterranean countries as a spice, herb, and medicine. Iranians use cardamom seeds in black tea, pastries, rice pudding, and desserts for its aroma and flavor. People use cardamom seed to relieve flatulence and to treat colic and indigestion. . One can also make cardamom infusion or tincture to use for indigestion. Add one tablespoon of cardamom pod powder to sixteen ounces of boiled water, then simmer for fifteen minutes. The above recipe is good for helping to release water retention and gas that causes menstrual pain. They also make an infusion with cardamon seeds, borage, cinnamon, and clove and then add honey to treat bronchitis, colds, and asthma.

Carrot: (Daucus carot)

parts used: Root, seeds

Bio-Chemical content: Tannin, carbohydrate, sugar, vitamins (A beta - carotene, B1, B2, B3, C) minerals (Iron, Phosphate, Calcium, and potasium), glycoside and alkaloid in leaf, essential oil, and tiglic acid in seeds.

Energy: Neutral

Country of oringin: WorldWide

Harvest time: Carrot root is harvest from early summer through fall. Some fast-growing are planted in early fall and harvested early spring.

Properties: Carrot has soothing, healing, anti-inflammatory, nutritious, and anti-cancerous properites.

Cosmetic uses: Carrot contains large amount of Vitamin A (Beta-Carotene). It makes it a great ingredinte in beauty creams, especially wrinkle cream, because it contain anti-wrinkle properties, its soothing, healing properties makes carrot especailly good for dry, damaged and sensitive skin. Carrot oil is ideal to prevent skin cancer.

Medicinal uses: Carrot has been consumed worldwild since ancient times, and have great medicinal and nutritional values, Carrot can be used in variety of soups, meals, salads, jams, and pastries. It has high amount of Vitamin A (beta-carotene), which make this plant especially useful in cancer-prevention. It may even help cure certain cancers.

Chinese use all parts of carrot. They use extract of its root for external treatment of cuts, burns, and they use its seeds to treat diarrhea, and flatulence, and to cleanse the liver.

Old World physicians used carrot to increase sexual desire, and aid the flow of urine. Carrot was also widely used to treat coughs, colds, stomatch aches, chest pain, and indigestion, and to aid in excreting bladder and kidney stones. To excrete kidney and bladder stones, and to increase the flow of urine, hollow out a radish and fill the hollow with equal amount of carrot seed turnip seed, then bake it and consume it.

Iranians make a delicioius jam with honey, which they believe helps in reproduction by increasing sperm volume and reduce uterus muscle tension.

The French drink carrot juice on an empty stomatch for blood production.

Carrots are rich in beta-carotene (Vitamin A), and anti-oxidant that inhibits free radical oxidant cells, Scientific research has proven that fruits and vegetables high in beta-carotene greatly help to prevent cancer, and individuals whose diets are deficient in beta-carotene are at increased risk, particularly for incurable cancers of the lungs and stomach.

In 1986 Swedish researchers proved that carrot plays a major role in preventing stomach cancer, so including carrot in your daily diet may ensure your stomach's health.

Dr. Marilyn Menkes, famous cancer researcher has observed that cigarrette smokers with little beta-carotene in their blood have four times the risk of lung cancer than individuals with ample beta-carotene in their blood.

Another group of scientists at New York State University in Baffalo, discovered that the men who consume beta-carotene daily show a 50% reduction in the incidence of lung cancer, and that one extra carrot a day may produce a 15-20% reduction of lung cancer risk.

In 1981 Dr. Richard Shekelle announced results of his extensive cancer research into the relationship between diet and lung cancer. In a 19 years longitudinal study of 2000 people, he determined that men addicted to cigarette smoking who did not include beta-carotene in their daily diet increased their risk of lung cancer eight time over similar men (including smokers with a 30-year habit) who did consume adequate beta-carotene. Since cancer may take 30-40 years to manifest itself, increasing beta-carotene in the diet seems to decrease the risk of the damaged cells turning cancerous, Longterm smokers who quit can reduce the risk of cancer by including large amounts of carrots in their diet, since bera-carotene fights against the free radicals that promote unhealty cell growth. In the most recent research, Regina G. Ziegler of the National Institute of Lung Cancer studied men who reside in New Jersey. She discovered that carrots, pumpkins, and sweet potatoes are very rich in beta-carotene and should be consumed daily to reduce the risk of cancer of the pros-tate, larynx, lung, and stomach.

Carrot reduce blood cholesterol and increase bowl movements. Carrot juice consumed in the morning on an empty stomach serves as an excellent colon cleanser. Carrots should be consumed daily, To get the most benefits from them and release their anti-cancerous properties, it is best to steam them, since steaming them increase the body's absorption of their beta-carotene by 400-500%

Cascara Sagrada (Rhamnus prushiana)

Parts used: Bark.

Biochemical contents: Glycosides, bitter principle, tannin, resin, and many minerals such as calcium, potassium, manganese, and vitamin B complex.

Energy: Cool.

Country of origin: India, Iran.

Harvest time: Cascara Sagrada bark is stripped from the tree's trunks and branches from mid-April to August. It is dried with the outer surface up and stored for one year before use.

Properties: Cascara sagrada has purgative, cleansing, soothing, and anti-inflammatory properties.

Medicinal uses: Cascara sagrada is a laxative and promotes a squeezing motion in the intestinal canal which causes bowel movements (peristalsis), helps in painless evacuation, and also helps to restore natural tone to the colon. American Indians call this plant "colon cleanser." They use the bark for cleansing the colon and get excellent results from it. Cascara sagrada helps to promote secretion of bile in the stomach, liver and gallbladder.

Iranians use this plant for liver detoxification and stomach pain. They combine it with psyllium and parsley to cleanse the blood and also to release warm energy from liver which may cause rashes and acne.

Caution: Fresh bark may cause vomiting.

Castor Bean (Ricinus communis)

Parts used: Oil extracted from the bean.

Biochemical contents: Fixed oil, glycosides, and linoleic acid.

Energy: Warm.

Country of origin: Iran, India

Harvest time: Castor beans can be collected from early summer to late fall.

Properties: They have laxative and diuretic properties.

Cosmetic uses: Castor oil is an emollient and can be used in most skin lotions and cleansers. If losing eyelashes or desiring longer and thicker lashes, apply castor oil at night after removing make-up. It can also be used on skin disorders, such as warts, corns, and cysts.

Medicinal uses: It is one of the most reliable cathartics known and is especially useful for treating food poisoning. In Iran, castor oil is given to hospital patients before surgery to cleanse and detoxify the body. Castor oil is also used to decongest the liver as a fomentation. Warm castor oil is to be applied generously over the entire abdomen, covered with a towel soaked in hot ginger tea, wrung out, and placed with a heat source over the region of the liver.

Caution: The castor oil is safe, but the beans and the rest of the plant are poisonous.

Catnip (Nepeta cataria)

Parts used: Dried aerial parts, leaves.

Biochemical contents: Volatile oil, tannins.

Energy: Warm.

Country of origin: Iran.

Harvest time: Catnip's flowers are gathered from summer to early fall.

Properties: Catnip has astringent and antispasmodic properties.

Medicinal uses: Catnip is a very popular plant in Iran. They use it to treat nervous tension, insomnia, and flatulence. Because of its antispasmodic property, this plant can ease stomach pain and stomach flu. Another name for this plant is cat grass. Cats love the smell of this herb, and catnip toys are their favorite playthings.

Cayenne (Frutescens)

Parts used: Fruit and leaves.

Biochemical contents: Alkaloid, volatile oil, vitamins A and C, iron, calcium, and B complex.

Energy: Hot.

Country of origin: India, South America.

Harvest time: Cayenne fruit should be collected when is it fully ripe which occurs from summer to the end of fall.

Properties: Cayenne has stimulating, anti-catarrh, antimicrobial, and tonic properties.

Principle uses: In cooking, it's found in a variety of dishes and salads. Cayenne fruits help to promote blood circulation. It is an excellent internal disinfectant and helps in relieving cramps. Cayenne is also antibacterial and is thus an excellent remedy for chills and colds. Because of its large percentage of vitamins C and A, it supports the body's defense and immune systems. It is especially helpful in wintertime.

Cayenne can stimulate and increase the appetite and help digestion. It is an excellent promoter of peripheral blood circulation. Cayenne fruit can be massaged on muscles that have poor circulation; it helps to restore normal circulation. Indians and South Americans use cayenne everyday with variety of dishes and salads. They also use it to treat sinus infections and rheumatic pains.

Iranians make a variety of soups and salads with cayenne especially during wintertime because it has warm energy and is also antibacterial. It keeps the body temperature warm and prevents bacteria from entering the body.

Medicinal uses: Chinese and Indians season many dishes with cayenne, partly because it help to kill any bacteria in fish, poultry, and meat. They also use cayenne to treat indigestion, vomiting, bloody diarrhea, bronchitis, and sinus infection. They smash fresh cayenne and apply it on sore joints to reduce muscle and arthritis pain.

Cayenne has anti-bacterial properties, which make this plant very useful for treating internal bleeding. It is an expectorant, hence excellent for treating bronchitis. Take 10-20 drops of cayenne with a glass of water three times a week prevent cold, flu, and bronchitis. Taking two teaspoons of red Mexican cayenne will stimulate the body to dissolve blood clots, and so reduce the risk of heart attack.

Dr. Irwin Ziment, a famous specialist in pulmonary diseases, calls red cayenne"natural Robitussim" he find the active substance in cayenne, named "capsaicin", very beneficial against bronchitis. As soon as cayenne enters the mouth, he reports, the burning on the tongue stimulates the stomach. This, in turn stimulates the bronchi cells to produce a substance that helps to release mucus from the throat and chest. Dr. Ziment indicates that red cayenne also cleanses the sinuses, furnishing relief from cold and flu symptoms.

through laboratory experiments on animals, Swedish scientists discovered the power of cayenne. They found that a daily does of "Capsaicin" reduce the sensitivities of the lungs. It diminished the muscle spasms of coughs and the damage to the bronchi cells produced by cigarette smoking. Their finding indicate that red cayenne may be helpful to individuals who suffer from asthma or other upper respiratory problems.

The ancient physicians of the old world used extracts of cayenne for local anesthesia during tooth surgery. Ancient Persian physicians combined an extract of cayenne with powered lentils to reduce local pain and inflammation. Interestingly, after many experiments, present-day century scientists have re-discovered cayenne's effectiveness as a pain-killer, whether applied topically or taken internally. "Capsaicin", substance that makes cayenne taste hot, rerduces the activities of the nerve cells which transmit the "pain" massages to the central nervous system.

Additional research indicates that cayenne ointment, applied on the skin or massaged into sore muscles, reduces arthritis and joint pain.

According to Dr. Paul Rosen, a psychologist at the University of Pennsylvania, the heat from cayenne makes the mouth burn with joy! That is, the sense of burning in the mouth stimulates the brain to produce chemical substances called "endorphins", which serve as the body's natural morphine. "Endorphins" not only reduce pain, but they also produce a sense of pleasure and satisfaction, and they help the body to burn fat.

Consuming cayenne with honey increases sexual desire. This mixture can also be used as a local anesthetic to numb an area.

Caution: Avoid excess consumption. It may cause liver disorder.

Cayenne is not recommended for in-

dividuals who have warm energy unless it is mixed with cool energy foods
to balance its heat.

Centaury (Erythrea centaurium)

Parts used: Dried leaves and flowers.

Biochemical contents: Bitter
glycosides, alkaloid, and phenolic
acids.

Energy: Cool.

Country of origin: Iran, Asia.

Harvest time: Centaury should be
collected from midsummer to fall.

Properties: Centaury has anti-catarrh,
tonic, antibacterial, and cleansing
properties

Cosmetic uses: It is good for all skin
types and conditions. Centaury is
highly antiseptic and also soothes the
skin. It works on all skin types and
conditions, especially on oily and
sensitive skin and skin with poor circulation, because it stimulates the circulation as well.

Medicinal uses: Centaury is one of
the most valued plants to treat liver
complaints. It is excellent for helping digestion and liver detoxification.
Centaury has a high percentage of
glycoside, which makes this plant
very valuable for digestion and ab-

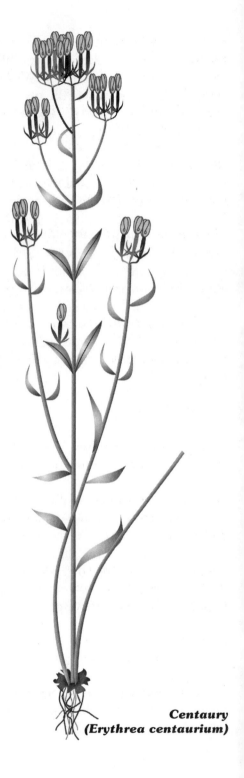

**Centaury
(Erythrea centaurium)**

sorption of nutrients. Iranians use tincture of centaury with cardamom before meals for digestion and to simulate gastric secretions of the liver and gallbladder. Centaury has been used to rid children of parasitic worms. Its phenolic acid content makes centaury effective in reducing fevers. Iranians use this plant to reduce high blood pressure.

Chamomile (Chamomilla Recutita Syn.)

Parts used: Leaves, flowers, and root.

Biochemical contents: Tannins, salicylic acid, mucilage, azulene oil, volatile oil; essential oil contains 3% glucose.

Energy: Neutral.

Country of origin: Iran, European countries, it grow worldwide

Harvest time: Chamomile flowers should be gathered between summer and spring.

Properties: Chamomile has antispasmodic, antiseptic, anti-inflammatory, sedative, and tonic properties.

Cosmetic uses: For thousands of years, people have known chamomile to be a very healing plant. It is good for all skin types and conditions, especially sensitive and irritated skin. Chamomile flowers contain blue

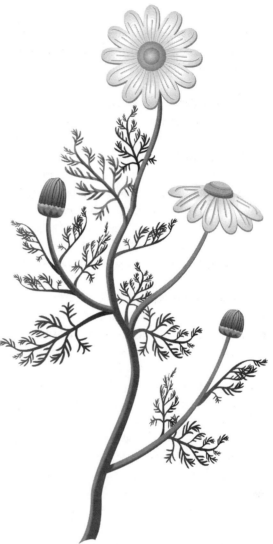

**Chamomile
(Chamomilla Recutita Syn.)**

azulene oil which is a very powerful wound healer. It is anti-inflammatory and promotes the healing of burns and skin conditions, such as rosacea, eczema, and skin with couperose (broken capillaries). Chamomile oil is used in aromatherapy to calm nervous tension and anxiety. It can be used in baths, vapor steam and massage.

Medicinal uses: Ancient Iranians and Mediterraneans valued this plant as one of the most powerful healing plants in herbal medicines, and today it is used in many parts of the world. Iranians use chamomile tea to soothe stomach ulcers and to reduce muscle tension and migraine headaches. They use chamomile tea with honey, cardamom, and cinnamon after childbirth to reduce the anxiety and muscle tension. Chamomile tea has a sedative property, enabling sleep and relaxing muscles spasm. Its essential oil contains 3% glucose, which has antispasmodic action. It also contains chamazulene, used as an antihistamine for allergy problems and pain reduction. Chinese and Japanese use its infusion of dried leaves as a gas and colic remedy. Indians use it for digestive disorders and fever problems. Steamed flowers are good for hair coloring. It enhances color and is used for highlighting brown hair.

To make chamomile oil :
16 oz. chamomile flowers
64 oz. sesame oil or olive oil

Leave in the sun for 40 days or steam. The residual oil can be used as ear drops to relieve earaches and to relieve muscle tension.

Caution: Long usage may cause vomiting.

Chickweed (Stellaria media)

Parts used: Aerial part, leaves.

Biochemical contents: Saponin, mucilage, proteins, carotene, many minerals such as potassium, calcium, phosphorus, aluminum, copper, iron, magnesium, manganese, silicon, zinc, vitamins B1 (thiamine), B2 (riboflavin), and B3 (niacin).

Energy: Warm.

Country of origin: Asia, Europe.

Harvest time: Chickweed can be picked all winter long.

Properties: Chickweed has emollient, soothing, antibacterial, antipyretic, antibiotic, healing, and antispasmodic properties.

Cosmetic uses: Chickweed is a superior medicinal plant for healing most skin types and conditions. It has strong anti-inflammatory properties on the skin, therefore it is excellent for skin disorders such as eczema and psoriasis. Chickweed can be used as an ointment and is an effective remedy for skin rashes and irritations. Because of its saponin content, chickweed can be used in most skin cleansers and shampoos.

Medicinal uses: Chickweed's saponin content increases the absorption of nutrients and helps increase metabolism. Saponin dissolves and eliminates fat, thereby affecting the thyroid and possibly helping with weight control. Indians make an infusion of chickweed and horsetail to treat lung congestion, blood purification, and bones. In Japan and China it is used to increase menstrual flow and blood circulation. In Spain, its infusion is used for bleeding. In Iran, chickweed is used as an anti-inflammatory plant. Its healing and soothing properties are similar to cortisone. Iranians use it for rheumatic pain and stomach ulcers.

Chickweed is extremely helpful for those with digestive system problems. It eases and helps those with stomach ulcers, constipation, and hemorrhoids. Drink an infusion of chickweed everyday for healthier, more beautiful skin and thick, healthy hair and nails. Chickweed is ideal for nursing mothers as it increases milk flow. Saponin in chickweed is good for diarrhea and urinary tract stones. Iranians drink infusions of chickweed with echinacea, horsetail, and ginseng to increase their immune systems, especially during the winter as the above combination increases the production of white cells and protects the body against bacteria and viruses. One scientific research study in Iran showed that chickweed may prevent and even cure some carcinomas, such as breast cancer.

Chicory (Cichorium intybus)

Parts used: Fresh roots and leaves.

Biochemical contents: Tannins, sugar, insulin (58 percent), alkaloids, and pectin.

Energy: Neutral.

Country of origin: Iran and India.

Harvest time: Chicory leaves can be gathered in the late spring, and the root is unearthed in late fall.

Properties: Chicory has tonic, soothing, and antispasmodic properties.

Cosmetic uses: The tannin content in this herb helps it to make a good lotion for all skin types, especially sensitive and irritated skin. It has emollient properties that make this plant work well for dry and mature skin.

Medicinal uses: Chicory is a plant of ancient usage in most countries. Iranians use it as a liver cleanser, laxative, and for treatment of rheumatism and gout. This is because chicory can eliminate uric acid from the body. Chicory contains alkaloid which helps to regulate rapid heartbeat and lower high blood pressure and fever. In general, chicory resembles dandelion in its medicinal properties. It is good to include in the evening diet. Its extract, combined with watercress and honey and taken on an empty stomach during spring, is very beneficial for both liver and kidneys and enhances the immune system. In India, it is taken to stop diarrhea, reduce fever, and increase flow of menstruation. Chicory can reduce high blood sugar. It is best to be included in daily meals for those who are suffering from high blood sugar and high blood pressure.

To reduce headache an extract of the leaves mix with vinegar is used to massage around the eye, forehead and temple. A combination of chicory extract with vinegar, and rosewater is beneficial for skin disorders, treating diarrhea, and to increase the production of bile and to cleanse the liver and gallbladder.

Chives (Allium schoenoprasum)

Parts used: Leaves.

Biochemical contents: Essential oil, sulfur.

Energy: Warm.

Country of origin: Iran, Asia, then worldwide.

Harvest time: Chive can be picked all year round, especially in spring and summer.

Properties: Chives has tonic and antibacterial properties.

Main uses: Chives are very popular with Iranians, and it is widely used in Iran and Asian countries for many dishes like soups, salads, quiche, soufflÈ, omelets, or herbal rice. Chive can be mixed with other herbs for soufflÈ or rice. Chives can be taken before meals to increases the appetite and saliva secretion. (See recipe on soufflÈ and herbal rice)

Cilantro (Coriandrum Sativum)

Parts used: Leaves, stalks, roots.

Biochemical contents: Fatty essential oil, flavonoid, mucilige, phosphate, vitamins A and C.

Energy: Cool.

Country of origin: Worldwide.

Harvest time: Its leaves are harvested from early summer through fall.

Properties: Cilantro has strong soothing, anti-inflammatory, aromatic, and antispasmodic properties.

Cosmetic uses: Its mucilige content makes it useful for all skin type creams and cleansers, especially sensitive skins. The oil of its seeds is very moisturizing and is ideal for dehydrated and mature skins.

Medicinal uses: Cilantro seeds as spices, are used throughout Asia to soothe stomach indigestion and colic. Japanese and Chinese people use it as a remedy for toothache, upper respiratory inflammation, and fever reduction. Its infusion is used for coughs, colds, measles, and insomnia. Its smoked roots and leaves are applied over children's measles for faster healing. Its seeds and essential oil are good for asthma and flu, as well as increasing menstrual flow. Ancient physicians believed that 30 gm. of cilantro before bed is soporific. Chewing cilantro increases appetite, stops bleeding of the gums (and even strengthens them), and reduces sexual stimulation. Iranians make cilantro soup for coughs, cold, flu, and sore throat. It is also suitable for bloody diarrhea and urinary inflammation.

Cleavers (Galium aperine)

Parts used: Aerial parts.

Biochemical contents: Flavonoid, tannins, and volatile oil.

Energy: Cool.

Country of origin: North America, and European countries.

Harvest time: Cleavers are gathered when in bloom in the springtime.

Properties: Cleavers has soothing, purgative, and diuretic properties.

Cosmetic uses: Cleaver is an excel-lent remedy for most skin disorders and diseases, such as acne, eczema, seborrhea, and psoriasis.

Medicinal uses: Cleaver is very diuretic and soothing. In Europe, they use it to treat bladder and kidney infection. They combine cleaver with horsetail and goldenrod to crush kidney and bladder stones. Cleavers may also lower high blood pressure. In Iran, people make an infusion with cleaver and burdock root to treat skin disorders such as acne because cleavers and burdock both have the ability to purify and cool the blood for better skin healing.

Clove (Caryophyllus aromaticus)

Parts used: Dried flowers and buds.

Biochemical contents: Volatile oil and phenols.

Energy: Warm.

Country of origin: Indonesia.

Harvest time: Clove bud should be gathered when the lower part turns from green to purple.

Properties: Clove has analgesic, soothing, antimicrobial, and stimulant properties.

Cosmetic uses: Clove is used in perfume, soap, and the dental industry and is good for all skin types and conditions because it has the ability to heal and cleanse the skin. The phenol content of this plant makes it highly antiseptic for toning and conditioning skin of all types, especially oily skin.

Medicinal uses: Clove is a traditional remedy in Iran and Mediterranean countries for colds, flu, and bronchitis, and toothache. Its antiseptic properties make it useful for cuts and burns. Clove buds are a good remedy for colds. In Iran, a combination of dried powdered clove, rose, and borage, soaked in rose water for 24 hours, is used for stomach upset, liver detoxification and removal of toxins from the system. Also, 2 tablespoons of dried powdered clove, a cup of pomegranate juice, and 2 tablespoons of honey, mixed and stored in a tight dark glass jar for a week, then mixed with sugar and boiled, produces a syrup which is ideal for cold energy diseases. As soon as one feels heavy or like one is coming down with the flu, prepare the following remedy: one tablespoon of clove, one fourth teaspoon of fresh or dried ginger, two squeezed fresh lemons, and one tablespoon of natural honey. Soak in sixteen ounces of hot water, simmer for ten minutes, and drink three to four cups a day. It is the greatest and fastest remedy for common colds and flu. Essential oil of clove contains 80-90% eugenin which is aromatic with the chemical formula $CH_{12}O_2$. It is also used as a substitute for vanilla. Indonesians smoke dried clove instead of tobacco.

Coltsfoot (Tussilago farfara)

Parts used: Flowers and leaves.

Biochemical contents: Saponins, mucilage, tannins, alkaloid, zinc, potassium, calcium, and bitter glycoside.

Energy: Neutral.

Country of origin: Iran, India.

Harvest time: Coltsfoot flowers should be gathered from the end of winter to mid-spring, and leaves are gathered in June and July.

Properties: Coltfoot has diuretic, tonic, emollient, anti-catarrh, and anti-inflammatory properties.

Cosmetic uses: It is an excellent plant for cleansing all skin types because of its saponin content. It is anti-inflammatory and has healing properties to soothe sensitive skin and to reduce irritation and acne.

Medicinal uses: Coltsfoot contains high percentages of mucilage and tannin, which are all soothing. Iranians value this plants for its healing properties. They make infusions with combinations of coltsfoot, elder, ephedra, and ginger sweetened with honey to treat colds, flu, coughs, and other respiratory problems. If the fresh leaves are applied to the sore area, the zinc content in coltsfoot will be healing to the sore area and soothe the pain. When I was a little girl, my grandfather made pipe cigarettes with coltsfoot, juniper, and mint. He used the dried herb, ground together until finely powdered, and smoked it in pine.

Caution: Excess consumption may damage the liver.

Comfrey (Symphytum officinale)

Parts used: Fresh or dry root and leaves.

Biochemical contents: Mucilage, allantoin, saponins, tannins, essential oil, sugar, protein, alkaloids, carotene, glycosides, vitamin B12, zinc, essential oil, starch.

Energy: Cool.

Country of origin: Europe and Asia.

Harvest time: Comfrey root is gathered during the spring or fall when the allantoin content of the leaves is at its highest.

Properties: Comfrey has astringent, emollient, anti-inflammatory, healing, soothing, expectorant, homeostatic, and tonic properties.

Cosmetic uses: Comfrey is one the most reputable healing plants, because of its allantoin content. Allantoin is a

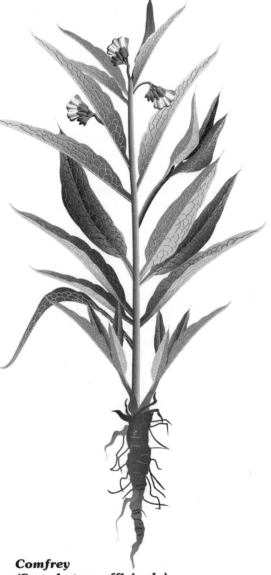

**Comfrey
(Symphytum officinale)**

great ingredient which stimulates and accelerates the cells in the skin. It helps in the healing process and the growth of new skin through a process called cell reproliferation. Comfrey is great for all skin types and conditions, especially for those dry, sun-damaged skins which are associated with wrinkles. It helps to regenerate this wrinkled, damaged skin. It soothes sensitive, aggravated, and irritated skin. Its anti-inflammatory properties give it the power to heal skin tissues. It breaks down the red cells trapped in bruises and also heals the inflammation of acne. Its allantoin content also enables cell reproduction. It moisturizes the skin and aids in absorption of nutrients.

Medicinal uses: Comfrey is one of the most valuable and superior plants. Its strong healing and anti-inflammatory properties are used to treat internal hemorrhaging, whether from lungs, stomach, or bowels. Comfrey root is popular in France for treating stomach ulcer. Fresh root is used topically to heal bruises, wounds, cracking nipples and scratches. Infusion of dried root helps to stop diarrhea.

Ancient Greeks used extract of comfrey to heal topical wounds, repair fractured bones, and help in knitting of bones. Iranians and western Europeans use comfrey to treat stomach ulcer and inflammation of the small intestines. They combine comfrey root with marshmallow root, slippery elm, and honey, then steam for fifteen minutes and drink for stomach pain and upper respiratory disorders.

Greeks soaked comfrey in boiling water for fifteen minutes to release a sticky substance, and then applied this material over wounds or broken bones. After a few minutes, this substance becomes solid. They also soaked piece of fabric in the prepared substance, then wrapped it around the broken bone to accelerate the healing process. This system of healing is called "knit bone."

Dr. Nicholas Culpepen, a British herbalist who used extract of comfrey root for topical and external healing, also believed that infusion of comfrey root is a great remedy for lungs disorders, fever, and reducing hemorrhoidal inflammation.

Caution: Avoid excessive consumption of comfrey. It may damage the liver. The International Institute of Cancer in the USA states that the results of internal use of comfrey on animals after two years of continuous use show liver cancer can develop. Other experiments show that the root is more carcinogenic than leaves.

Coneflower (Echinacea amgistofpoa)

Parts used: Dried root and rhizome.

Biochemical contents: Essential oil, glycoside, insulin, polysaccharide.

Energy: Warm.

Country of origin: European countries.

Harvest time: Coneflower roots are collected in the fall.

Properties: Coneflower has diuretic and soothing properties.

Cosmetic uses : It is used for cleansing problems of skin and other conditions, such as boils and acne, that are associated with impure blood. It is also a wound healer.

Medicinal uses : Coneflower is famed to be one of the most powerful plants to enhance the immune system and increase energy. Research shows, due to the polysaccharide content, it can stimulate the production of white cells and enhance the immune system, thus it is useful for treating infections and allergies. One can combine coneflower (echinacea) with ginseng to fight infections of all kinds, and possibly including cancer of breast. Europeans use coneflower to reduce the inflammation of lungs and sinus infection. Iranians make an infusion with coneflower, clove, and ginger to treat colds and flu. They drink the infusion during wintertime to prevent bacteria from entering the body.

Corn (Zeamaus)

Parts used: Stigmas, leaves, starch meal, and oil.

Biochemical contents: Volatile oil, saponins, alkaloids, glycosides, vitamins C, A, and K, allantoin, tannins, potassium, calcium, and sugar.

Energy: Neutral.

Country of origin: Iran, European countries, then worldwide

Harvest time: Corn can be harvested from summer to the end of fall. Corn silk is best harvested in summer, then separated and dried.

Properties: Corn has laxative, diuretic, demulcent, soothing, cleansing, antiseptic, antispasmodic, and anti-inflammatory properties.

Cosmetic uses: Its saponin level induces cleansing properties affecting both skin condition and body cleansing. Its healing and moisturizing actions are due to tannins and allantoin. Corn is an antioxidant because of its high content of vitamins C and A. Corn is very soothing and can be used in soothing cosmetic masks. Corn can increase the elasticity of the skin. Cornmeal is also used for cake and breads. Cornstarch is generally used as a thickener in cooking.

Medicinal uses: Corn helps in the passing of stones, lowers blood pressure, and increases the flow of bile. If used before bedtime along with other steamed vegetables, such as asparagus, it is very cathartic. Iranians make barbecued corn for an afternoon snack and also for internal cleansing.

Corn Silk (Zea Mays)

Parts used: Silk.

Biochemical contents: Flavonoid, mucilage, organic saponins, allantoin, volatile oil, alkaloid, vitamins A, C, K, and minerals.

Energy: Neutral.

Country of origin: Iran, South America.

Harvest time: Corn silk is harvested in the summer, separated and dried.

Properties: It has anti-inflammatory, soothing, cleansing, antiseptic, antispasmodic, and demulcent properties.

Medicinal uses: The Chinese have used corn silk from ancient time to reduce high blood pressure and alleviate urinary problems. Corn silk is very diuretic, and its high potassium content makes it a great remedy for urinary infections and stones. It soothes and relaxes the lining of the bladder and helps improve urine flow. Corn silk can be combined with horsetail, bearberry, and couch grass to help decrease the pain and discomfort of kidney stones. Iranians make infusions with corn silk and parsley to cure bladder infection. They also use corn silk in salads and a variety of soups, especially during cold and flu season.

Couch Grass (Agropyran repens) (L.)Beauvois)

Parts used: Rhizome.

Biochemical contents: Volatile oil, glycoside, mucilage, saponin, silica, iron, potassium, vitamins A and B.

Energy: Warm.

Country of origin: Iran, European countries.

Harvest time: Couch grass can be harvested from spring to early fall.

Properties: Couch grass has diuretic, antimicrobial, antiseptic, anti-inflammatory, and soothing properties.

Medicinal uses: Couch grass is a very powerful medicinal plant to treat urinary tract infections and kidney diseases. Europeans use couch grass to reduce the pain and inflammation of rheumatic joint pain, fever, and liver detoxification. Couch grass has antibiotic and soothing properties. Because of its volatile oil and mucilage content, it is a great remedy for cystitis/ bladder infections and stones. Iranians make an infusion with two parts dried couch grass and one part of each corn silk, horsetail, and parsley in thirty-two ounces of boiling water. Simmer for twenty minutes. The above recipe should be taken one full glass three times a day to treat bladder and kidney infections.

Cowslip (Caltha palustris)

Parts used: Root, leaves, and flowers.

Biochemical contents: Volatile oil, saponins, flavonoids, glycosides, and essential oil.

Energy: Neutral.

Country of origin: Iran, Egypt, India.

Harvest time: Cowslip leaves and flowers are harvested from March to May, and roots are harvested in the fall.

Properties: Cowslip has expectorant, diuretic, antiseptic, and sedative properties.

Cosmetic uses: Cowslip can be used in most skin cleansers and conditioners because of its volatile oil and saponin content. The flowers, containing most of the essential oil, are ideal for oily skin. Cowslip ointment can be used for sunburn and inflammation of the skin.

Medicinal uses: Cowslip is a most valuable plant due to its soothing and healing properties. It is best used for nervous tension, insomnia, and nervous headaches. Because of the salicylate present in its roots, Egyptians made cowslip tea and decoctions with the root to treat arthritis pain. They also made a special wine with cowslip to help digestion. Cowslip roots contain a high percentage of saponin, which makes it ideal for treating bronchitis and whooping coughs.

In Iran, people make tea with cowslip, peppermint, cardamom, and honey to reduce muscle tension and menstrual pain.

Cramp Bark (Viburnum opulus)

Parts used: Bark.

Biochemical contents: Bitter principles, tannin, hydroquinones.

Energy: Warm.

Country of origin: Iran.

Harvest time: Cramp bark can be collected from mid- to late spring.

Properties: Crampbark has antispasmodic, sedative, and astringent properties.

Medicinal uses: Cramp bark is one of the most qualified plants for comforting cramps, menstrual pain, and female reproductive problems. Ancient Iranians combined cramp bark with ginger and black haw to prevent miscarriage. Cramp bark is an excellent relaxant for muscle tension and arthritis pain.

Caution: The fresh berries are poisonous.

Cucumber (Cucumis sativus)

Parts used: Seeds, oil, and the whole fresh fruit and juice.

Biochemical contents: Tannins, mucilage, vitamins, and minerals.

Energy: Cold.

Country of origin: Iran, Asia, U.S.A, then worldwide

Harvest time: Cucumber can be harvested from end of spring to fall.

Properties: Cucumber has diuretic, cooling, and soothing properties.

Cosmetic uses: Cucumbers can be used in creams for all skin types and are a cooling remedy for sensitive, inflamed skin and puffiness around the eyes. Slice a cucumber and place slices around the eyes for ten minutes; this will relieve both the puffiness and inflammation of sun-damaged and irritated skin. It is a quick remedy especially if one is short on sleep.

Medicinal uses: Iranians use cucumber to cleanse and soothe stomach inflammation. Its seeds are very nutritious and unblock the urinary system. Its smashed form is very useful for skin disorders. Infusion of its roots is useful for beri-beri disease. The extract of its leaves is good for infant indigestion. Its end contains bitter glycoside, highly recommended for bladder pain, stomach pain, liver and gallbladder cleansing, and increase of bile flow. They also use cucumber like a fruit or in salads, also as a summer afternoon snack with tomatoes, feta cheese, and other herbs. Iranians make cold summer soup with cucumber (See the recipe on Cold Summer Soup).

Cumin: (Nigella Satival.)

Parts used: Seeds

Biochemical contents: 2% essential oil, glycosides, saponin, 35% fixed oi.

Energy: Warm

Country of origin: Europe, N. Africa, Iran, Asia

Harvest time: Cumin seeds are harvested from late summer to fall.

Properties: It has antiseptic, anti-inflammatory, and cleansing properties.

Cosmetic uses: Cumin seed oil contains essential oil and saponin which make this plant qualify as ingredients for all skin types cleansers and conditioners. It has anti-inflammatory properties which make it very good for skin disorders such as couperose. It reduces the redness and blisters from the skin.

Medicinal uses: Indians used cumin for digestion and gas release from the stomach. Cumin increases menstrual flow and also increases milk flow in nursing mothers.

Cumin seed oil with sesame oil is good for external applications such as to cuts, burns, and stings, as it reduces inflammation on the skin.

Iranians use cumin seeds over breads and cookies, and they use it with rice pudding and butter for women after childbirth for rejuvenation.

Infusion of cumin seeds are good for coughs and upper respiratory problems, hepatitis, arthritis, and if is used with honey, it help to excrete bladder and kidney stones.

Caution: Overdosage may cause miscarriage.

Cypress Tree (Cupressus sempervirens L.)

Parts used: Fruits, leaves, branches.

Biochemical contents: Fatty essential oil 2% and pinene 80%.

Energy: Warm.

Country of origin: Iran.

Harvest time: Summer through fall.

Properties: Cypress tree has antiseptic, antispasmodic, antibacterial, and aromatic properties.

Cosmetic uses: Because of its antiseptic properties, this plant is ideal for all skin types as a conditioner and oily skin cleanser. It can also be used as a main ingredient for treating skin disorders such as acne and boils.

Medicinal uses: Cypress leaves and its essential oil are used for treating urinary infection and gastrointestinal disorders. In India, they chop the fruit and branches and use them for treating intestinal worms and to stop bleeding. In Iran, they use the leaves for gastrointestinal problems and to increase urine. Some individuals use the leaves as a gargle and chew the fruit for gum diseases. Cypress dried leaves mixed with honey are great to treat coughs and flu. To treat baldness and hair loss, cypress fruits can be boiled in vinegar until cooked, then sesame oil added. If henna is added to this combination and applied to skull and hair, it makes the hair black, and hair root becomes strong. Some people in Iran boil the cypress in water to use before meals to stop diarrhea and internal bleeding, especially of the uterus, and to heal hemorrhoids.

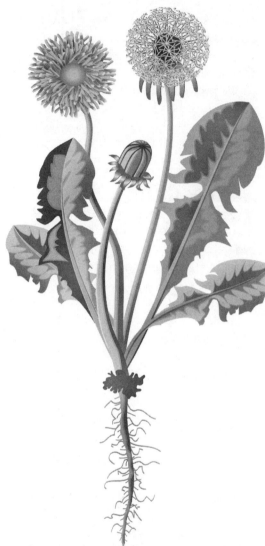

**Dandelion
(Taraxacum officinale)**

Dandelion (Taraxacum officinale)

Parts used: Root, leaves, or whole plant.

Biochemical contents: Bitter glyco-side, inulin, pectin, phenolic acid, vitamins A, B, C, and D, potassium, and iron.

Energy: Cool.

Country of origin: Iran, China, India.

Harvest time: The best time for gathering is from spring to late summer, and roots are gathered in late fall.

Properties: It has diuretic, tonic, digestive, stimulant, antispasmodic, and sedative properties.

Cosmetic uses: A remedy for many skin diseases, dandelion is excellent for excessively oily skin, pH balancing, and a fine skin toner and conditioner. The vitamin A in dandelion is higher than that of carrots, therefore this plant is best qualified for acne and for maintaining a healthy and beautiful complexion.

Medicinal uses: Dandelion is the best friend for all internal organs especially the liver. It cleans the liver and blood, and stimulates the production and flow of bile from your liver and gallbladder. It increases one's metabolism and control weight. Dandelion is best taken fresh every day with your salad. It is very rich in most vitamins and minerals especially vitamin A. It increases energy and immune system.

In China, they dig out dandelion by root, and dry it. After six month they make syrup. They use its syrup to increase the milk, and stimulate the production of bile. They also use it for wounds, toothache, acne, and eczema. Dandelion is an excellent blood purifier. Its leaves and root can be soaked to release bio-chemical properties and to reduce the inflammations on breast, itchy skin and stomach inflammation.

In India, dandelion root is used to treat liver disorders, and to crush kidney stone, and to stop internal bleeding.

In Iran dandelion is used to treat kidney and bladder infection. They also use it to increase the milk in nursing mother. The extraction from the leaves is used around the eye to increases the vision. Iranian use dandelion as a suppository to reduce uterus pain and inflammation. They also make a compress with dandelion leave and is used to reduce arthritis pain and inflammation.

Dandelion syrup recipe:
Sixteen ounces of dried dandelion leaves with 68 ounces of boiled water, soak the leaves in water and using a lid let it simmer for twelve hours, then strain it. add honey and boil the extract until is thick, drink one tablespoon every day before meal, to increase the appetite, and tone stomach tissue.

Devil's Claw (Charpagophytum Procumbens)

Parts used: Tuber.

Biochemical contents: Glycosides, resin, salicylic acid.

Energy: Cool.

Country of origin: Africa, Iran.

Harvest time: Devil's claw's roots and trunk are collected at the end of the rainy season in its native Africa.

Properties: Devil's Claw has a powerful anti-inflammatory property.

Cosmetic uses: Devil's claw has a reputation for treating most skin diseases, such as eczema and psoriasis.

Medicinal uses: Devil's claw is an African plant with strong anti-inflammatory and pain-relieving properties comparable to cortisone. Africans use this plant to reduce and ease arthritis and joint pains. Europeans use devil's claw to lower blood sugar. In Iran, people use devil's claw for tension headaches and muscle tension. They combine devil's claw with marjoram and borage and infuse for fifteen minutes. Drink daily for arthritis pain and to stop menstrual pain.

Caution: Devil's claw should be avoided during pregnancy since it stimulates uterine muscles.

Dill Weed (Aniethum graveolens)

Parts used: Leaves, stem, aerial portion.

Biochemical contents: Essential oil, glycosides, and fatty oil.

Energy: Warm.

Country of origin: Iran.

Harvest time: Dill weed can be harvested from late spring to late fall.

Properties: Dill weed has diuretic and tonic properties.

Main uses: Dill makes a good tea for the digestive system. Its leaves are used in salads and a variety of other dishes. In Iran, dill weed is used in many dishes and salads (see recipe on dill weed dish).

Medicinal uses: Dill weed is primarily used for stomach ache and insomnia caused by indigestion. It is a good remedy for children's colicky stomach. Dill can be taken by nursing mothers as a tea to increase the flow of milk. In most Asian countries it is used for indigestion and colic. Ancient Iranians used it to increase menstrual flow, as well as urination, and to crush kidney and bladder stones. Its infusion with honey is good for internal detoxification.

Echinacea (Echinacea Angustifolia)

Parts used: Leaves and root.

Biochemical contents: Essential oil, polysaccharides, echinacoside.

Energy: Cool.

Country of origin: Asia.

Harvest time: Echinacea root should be unearthed in fall; the root is best when used fresh.

Properties: Echinacea has tonic, antimicrobial, anti-catarrh, and anti-inflammatory properties.

Cosmetic uses: Echinacea can be used on most skin conditions, especially boils and acne, since it is effective against both bacterial and viral attacks.

Medicinal uses: Echinacea is perhaps the greatest herbal medicine known to date. Native Americans have used it for centuries. It can be used for any kind of infection anywhere in the body. Echinacea is one the superior plants for immune system, helping the production of white blood cells and body's ability to resist infection. Iranians have used echinacea for centuries. They use it in soups and rice to enhance the immune system, especially during illness and after surgery. They drink echinacea tea for arthritis pain and blood cleansing. Since echinacea is

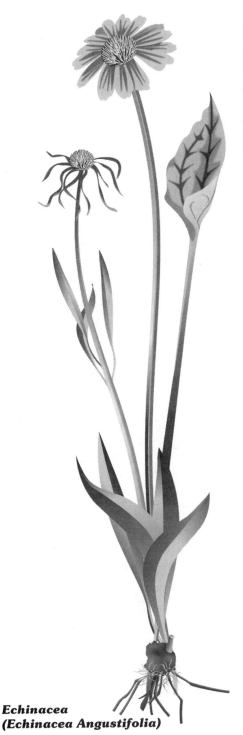

effective against both bacterial and viral attacks, it may be used for diseases like cancers, and possibly treatment of AIDS. Echinacea is the best herb for all acute inflammatory conditions. It is very mild, and there are no reports of side effects. Echinacea can be combined with other herbs, like ginger, chickweed, and ginseng, to treat upper respiratory problems such as tonsillitis, and sinus infections.

Iranian make tea with echinacea, ginseng root, horsetail, chickweed, and ginger root. Add honey and drink everyday during the wintertime to prevent colds and upper respiratory infections.

Elder (Sambucus)

Parts Used: Flowers, berries, leaves, root, bark.

Biochemical contents: Mucilage, sugar, pectin, glycosides, fruit acid, vitamin C linoleic acid, tannins, vitamin C, and fatty acid.

Energy: Cool.

Country of origin: Iran, Asia, and Europe.

Harvest time: Elder flowers are gathered in the spring to summer. Bark and berries are best harvested in the fall.

Properties: Elder flowers have anti-catarrh activity, the berries are diuretic

Echinacea
(Echinacea Angustifolia)

and cathartic, and the leaves are diuretic and expectorant.

Cosmetic uses: The mucilage and tannins in the plant are helpful in skin inflammation, irritation, and other conditions. Elder soothes and heals irritated skin and makes a good cream for sensitive and irritated skin.

Medicinal uses: Elder is one the most famed and powerful plants used in Iran to treat colds, coughs, headaches, and any inflammation of the upper respiratory tract or sinuses. Iranians make an infusion with elder leaves and salt for gargling Egyptian used an infusion of leaves and applied it to the forehead to release headaches. They also used an ointment from the leaves for bruises and sprains. Elderberries make wonderful pies and wine. They also act as a laxative and help to eliminate toxins from the system. In general, elder is a superior plant for treating flu, colds, and upper respiratory problems. In France, people use elder in salads for internal cleansing and constipation. Ancient physicians prescribed two ounces of elder leaves boiled in water or milk as a drink daily to relieve constipation. Chinese use elder leaf infusion for colds, fevers, and sore throat.

Ephedra (Ephedra sinica)

Parts used: Stem, twigs.

Biochemical contents: Alkaloid, ephedrine.

Energy: Warm.

Country of origin: Iran, Asia.

Harvest time: Ephedra is best gathered in the fall, before the frost, when the alkaloid content is at its highest.

Properties: Ephedra has stimulant and anti-allergy properties.

Medicinal uses: Ephedra is used with the greatest success for the treatment of asthma, bronchitis, lungs, coughs, and sinus problems. Ephedra is one of the oldest known medicines, used by the Chinese for thousands of years to treat upper respiratory problems and arthritis pain. American Indians used ephedra and other spices, such as ginger and cinnamon, for treatment of rheumatic pain, whooping coughs, and fever. Ephedra is a very popular herb in Iran for treating colds, and sinus pain. They make an infusion with ephedra, peppermint, and elder to relieve sinus pain and sore throat. They also use it as a steam inhalation with eucalyptus and sage to kill bacteria around the home and unblock nasal and sinus passageways.

Eucalyptus (Eucalyptus globulus)

Parts used: Leaves and oil from leaves.

Biochemical contents: Volatile oil, sesquiterpene alcohol, essential oil.

Energy: Warm.

Country of origin: Iran, India.

Harvest time: Eucalyptus can be gathered all year round.

Properties: It has tonic and antibacterial properties.

Cosmetic uses: The volatile oil in the plant is highly antiseptic. It is most useful for acne, skin conditions, and boils.

Medicinal uses: Eucalyptus is a most powerful plant to treat colds, coughs, and lung and sinus congestion. Eucalyptus leaves or oil can be steamed to kill bacteria at home, and inhalation of this herb or oil is effective for improving lung diseases. To relieve sinus pain and pressure, pour a few drops of eucalyptus oil and put some fresh leaves into a pot of hot water and let it boil; inhale through the nose while applying accupressure massage around the sinus area. Excess mucus that causes the pain will be released through the nasal passage. Eucalyptus also combats lung infections. The volatile oil passes through the lungs and is exhaled. Eucalyptus is one of the most popular plants in Iran for sinus pain and infection. They steam eucalyptus leaves everyday during the winter to kill bacteria around the home and to unblock nasal and sinus passageways.

Caution: Never take this plant internally.

Evening Primrose (Oenothera biennis)

Parts used: Extracted seed oil, leaves, and root.

Biochemical contents: Essential fatty acid and gamma linoleic acid (GLA).

Energy: Warm.

Country of origin: Europe, Asia.

Harvest time: Evening primrose does not open until the second year, and the seeds can be collected the second year in spring.

Properties: It has anti-inflammatory, antispasmodic, astringent, and sedative properties.

Cosmetic uses: Evening primroses contain anti-inflammatory property that makes this plant very good as an ingredient for all skin type moisturizer especially sensitive skin.

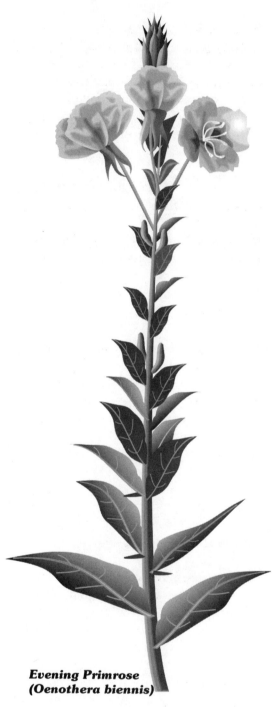

Evening Primrose
(Oenothera biennis)

GLA contain in evening primrose make this plant very beneficial for all skin type cleansers, because GLA has ability to keep the complexion pH balanced.

Principle uses: After boiling, evening primrose's root and leaves can be used for blood cleansing and are considered delicious. French call this plant "gardener's ghambone." The fatty acid GLA (gamma linoleic acid) can be found in beauty products and is very beneficial for regulating blood pressure, keeping complexion balance, and treating menstrual pain. Evening primrose contains 10% GLA. It is a most powerful plant for treating PMS and hormonal disorders. It has beneficial effects in calming hyperactive children. Because evening primrose contains a large percentage of GLA and the body converts GLA into a very important substances like progesterone, evening primrose can be very beneficial to the body and play an important role in regulating menstruation, blood pressure and the health of the skin. The production of progesterone in some people may stop, therefore it is necessary to take plants such as evening primrose and borage to help encourage its production.

Eyebright (Euphrasia officinalis)

Parts used: Aerial.

Biochemical contents: glycosides, phenolic acid, tannin, saponins.

Energy: Cool.

Country of origin: Iran

Harvest time: Eyebright is gathered from late summer to fall.

Properties: Eyebright has tonic, astringent, anti-inflammatory, and anti-catarrhal properties.

Cosmetic uses: Eyebright is useful in many skin conditioners and toners. Its combination of astringent and anti-inflammatory properties makes it relevant for many skin conditions, especially sensitive and irritated skin.

Medicinal uses: Eyebright is an excellent remedy for mucous membrane irritation, sinusitis, and other congestive states. Eyebright has cooling and detoxifying properties and is especially good for inflammation of the eye and sinus. Eyebright is a frequently used plant in Iran for fever, colds, sore throat, and sinus congestion. Ancient Egyptians used it in a hot compress over sore and infected eyes and as an eyewash. Eyebright can be inhaled as a steam for sinus and nasal congestion.

False Unicorn Root (Chamaelirium luteum)

Parts used: Root, rhizome.

Biochemical contents: Glycosides, saponins.

Energy: Cool.

Country of origin: Iran

Harvest time: The underground part of false unicorn is gathered in the fall.

Properties: It has diuretic and uterine tonic properties.

Medicinal uses: False unicorn is one of the most famous plants in Iran used for the female reproductive system. It has been used for treating absence or delay of periods, miscarriages, and vomiting during pregnancy. Combine false unicorn with black cohosh and marjoram for amenorrhea. False unicorn is one of the best tonics and is a good remedy for toning sexual organs in particular. False unicorn can also be used for treating anorexia.

Fennel (Funiculum vulgare)

Parts used: Root, seed, and fresh leaves.

Biochemical contents: Volatile oil in seed, linoleic acid, vitamins, and minerals (calcium, and potassium).

Energy: Warm.

Country of origin: Iran, Asia.

Fennel leaves can be harvested from spring to summer, and the seed can be harvested in the fall.

Properties: Fennel has antispasmodic, tonic, and stimulant properties.

Cosmetic uses: Fennel seeds have antiseptic properties. It is a moisturizer, helping to increase the flow of oxygen to the skin and has a toning effect on skin tissue. It is ideal for smokers who don't have a normal circulation. Fennel has anti-wrinkle properties especially when combined with other herbs, such as parsley and lavender.

Medicinal uses: Fennel is an excellent stomach and intestinal remedy. It relieves colic and stimulates the appetite. Since ancient times in Iran, the seeds have been used for indigestion, and fennel tea is used for nursing mothers since it promotes the flow of breast milk. Fennel can be combined with parsley and horsetail to treat urinary infections and stones. Fennel can be used in a variety of soups and salads. Ancient Iranians used fennel tea with honey and a powder made from cardamom seeds after childbirth to increase flow of breast milk and also to tone the uterine muscles more rapidly.

Fenugreek (Trigonella Foenum)

Parts used: Seeds, leaves, and stem.

Biochemical contents: Volatile oil, glycosides, mucilage, essential oil, minerals, and vitamins.

Energy: Warm.

Country of origin: Iran, Africa, Asia.

Harvest time: The leaves are gathered late spring and summer, and the seeds are collected in fall.

Properties: Fenugreek has tonic, emollient, and expectorant properties.

Cosmetic uses: Skin toning and conditioning. Its antiseptic properties make it useful for skin conditions, such as acne. The seeds are used as an emollient for boils and as a skin-softening ointment.

Medicinal uses: Fenugreek can be a fine contraceptive. Fenugreek seeds increase the flow of milk in cows and may be a good source of diosgenin, the essential ingredient in birth control pills. There have been clinical investigations about fenugreek leaves as a source of birth control essential ingredients. Fenugreek is a very popular herb with Iranians. They make a variety of dishes, especially stews and soups, and use it as medicine to treat sore throat and upper respiratory problems. Fenugreek has a bitter taste and releases a delicious and strong aroma while cooking. Its infusion with honey opens mucous membranes. Its infusion with tamarin is good relief for tension after giving birth, for skin disorders such as eczema, for liver and gallbladder inflammation, and for reducing hair loss. Blended with vinegar and rose oil, it can cure headaches and help prevent brain stroke. Fenugreek is useful for the treatment of diabetes, gout, coughs, backache, and high blood pressure.

Overdoses of fenugreek can decrease sperm production and sexual desire.

(see recipe on Fenugreek Stew).

Feverfew (Chrysanthemum parthenium)

Parts used: Leaves and flowers.

Biochemical contents: Volatile oil, tannin.

Energy: Cool.

Country of origin: Europe, Asia.

Harvest time: Feverfew leaves can be picked during the spring, and the flowers are gathered in the summer.

Properties: Feverfew has anti-inflammatory and relaxant properties.

Medicinal uses: Feverfew is one of the best herbal remedies for migraine headaches. In 1978, clinical investigations proved that feverfew leaves can cure migraine headaches. In 1988, a study again proved its effectiveness. Feverfew dried flowers are a good remedy for fever and muscle spasm. Feverfew has anti-inflammatory properties. It relieves the inflammation and pain of arthritis. If migraine headache is associated with menstrual pain and PMS, feverfew may help the depression and dysmenorrhea, especially in combination with borage, valerian, and passion flower. Ancient Iranians used it for liver and urinary disorders. It increases the secretion of sweat glands and urination, and it is also good for stomach pain. For insomnia, boil feverfew with barley and lavender oil, then massage it on the forehead to relax the mind. Massage the recipe over eyes to improve the sight. Some people believe that it may cure eye cataracts. Feverfew has become popular in Europe since 1970, for the treatment of migraine headaches, indigestion, and reducing blood pressure. It has been used traditionally within Iran for the past few centuries. Smelling the feverfew flower is a relaxant and soporific.

One famous British physician name John Parkinson in the 7th century the after long research had claimed feverfew is great for all kinds of headaches.

A hundred years afterward physician name John Hill claimed feverfew is great for migraine headache as well as female problems.

Caution: Some users of feverfew have developed mouth ulcers. Should this occur, discontinue. It also increases menstrual flow and should be avoided during pregnancy.

Figwort (Scrophularia Nodosa)

Parts used: Aerial parts.

Biochemical contents: Saponins, flavonoids, resin, cardioactive glycosides, pectic acid. Figwort root contains some toxin alkaloid.

Energy: Neutral.

Country of origin: Asia, North America, and most European countries.

Harvest time: Figwort leaves are gathered in the summer when it is flowering.

Properties: Figwort has diuretic and cardiac stimulant properties.

Cosmetic uses: In Iran, figwort has been used topically since ancient times. Figwort root and leaves are mostly used for skin disorders, such as eczema, psoriasis, acne, and itchy irritated skin. It is also very useful for treating baldness. Because of its cleansing properties, figwort is used as a general skin cleanser. It also stimulates the lymphatic glands.

Medicinal uses: Its cleansing effect is caused by the diuretic and purgative properties. It may be used as a laxative in combination with other purgative herbs, such as gentian and dandelion.

Caution: Poisonous in large doses (Restricted). Should not be taken if there is abnormal heartbeat.

Flax (Linum usitassimum)

Parts used: Seed and oil.

Biochemical contents: Linoleic acid, mucilage, protein, and glycoside, fatty acid.

Energy: Cool.

Country of origin: Iran, Asia, Europe.

Harvest time: Flax seeds are collected in the fall when fully ripe.

Properties: Flax has emollient and laxative properties.

Cosmetic uses: Its mucilage content gives soothing, healing, and firming effect to skin tissues. Its high levels of protein and linoleic acid make flax oil very good for burns and inflamed skin, especially for psoriasis and boils.

Medicinal uses: Flax seed is a laxative, emollient, and demulcent. It is used for coughs, colds, and bronchitis. Flax is mostly known for its stem fiber, which is what makes it an excellent remedy for constipation. It helps to increase the flow of bile and cleanses the system. Iranians use one tablespoon of flax seeds with their meal to prevent constipation and also to cleanse the liver.

Caution: Three ounces of seed or more taken at once can cause poisoning.

Foxglove (Digitalis purpurea)

Parts used: Leaves.

Biochemical contents: Several glycosides including digitoxin, which acts on the heart muscles.

Energy: Cool.

Country of origin: Iran, European countries

Harvest time: Foxglove leaves are picked from the second year of growth.

Properties: Foxglove has a cardiotonic property.

Medicinal uses: Foxglove should be taken as a medication only under the direction of a physician. Foxglove has delightful flowers and grows on roadsides. Foxglove is used for palpitations of the heart and as a cardiac stimulant. Ancient Egyptians used foxglove for asthma attacks. Ancient Iranians used steam from

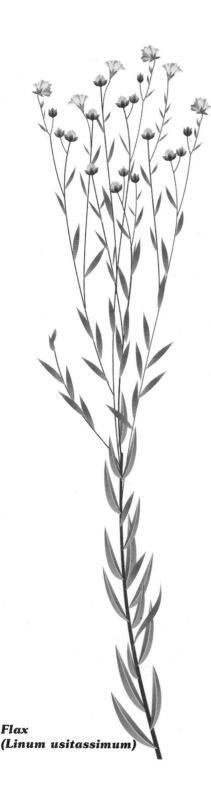

Flax
(Linum usitassimum)

foxglove to regulate heartbeat and to reduce anxiety attacks. Do not take foxglove internally, unless under a doctor's supervision.

Caution: This plant is extremely poisonous and can cause paralysis and sudden death (Restricted).

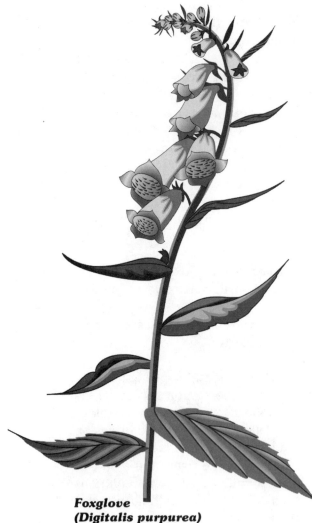

**Foxglove
(Digitalis purpurea)**

Garlic (Allium sativum).

Parts used: cloves.

Biochemical contents: Volatile oil, vitamins A, B2, and C, potassium, magnesium, and amino acids.

Energy: Hot.

Country of origin: Mediterranean countries, Iran and then worldwide.

Harvest time: Garlic is harvested in early fall.

Properties: Garlic has antiseptic, anti-inflammatory, antispasmodic, anti-catarrh, antibacterial, antimicrobial, stimulant, and tonic properties.

Cosmetic uses: Garlic has strong anti-bacterial and antiseptic properties caused by the volatile oil. Garlic can be used in most skin cleansers and toners.

Medicinal uses: Garlic is a superior herbs that can be taken ever day for better health and to enhance the immune system. Garlic is a useful remedy for colds, coughs, high cholesterol, high blood pressure, blood sugar and control of mild diabetes. Garlic also helps digestion. Garlic's ability to control blood clotting makes it useful in cardiovascular disease.

Syrup of garlic is a powerful expectorant, valuable for asthma, coughs, and chronic bronchitis. In Iran, garlic syrup is made by adding vinegar to fresh garlic in a glass jar, sealing the top, and letting it sit for many years to age. The product turns into a brownish, thick, sweet and sour syrup that makes a great remedy for arthritis, rheumatism and cold. In Iran, people who live in the north, with its high humidity use garlic and garlic syrup every day to prevent muscle ache and arthritis. There are garlic syrups available in Iran that are forty years old. Research shows that in China, 80 percent of people who add one clove of garlic daily to their diet do not get stomach cancer. One report from a Chinese medicinal journal indicated that Chinese physicians in Changsha due to a tight financial budget could not supply an antibiotic named amphotericin to treat brain disease and meningitis infection. They instead used garlic orally and by injection to cure diseases. Eleven out of 16 patients were cured by garlic instead of antibiotics. This result make one consider the utility of garlic when it appears to be able to cross the blood-brain in order to treat disease, which is something that many of the strongest antibiotics cannot do. In fact, in early time before antibiotics were discovered, physicians prescribed garlic to kill infectious bacteria. Ancient Egyptians worshipped garlic. Pliny, a famous Italian scientist who lived one century before Christ prescribed and recommended garlic for treating sixty-one diseases. In 1858, Pasteur, a famous bacteriologist, discovered the power of garlic by experimenting and observing that bacteria were destroyed in extract of garlic.

In Iran, some people eat garlic everyday for weight reduction. Garlic is a routine part of the Iranian diet. It can be used fresh, baked, sautÈed, or cooked in variety of soups and other dishes. It is a powerful antibacterial and anti-fungal herb. Iranians also use garlic to treat coughs, flu, and sinus and throat infections. It has also been used successfully to control diarrhea, diphtheria, whooping cough, typhoid, and hepatitis, and weight. One clove of garlic a day keeps the cancer and bacteria away. Garlic liquefies the blood and prevents heart attacks. Some research even shows it is also an anti-cancer agent, especially for breast cancer.

Gentian (Gentiana)

Parts used: Dried root and rhizome.

Biochemical contents: Bitter glycosides, alkaloids, volatile oil, and sugar.

Energy: Warm.

Country of origin: Asia.

Harvest time: Gentian roots are dug up in fall.

Properties: Gentian has antimicrobial, tonic, and gastric stimulant properties.

Medicinal uses: Gentian has been

used as an appetizer and for internal detoxification since ancient times.

Gentian's glycoside content helps to promote digestive secretion. Its bitter root helps the flow of bile and detoxifies the liver and gallbladder. Ancient physicians believed gentian, used after surgery or sickness, to be highly effective in reducing fever. Gentian tincture improves appetite and, if taken before meals, promotes digestion and absorption of nutrients. Gentian's alkaloid content is useful for gastric and intestinal inflammation and also reduces fever. Iranians make a tincture with a combination of gentian, dandelion, rosemary, and cardamom. This is used for arthritic and rheumatic joint pain. They also take it before meals to increase the appetite and digest food better. It is a good appetizer. Chinese drink its tea to purify blood and cure acne and boils. Its root is good for bloody diarrhea, fever, tuberculosis, and faintness. It also reduces weakness in knees and joints. The most recent scientific research shows that gentian root strongly stimulates the digestive system. Ancient Egyptians and Greeks used gentian root syrup to stimulate the appetite and to kill worms of all kinds in the stomach and intestine. It cures liver disorders and heals wounds. No research shows that gentian root stimulates uterus muscle, yet for the last hundred years it has been used to increase menstrual flow. Pregnant women should avoid it, and it is also not recommended for patients with high blood pressure.

Caution: Long doses may cause vomiting.

Ginger (Zingiber officinale)

Parts used: Root fresh or dried.

Biochemical contents: Volatile oil, glycoside, alkaloid, minerals ,essential oil.

Energy: Warm.

Country of origin: Iran, Asia, India.

Harvest time: Ginger roots are dug out after the leaves have dried.

Properties: This plant has stimulant and antispasmodic properties.

Principle uses: Ginger settles the digestive system, strengthens and dilates the blood vessels and increases blood circulation. It also eases morning sickness and motion sickness. Ginger may be good for hangovers. If suffering from bad circulation, try hand and foot baths with fresh ginger, cinnamon stick, and warm water. In the mornings, soak hands and massage for a few minutes; soak feet in the evenings and massage. This treatment will dilate the blood vessels and increase blood circulation. Since ginger has a warm energy, it is best taken after eating cold energy foods for balance. Ginger is a treatment of colds, flu, and coughs. For flu or colds, make an infusion of ginger by adding one teaspoon of fresh ground ginger root, three tablespoons of fresh squeezed lemon juice, one tablespoon of honey, one tablespoon of elder flower, and one glass of water. Boil the water, add the ginger and elder, let it simmer for ten minutes and then add honey and lemon juice. This is a time tested remedy for colds and flu. Repeat every four to six hours.

The Chinese use fresh ginger in a variety of dishes, and Iranians use ginger in cakes, cookies, candies and drinks as well. I remember as a little girl, my grandmother would eat ginger candy on the days that her diet consisted of many cold energy level foods. She would use ginger candy to balance cold energy.

Ginseng (Panax)

Parts used: Root.

Biochemical contents: Saponin, ginsenin, fatty essential oil, alkaloid, bitter principle, and vitamin B complex.

Energy: Warm.

Country of origin: China.

Harvest time: Ginseng root is harvested six months after planting when the active principle is concentrated.

Properties: Gensing has healing, soothing, antibacterial and antimicro-bial properties.

Medicinal uses: Ginseng root has healing properties, increases energy, and supports the immune system. Scientific research in 1947 showed that ginseng root and other parts amazingly cure nervous tension, enhance the immune system, and give energy. Today scientists are still researching and so far have found many physiological substances from ginseng, one of which is called panaxin, which strengthens muscles, as well as controls metabolism and sweat glands. Most recent research shows that individuals who use ginseng root tea are physically, emotionally, and psychologically healthier, happier, and stronger. Ginseng root contains adaptogenic properties which balance physiological functions and blood pressure. Also, its antioxidant content increases the power of adaptogenic properties. The most recent research by American agriculturists shows that ginseng root normalizes blood sugar eventually.

Ginseng has been used in many countries, especially China. Chinese strongly believe in its efficiency to give energy and increase white cells, relieve exhaustion and nervous tensions, and normalize the digestive system. Ginseng root increases the metabolism of sugars and hydrocarbons, regulates and normalizes oxygen, and is very beneficial for brain and nerve relaxation. Chinese use this herb to relieve stress, increase energy level, and reinforce the immune system. They believe it works directly on the central nervous system and helps resist bacteria, viruses, and physical and mental stress. Since it has a sedative effect, it is useful for insomnia. Ancient Iranians used this plant for alleviating physical stress, providing vitality and energy, and relaxing exhausted minds. Iranians make an infusion with ginseng root, chickweed, and echinacea. They add honey and drink this during wintertime to prevent bacteria and viruses from entering the body. They also drink the same combination during sicknesses, after surgery, and after childbirth. They make a soup with ginseng root, spinach, chickweed, echinacea and nettle during illness and after surgery to increase the production of white cells and faster healing.

Goat's Rue (Galega officinalis)

Parts used: Aerial.

Biochemical contents: Alkaloid, saponin, flavonoid, tannins.

Energy: Neutral.

Country of origin: European countries, the northern part of Iran.

Harvest time: Goat's rue grows in damp areas, mostly continental Europe and is harvested mainly in the summer.

Properties: It has anti-inflammatory, stimulant, cleansing, anti-diabetic, and antispasmodic properties.

Cosmetic uses: Goat's rue can be used in most skin cleansers and conditioners because of its saponin content. It also helps to reduce inflammation of acne and sensitive skin.

Medicinal uses: Goat's rue is one of the most common anti-diabetic herbs, able to decrease the blood sugar level and maintain it. Iranians use an infusion of goat's rue for nursing mothers to increase the flow of milk and also use it after birth for internal cleansing.

Caution: To be used by diabetics only under medical supervision.

Golden Seal (Hydrastis canadensis)

Parts used: Root, rhizomes.

Biochemical contents: Alkaloids including berberine, essential oil, volatile oil, fatty oil, resin, sugar.

Energy: Warm.

Country of origin: Iran, India.

Harvest time: Golden seal roots are unearthed from three year old plants in the fall.

Properties: Golden seal has anti-inflammatory, antiseptic, and stimulant properties.

Cosmetic uses: Golden seal is highly antiseptic and can be used in most skin cleansers and astringents. It works well on infected skin, as a lotion or toner, and to disinfect and soothe the area.

Medicinal uses: Iranians use golden seal to enhance the immune system and fight flu, colds, and infections of the upper respiratory tract. They use it as a tea everyday during wintertime. North American Indians used golden seal to treat upper respiratory infections. Golden seal is one of the most powerful plants that can be used for a significant number of infections by helping the production of white cells and enhancing the immune systems. Alkaloid content in this plant lowers blood pressure and reduces fever.

Caution: Golden seal should not be taken during pregnancy due to alkaloid berberine content.

Golden rod (Solidago)

Parts used: Flowers, leaves.

Biochemical contents: Saponins, tannins, essential oil.

Energy: Neutral.

Country of origin: Iran.

Harvest time: Goldenrod stalks are collected from the summer to the fall.

Properties: Goldenrod has anti-in-flammatory, diuretic, anti-catarrh, and antiseptic properties.

Cosmetic uses: The saponin content gives goldenrod cleansing properties, therefore it can be used in shampoos and cleansers for all skin types. It is anti-inflammatory, reduces irritation, relieves itching, and promotes wound healing.

Medicinal uses: Goldenrod is one the best known herbs for treating urinary and kidney infections, crushing kidney and bladder stones, and easing backaches caused by kidney stones. Its tannins make it anti-inflammatory and a useful remedy for diarrhea and the cleansing of the intestinal system. Iranians use goldenrod in combination with other herbs, such as ginger and peppermint, to soothe the stomach and dispel flatulence. Ancient Greeks used goldenrod to treat colds and influenza.

Gravel Root (Eupatorium purpureum)

Parts used: Rhizome and roots.

Biochemical contents: Flavonoids, volatile oil, resin.

Energy: Neutral.

Country of origin: Iran.

Harvest time: Gravel root rhizomes and roots should be dug up in fall after the plant stops flowering.

Properties: Gravel root has diuretic, tonic, and anti-rheumatic properties.

Cosmetic uses: Because of its volatile oils, gravelroot is useful for most skin cleansers, toners and conditioners.

Medicinal uses: Gravel root is a powerful diuretic herb and is used to treat urinary infections and kidney stones. In Iran, it is not only used for the treatment of urinary infections and gravel, but it is also used for arthritis and menstrual pain and cramping. Because it encourages the excretion of excess uric acid, it is a prime remedy for gout and rheumatism. Iranians make gravel root infusion combined with borage and valerian to release the pain and discomfort of periods and arthritis. The dose is one cup four to five times a day.

Groomwell (Lithospermum officinale L.)

Parts used: Leaves, fruits, and roots.

Biochemical contents: Alkaloid, glycosides, carbonate calcium.

Energy: Warm.

Country of origin: India, Asia, and Iran. Scientific research shows that this plant is from the borage family.

Harvest time: Leaves and fruits are harvest in summer and roots are in fall.

Properties: It has antispasmodic, antiseptic and cleansing properties.

Main uses: In India, they make a syrup with this plant and use it for blood cleansing. They boil the root and use it externally for skin blisters, itchy skin, and measles. They also grind the seeds and mix it with honey to make a syrup for bladder disorders. There is a substance in the root and branches that reduces adrenal gland activity. Top branches are used for birth control. Europeans use groomwell for bladder and kidney stones, and in Spain, the plant is used as a tea or infusion as a relaxant for nervous disorders and as a pain

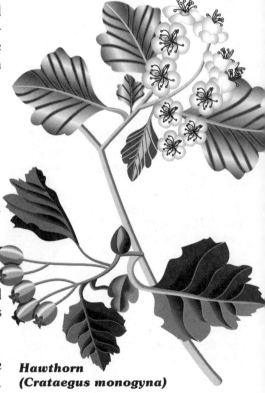

**Hawthorn
(Crataegus monogyna)**

killer. Since it kills and dries the sperm in men, excess use of this plant reduces sexual activities and desire. In Iran, two different kinds of groomwell grow, both containing medicinal properties and widely used.

Hawthorn (Crataegus monogyna)

Parts used: Flowers, berries, leaves.

Biochemical contents: Saponins, flavonoid glycosides, tannins.

Energy: Cool.

Country of origin: Iran, Asia.

Harvest time: Hawthorn berries are collected in the fall.

Properties: Hawthorn has diuretic, cleansing, and cardiac tonic properties.

Cosmetic uses: It has cleansing and soothing properties and can be used for sensitive skin and skin with poor circulation.

Medicinal uses: Hawthorn berries have been proven to be one of the best tonic remedies for the heart and circulation. Iranians strongly believe in hawthorn. They use it for depression, emotional stress, blood cleansing, high blood pressure, strengthening heart muscles, and regulating the heartbeat. The berries are chewed like dried fruits. They also make an infusion with haw-

thorn berries and other herbs such as borage and valerian for mental depression. They make jams and pies with hawthorn berries. Hawthorn's flavonoid content regulates heartbeats and dilates the coronary arteries. Hawthorn normalizes blood pressure and is a good remedy for insomnia. In France, hawthorn is used to help digestion. In China, it is a remedy for treating diarrhea. It is commonly used in Iran.

Heather (Calluna vulgaris)

Parts used: Fresh flowers.

Biochemical contents: Volatile oil, alkaloid, tannin, flavonoid, beta carotene, and citric acid.

Energy: Warm.

Country of origin: Europe, Far east.

Harvest time: Heather flowers are gathered in fall.

Properties: Heather has tonic, diuretic, antiseptic, and anti-inflammatory properties.

Cosmetic uses: Heather is excellent for toning, conditioning, and balancing the pH of skin. It is highly antiseptic and soothing for most skins, especially sensitive and inflamed skin.

Medicinal uses: Heather is recommended for treatment of urinary infections and disorders because of its antiseptic properties. In Iran, people use heather to relieve rheumatism, joint pain, and gout. They prepare an ointment of two cups of heather blossoms to one cup of sesame oil, soak for 3-4 weeks while keeping it in the sun, then apply it to painful areas. They also make infusion of heather in combination with other herbs, like marjoram and peppermint and drink one cup three to four times a day. As it has anti-inflammatory and soothing properties, it can also be used for insomnia. Eating heather seeds mixed with honey is good for killing worms. Its infusion (seeds and blossoms), is good for treating bladder inflammation and infection.

Henna (Lawsonia inermis)

Parts used: Leaves, powdered leaves.

Biochemical contents: Essential oil, natural dye, mucilage.

Energy: Warm.

Country of origin: Iran, India, Egypt, Morocco, and Asia.

Harvest time: Henna leaves are collected in the fall.

Properties: It has soothing, moisturizing, and coloring properties.

Principle uses: Henna leaves contain hennotannic acid and a substance called lawsone (dye). Recent research show that lawsone has antibiotic properties. Henna flowers contain soothing properties which are very beneficial for insomnia. In China and India, they use henna leaves for treating dandruff. They make tea with henna leaves and use it for labor pain. In Malaysia, they smash the leaves and use it for burns, skin disorders (such as acne and boils), and rheumatic pain. Since ancient times, henna has been a very popular natural dye;. It has been used in Iran and Egypt to dye hair and nails and to cleanse and nourish the skin and hair. I remember my grandmother dyed her hair with henna twice a month to give color and nourish her hair.

Henna is also getting popular in western countries for tattooing, natural hair coloring, and body cleansing. The following recipe demonstrates the method of making natural hair dye with henna. The amount of henna used depends on length of hair and its thickness.

For medium length hair use:
1 cup of henna (if redder hair is desired, add more henna)
1 cup of Turkish coffee
1/2 cup of lemon juice
1 cup of hot water

Pour coffee, henna, and lemon juice in a bowl, add hot water to it, and stir with a plastic spatula to make a medium paste. Paint the paste on the hair working down to the root. Cover the hair with a plastic shower cap and leave it on for two to three hours. Shampoo and rinse.

Note: Test the color after one hour by rubbing a small portion of hair and rinsing. If it has achieved the desired color, rinse it; if not, leave the dye on longer.

Honeysuckle (Lonicera caprifolium)

Parts used: Aerial parts.

Biochemical contents: Mucilage, salicylic acid, glycoside, essential oils.

Energy: Warm.

Country of origin: Iran.

Harvest time: Honeysuckle flowers and aerials are harvested from mid-May to September.

Properties: It has anti-inflammatory, soothing, and aromatic properties.

Principal uses: Honeysuckle has a sweet-smelling essential oil that makes it useful for treating skin infections. In Iran, this plant is very popular for its fragrance. They use it for aromatherapy to release the physical and emotional tension through steam inhalation.

Honeysuckle is a summer plant and one of the most popular plants in Iranian countries. Most people grow it in their backyard. In summer, families gather in backyards for their afternoon snack and enjoy the aroma and beauty of their honeysuckle as the honeysuckle releases its aroma, especially after it has been watered. Iranians use honeysuckle in black tea for its fragrance and drink after a meal for digestion. They also make jams and cakes with honeysuckle.

Hops (Humulus lupulus)

Parts used: Dried female cones.

Biochemical contents: Alkaloids, glycoside, resin, fat, volatile oil, essential oil, flavonoid, amino acids.

Energy: Warm.

Country of origin: Iran; also planted worldwide for lupuline production.

Harvest time: Female hop cones are gathered in late summer before they are fully ripe and are dried in the shade.

Properties: Hops have sedative, soothing, anti-inflammatory, antispasmodic, and antiseptic properties.

Cosmetic uses: It has soothing and antiseptic properties and can be used as toners and conditioners for sensitive and irritated skins.

Medicinal uses: Hops are mostly planted to produce lupuline to be used by beer industries. Lupuline is a substance which gives aroma and bitter flavor to beer and has a tranquilizing and soothing action. For many centuries, physicians did not believe in hop as a sedative and tranquilizer, but in 1983, a chemical substance named 2-methyl-3-butene-2 was discovered. This substance exists in hop leaves, and it become stronger as it ages. If one wants to use hop leaves as a pain killer and tranquilizer, it is best to use the old and dried leaves as they contain stronger chemical property. Female hop pickers should wear protective gloves. Some individuals who use hop as medicine might develop skin rashes and itches

Hops have been used for their medicinal value since ancient time. Ancient Iranians prescribed hops for blood cleansing and liver detoxification. Hops are used in Iran for treatment of insomnia and nervous tension. Iranians make a pillow with hops, lavender and orange blossom. It has sedative effects due to its volatile oil and soothing properties. When used as pillow, volatile oil is released and affects the brain directly. They also use it in a hot tub for relaxation and steam inhalation. From 1831-1916 hops were widely used as a tranquilizer and pain killer in America. Recently herbalists have prescribed hops as antibacterial. It fights infection of the upper digestive tract, and soothes and reduces the inflammation and spasms of the gastrointestinal tract. There is a chemical substance in hops which prevents infection. Hops flowers can be smashed for external appli-cation to cuts and burns for faster healing and to prevent infection. Scientific research in Germany shows that hop has estrogenic properties, and this substance can regulate delay periods.

Caution: Hops are not recommended in the treatment of depressive illness because of its sedative effects. According to the FDA, hops is a safe plant, except for pregnant women, nursing mothers, and children under twelve. Use hops under physician care.

Horehound (Murrubium vulgare)

Parts used: Leaves.

Biochemical contents: Alkaloid, volatile oil, flavonoids, glycoside, and bitter principle.

Energy: Cool.

Country of origin: Iran, Egypt.

Harvest time: Horehound leaves are gathered from late spring to summer.

Properties: The plant has expectorant, antiseptic, antibiotic, and cleansing properties.

Medicinal uses: Horehound is famous for treating coughs and upper respiratory disorders. Ancient Greeks, Iranians, and Egyptians used horehound for chest and sinus pains, coughs, and whooping coughs. They made tinctures with horehound, peppermint, and sage, then added honey and used it for coughs and whooping cough. It causes the secretion of a mucus which is readily cleared by coughing. Horehound contains large amounts of volatile oil. This oil is highly antiseptic, antibacterial, and is very useful for treatment of throat and upper respiratory infections. One can gargle a combination of horehound, sage, salt and vinegar to soothe inflammation of the throat and retard or kill bacteria that cause the infection. The bitter principle in horehound increases the appetite and cleanses the liver and gallbladder.

Horse Chestnut (Aesculus hippocastanum)

Parts used: Fruit and bark.

Biochemical contents: Saponin, tannin, essential oil, flavonoid, fatty oil, sugar.

Energy: Warm.

Harvest time: Horse chestnut fruit ripens and is gathered in the fall from September to October. Bark is collected in spring or fall.

Properties: Horse chestnut has expectorant, anti-inflammatory, soothing, cleansing, and stimulant properties.

Cosmetic uses: Horse chestnut is excellent in cosmetics. Its saponin content makes it great as cleansers and toners for all skin types. It has anti-inflammatory and soothing properties on irritated, sensitive and diseased skin, such as eczema and boils. It has a moisturizing factor that makes it a great ingredient for use on of all skin types, especially dry skin.

Medicinal uses: Horse chestnut contains saponins, tannins, and flavonoids, which qualify it as a treatment for hemorrhoids and prostate enlargement. Iranians use horse chestnut with other plants, such as wild yam and borage, to treat female problems, including absent period, uterus pain, and discomforts. They make ointments with horse chestnut and lavender and apply it on hemorrhoids to stop bleeding and to soothe.

Horseradish (Amoracia lapatifolia)

Parts used: Fresh root, leaves.

Biochemical contents: Vitamin C, glycosides.

Energy: Warm.

Country of origin: Iran, Mediterranean countries.

Harvest time: Horseradish roots are dug in the winter.

Properties: Horseradish has stimulant, diuretic, and laxative properties.

Cosmetic uses: Horseradish is highly antiseptic and stimulating. It is excellent for general skin toners and masks, especially oily skin. It is refreshing and stimulating, particularly for skin with poor circulation.

Medicinal uses: Horseradish is from the radish family, and like radish, it is a very good remedy for bladder stones or urinary infections. Iranians use horseradish for many different purposes. Its juice is ingested in the morning on an empty stomach to crush or dissolve bladder stones, to control weight, to increase the metabolism, and to cause fat to burn. In the winter, the juice is used to stimulate the circulation and keep the body temperature warm. Horseradish has antibiotics properties that make it healing for lung and throat infection. Horseradish can also increase the circulation, if used externally. By rubbing horseradish with olive oil on rheumatic joints, blood flow and circulation are maintained. Horseradish is ideal for people who have low appetite because it stimulates the digestive system.

Horsetail (Eguisetum arvense)

Parts used: Aerial parts.

Biochemical contents: Silica, saponins, alkaloids, tannins, sulfur, potassium, magnesium, and flavonoids.

Energy: Neutral.

Country of origin: Iran.

Harvest time: Horsetail is gathered in early summer and hung in an airy place to dry.

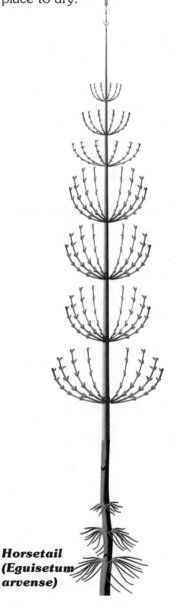

Horsetail (Eguisetum arvense)

Properties: Horsetail has diuretic, tonic, anti-inflammatory, soothing, and astringent properties.

Cosmetic uses: Horsetail is a wonderful ingredient for skin cleansers and conditioners and for hair products because of its saponin content. It is pH balanced, soothing, and healing because of its tannins. It can be an excellent ingredient for sensitive and inflamed skin and skin with poor circulation.

Medicinal uses: Horsetail is one of the most powerful herbs known for urinary infections and stones. Horsetail is a major source of silica, which is helpful for keeping the bones strong and healthy, promoting the formation of the cartilage, encouraging use and absorption of calcium, and helping to guard against hardening of arteries. Horsetail tea is best recommended for woman over forty and during menopause. Horsetail helps to thicken nails and hair, and helps calcium balance. Iranians make tea with horsetail, parsley, and comfrey to treat stomach ulcers, urinary infection, and prostate inflammation. Horsetail is a great remedy for lung and respiratory diseases. It is also useful for bedwetting children, especially in a combination of horsetail with ginger and honey to be given to children who lose control during sleep.

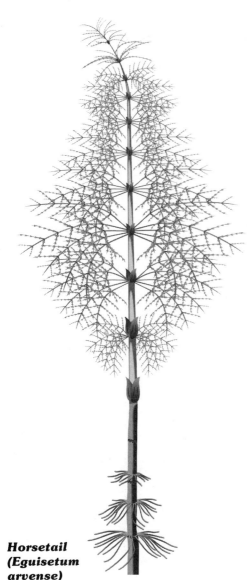

Horsetail (Eguisetum arvense)

Hyssop (Hyssopus officinalis)

Parts used: Flowers.

Biochemical contents: Volatile oil, tannin, glycoside flavonoids, phenol, bitter substance, resin, and essential oil.

Energy: Cool.

Country of origin: Turkey, India, Europe, Soviet Union, Iran.

Harvest time: Hyssop is a tall plant with purplish-blue flowers that are gathered in the summer.

Properties: It has antispasmodic, anti-catarrh, tonic, and sedative properties. *Cosmetic uses:* Hyssop is useful in most skin toners and conditioners because of its volatile oil. It has anti-inflammatory properties that make it perfect for use on sensitive and inflamed skins. The tannin content in hyssop makes it a useful ointment for treating burns, sunburns, and bruises.

Medicinal uses: Bitter glycosides and tannin content bring this plant into the medicinal arena. Iranians use hyssop to treat upper respiratory catarrh, colds, sinus infections, and coughs. They also combine it with other herbs, such as ginger and devil's claw, to relieve rheumatic pain. Volatile oil content makes it antispasmodic. Egyptians make an infusion with hyssop and other plants, like wormwood, to detoxify the liver and gallbladder and also to help expel intestinal worms. It is one the best remedies for respiratory infections and disorders such as influenza. Indians use it for treatment of asthma, stomach gas, colic, increasing menstrual flow, and stimulating the mucous membranes. Steamed hyssop with vinegar is beneficial for toothache,

and with honey, it is useful for lung inflammation, asthma and stomach worms. For a fresh infusion, put 20 gm. of hyssop flower in 1/2 gallon water. Boil for 15 minutes, then drink 2-3 cups daily for bronchitis. A compress of hyssop tea is useful to prevent cold sores. In India, traditional use of hyssop has been for miscarriages.

Iceland Moss (Cetraria islandical)

Parts used: Whole plant.

Biochemical contents: Mucilage, bitter fumaric acid, iodine.

Energy: Cool.

Country of origin: North European mountains, North America.

Harvest time: Iceland moss may be gathered between spring and early fall.

Properties: It has anti-catarrh, expectorant, anti-inflammatory and tonic properties.

Cosmetic uses: High amount of muclige in Iceland moss makes this plant appropriate for all skin creams and conditioners, especially those for sensitive and dry skin.

Main uses: Iceland moss has high mucilage content, which makes it a fine remedy for respiratory disorders and digestive problems. It generally soothes mucous membranes. Iranians use Iceland moss to treat bladder infections. They also use Iceland moss for nausea during pregnancy by making an infusion. They add lemon and honey and drink one cup three times a day. Iceland moss has strong antibiotic properties and a reputation for killing intestinal worms and bacilli. It is a prime remedy for asthma and other respiratory disorders. In Germany, it is used for treatment of coughs, asthma, constipation, diarrhea, and hepatitis. If soaked in water for a day, it releases a substance which is highly nutritious. Its nutritional value is similar to wheat flower. Saccharure can be obtained from Iceland moss. This substance is therapeutic and a natural sugar which is highly beneficial to both body and brain, and it can be used as sweetener. Saccharure is also great for treating flu, lung inflammation, and bronchitis.

Indigo (wild indigo) (Baptisia tinctoria)

Parts used: Root.

Biochemical contents: Alkaloid, glycosides, resin.

Energy: Neutral.

Country of origin: European countries, Iran

Harvest time Indigo is best collected in the fall.

Properties: Indigo has tonic and anti-spasmodic properties.

Main uses: Wild indigo is best used externally for cuts and infected wounds and for skin inflammation and infections. Iranians make ointment with wild indigo and lavender to treat sore and cracked nipples of nursing mothers.

Caution: Strong doses of wild indigo may have purgative and emetic effects.

Irish Moss (Chondrus crispus)

Parts used: The dried plant.

Biochemical contents: Several mucopolysaccharides, mucilage, iron, iodine, sulfur, vitamins A and B1.

Energy: Cool.

Country of origin: Europe, Iran.

Harvest time: Irish moss is a seaweed harvested during summer from the rocks along the coastlines of Europe, especially Ireland.

Properties: Irish moss has emollient, anti-catarrh, anti-inflammatory, and expectorant properties.

Cosmetic uses: Irish moss has excellent humectant properties, which make it a fantastic moisturizer for dry skin and hair. It is also used for its emollient properties and makes an excellent anti-wrinkle cream. In cosmetic laboratories, they dissolve Irish moss in cold water to produce a viscous solution, combine it with milk protein, and form a thick gel which is used as an emulsifier in skin lotions and other cosmetic products. Irish moss can be used as an emulsifier for dry skin and is the best ingredient for wrinkle cream. The high mucilage content of this plant makes it a fine remedy for coughs, bronchitis, and stomach ulcers. Irish Moss is very nourishing and makes a delicious dessert when boiled with milk and spices.

Jasmine (Jasminum viminale salib)

Parts used: Flowers, leaves.

Biochemical content: Essential oil, alkaloid, salicylic acid.

Energy: warm.

Country of origin: Iran, Europe, Mediterranean countries.

Harvest time: Flowers are harvested from late spring to early fall.

Cosmetic uses: White jasmine has antispasmodic, soothing, and aromatic properties. It is mostly used in the perfume industry and aromatherapy. It releases muscle tension and mental stress. It can be used via steam inhalation or in a bath.

Medicinal uses: Indians use jasmine root for stomach gas and skin disorders. Essential oil is used for tensions, headaches, muscle pains, strengthening of gums, and also to increase menstrual flow. Its leaves are used as internal cleansers. Iranians blend the flowers with black tea for its aroma and drink it after meals for better digestion. They also pillow it with the combination of lavender, rose, and rosemary for tension headaches, depression, and anxiety. Its leaves contain bitter glycosides, making it valuable for indigestion and as an internal cleanser. Essential oil of jasmine is also used to decrease menstrual pain.

Juniper (Juniperis communis)

Parts used: Berries, new twigs.

Biochemical contents: Volatile oil, sugars, vitamin C, flavonoid, 83% essential oil, 36% juniperol, and camphor.

Energy: Warm.

Country of origin: Iran, India.

Harvest time: Juniper berries are collected in fall. If to be used for medication, it should be only ripe second year fruits.

Properties: Juniper has tonic, diuretic, and antiseptic properties.

Cosmetic use: Juniper is highly antiseptic and is a good remedy for skin conditions, such as boils and acne. It is also very good for conditioning and for pH balancing of oily skin and hair. Because of its volatile oil content, it is a good ingredient for all skin types cleansers and toners.

Medicinal uses: Juniper berries are excellent for treating rheumatism, gout, coughs, colds, and possibly gum infections. Juniper is one the most valued plants in Iran. They use juniper for many different kinds of treatments, such as bladder infection, throat infection, and arthritis pain. Juniper is known as a stimulant and diuretic, and infusion of juniper can relieve arthritis and bladder pain. A century ago, it was the fruit of juniper that was one of the most valuable and important treatments for dropsy and arthritis pain. Country people in Europe occasionally eat handfuls of berries or take an infusion of berries as a mild diuretic or laxative. The berries are good for digestion and help eliminate gas. In India, people use its fruits and essential oil to treat stomach gas and to stimulate the appetite. It increases the flow of urine and menstruation. Fresh berries are also good for treating coughs, stomach pain, and uterine pain. Infusion of fresh berries can crush urinary and kidney stones. After World War II, French hospitals used smoked juniper berries as an antibacterial and for cleansing hospitals. One 17th century herbalist discovered juniper to be an excellent remedy to treat lung diseases (such as liquid accumulation in lungs) and heart diseases.

Caution: Do not take this plant during pregnancy or kidney problems.

Kava Kava (Piper methysticum)

Parts used: Dried roots and rhizomes.

Biochemical contents: Alkaloid, mucilage, starch.

Energy: Warm.

Country of origin: Hawaii, Polynesia.

Harvest time: Kava kava rhizomes are unearthed in fall and dried in the sun.

Properties: Kava Kava has sedative and antispasmodic and anti-inflammatory properties.

Principal uses: Kava kava is one the most powerful plants known to relieve insomnia and soothe the nervous system. Kava kava tea is a remedy for insomnia. It first stimulates and then depresses the nervous system. Chemical substance name Dihydrokawain was discovered in the resin of kava kava by Dr. Wien in 1939 which is a strong tranquilizer. In 1959 Dr. Hansel discovered another substance in kava kava named Dihydrome Thysticin.

Kava kava contains antiseptic and anti-inflammatory properties which make it a great remedy for treating rheumatism and urinary infections. It may lower the blood pressure and reduce fever due to its alkaloid content. Ancient Chinese used kava kava tea with peppermint to relieve menstrual pain. Its root is good for the male reproductive system and for urinary and sexual disorders and its leaves are good for internal and external bleeding.

Caution: Overdoses of kava kava may cause accumulation of toxins in the liver.

Kelp (Laminaria)

Parts used: Whole plant.

Biochemical contents: Mucilage, tannin, vitamins A, B complex, C, E, and K, minerals such as potassium, calcium, magnesium, selenium, iodine, phosphorus, and manganese.

Energy: Warm.

Country of origin: Asian countries.

Harvest time: Kelp is found at sea coasts and can be collected from Japan, Australia, Korea, China, and Hawaii.

Properties: Kelp has cathartic, emollient, anti-stress, antibacterial, anti-rheumatic, antibiotic, antioxidant, anti-cancer, anti-toxic, and diuretic properties.

Cosmetic uses: Seaweed is an excellent ingredient for many skin creams and moisturizers because of its emollient properties. It contains large amounts of mucilage and tannin which make this plant useful for sensitive and irritated skin. It is also anti-wrinkle. Seaweed is an ingredient in most skin care products in oriental countries.

Medicinal uses: Brown seaweed, such as kelp, if used regularly in the diet, nourishes, ensures health, and prevents damage to tissues from chemical pollution. Kelp and other seaweed help us to stay in shape, keep the blood pressure and cholesterol low, restore sexual interest, and contribute to healthy skin and hair. Kelp enhances the immune system and is an excellent herb for muscle pains, rheumatism, arthritis, viral infections and nervous tension. Seaweed is great for getting in shape as it provides nourishment to the thyroid. It thus influences metabolism and helps weight melt by reengineering fat metabolism.

Lady's Mantle (Alchemilla vulgaris)

Parts used: Root.

Biochemical contents: Tannins, volatile oil.

Energy: Cool.

Country of origin: Iran, India.

Harvest time: Lady's mantle leaves and stems are gathered in the summer.

Properties: It has astringent, anti-inflammatory, and diuretic properties.

Cosmetic uses: Lady's Mantle is highly astringent and can be used externally on cuts and wounds. It has the ability to promote the healing process of any wound; therefore, it is useful for sensitive, irritated, and acne skins.

Medicinal uses: Lady's mantle can be used for menstrual disorders, cuts, and wounds in the ointment or cream form. The tannin content in this plant makes a good remedy for muscle tension and pain, especially menstrual pain. It helps eases muscle tension during period pain. Iranians use lady's mantle to reduce the inflammation and pain of arthritis, as well as for joint, throat, and back pain. They combine lady's mantle with peppermint, marjoram, and valerian and make an infusion, drinking one cup three to four times a day to reduce arthritis pain. Infusion of lady's mantle and sage is gargled to soothe sore throat. Egyptians used this plant for bladder infection and inflammation. The astringency of this plant provides a good treatment for diarrhea.

Lady's Slipper (Cypripodium calceolus)

Parts used: Dried root.

Biochemical contents: Volatile oil, tannins, glycosides.

Energy: Cool.

Country of origin: European countries.

Harvest time: Lady's slipper is a protected plant in the United Kingdom and the United States and should not be picked if it is found growing wild.

Properties: Lady's slipper has antispasmodic, antiseptic, tonic, and sedative properties.

Cosmetic uses: The volatile oil and tannins in this plant make it a good antiseptic and anti-inflammatory for skin conditions that need to be healed.

Medicinal uses: Lady's slipper contains antispasmodic properties for treating any muscle tension and spasms. American Indians use this plant root for muscle spasms and tension headaches. Europeans use this plant to ease muscle and menstrual cramping, arthritis pain, and discomfort. Lady's slipper may be used for combating emotional stress, tension, and anxiety. It will promote a tranquil mood; therefore, it is also a good remedy for anxiety associated with insomnia. Glycoside content in this plant qualifies it for internal and liver cleansing.

Caution: Long dosage can cause headache.

Lantana (Lantana indica roxb)

Parts used: Flowers, leaves.

Biochemical contents: Essential oil, lantanine, alkaloids in leaves.

Energy: Warm.

Country of origin: South America, Iran.

Harvest time: Late spring to mid-fall.

Properties: It has antispasmodic and aromatic properties.

Main uses: Lantana is highly colorful and is mostly used in garnishing and ground cover. Its oil and lantaning acid decrease blood circulation and reduce fever. The alkaloid content is helpful in reducing fever, decreasing blood pressure, and cleansing to the lungs and mucous membranes. Iranians use it topically for wounds. Its oil is good for muscle tension and joint pain. In India, it is used in detoxifying skin, especially after bee stings. Chinese also use it topically and steam it for use in the bath to treat skin disorders. Indians and Chinese also use it to kill worms and to stimulate the female system to increase menstrual flow. In the Philippines, it is used for detoxification and sanitation.

Lavender (Lavendula officinalis)

Parts used: Flowers.

Biochemical contents: Volatile oil, essential oil, tannins, flavonoids, bitter flavor.

Energy: Warm

Country of origin: Asia, Europe.

Harvest time: Lavender flowers are picked early summer to early fall.

Properties: Lavender has antispasmodic, antiseptic, antidepressant, antiemetic, anti-inflammatory, and soothing properties.

Cosmetic uses: Lavender is a unique plant that offers several therapeutic values to the skin and body. It soothes and relaxes sensitive skin. It is anti-inflammatory and heals skin conditions, such as eczema, psoriasis, and couperose (broken capillaries). Lavender oil is highly antiseptic and acts as an antibacterial for acne skin. Lavender oil is an excellent relaxant and is used in aromatherapy for emotional stress and anxiety.

Medicinal uses: Lavender has an aromatic flowers and leaves, and has a bitter flavor. It has small seeds dark yellow color, it releases a camphor like aroma when rubbed it in the palm of one's hand.

Lavender is an excellent remedy for treating chest pain, tention headache, coughs, migraine headache, and colds. It has a bitter taste which make it good for liver and gallbladder detoxification, and urinary infection. Dried and powderd flowers and leaves of lavender mixed with honey or brown sugar, taken every night to treat headache, forgetfulness, nervous tention, mental depression, fainting and stomach ulcer. An infusion of lavender with oregano, and celery seeds can be used to treat stomach gripe, hemmorrhoid, And flatulence.

In Europe dried lavender flowers are put into pillows to reduce mental depression. Lavender compresses are used to reduce arthritis pain.

In France lavender is used to reduce fever and sweating, and to treat flu. An infusion of lavender, borage, marigold, and sweat violets is used to treat cold, and flu. Three to four cups of infusion are taken daily.

In Iran, lavender has been used traditionally for upper respiratory infections, They also make an ointment with lavender and marigold to treat burns, cuts, and bee stings. Some Iranian burn lavender flower at home for its aroma.

Caution: Lavender oil should be taken internally only under supervision.

Lemon Balm (Melissa officinalis)

Parts used: Leaves, flowers, oil.

Biochemical contents: Volatile oil, tannins, flavonoids, and essential oil.

Energy: Warm.

Country of origin: Iran, S. America France, Asia.

Harvest time: Lemon balm leaves and stems can be gathered from early summer to fall.

Properties: Its has antispasmodic, antidepressant, antiemetic, astringent, and aromatic properties.

Cosmetic uses: Another name for lemon balm is melissa. The therapeutic essential oil is used in aromatherapy for emotional stress and to relieve depression. Lemon balm is used in cosmetics and skin care to relieve skin irritation. It is very effective for oily skins with large pores. It refreshes and balances the skin. Its anti-inflammatory property makes it good for sensitive skins.

Medicinal uses: In France, they make a syrup with melissa named eau de melisse for treating stomach gas indigestion and upper respiratory pain. It is great for increasing mental acuity and memory. Chewing melissa is mouth-refreshing and neutralizes the smell of liquor in mouth. It also stops hiccups. In India, people use melissa to reduce fever and to control liver, brain, and heart disease. Melissa is an excellent remedy for stomach gas, nervous tension, and insomnia. The volatile oil in this plant has a strong sedative effect. This plant is a powerful remedy for depression; it lifts the spirits. It is also an excellent infusion to be taken after meals for digestion and the removal of excess gas from the stomach. Iranians use lemon balm (melissa) for menstrual pain, colds, and flu. Because of its volatile oil and tannin content, it is used for sore throat and colds.

Lemon Verbena (Aloysia citriodora)

Parts used: Leaves and flowers.

Biochemical contents: Essential oil, volatile oil, tannin.

Energy: Cool.

Country of origin: Iran, Europe, S.America.

Harvest time: Lemon verbena leaves can be harvested any time often year.

Properties: It has stimulating, soothing, and antiseptic properties.

Cosmetic uses: Lemon verbena contains an essential oil used in aromatherapy for depression, physical stress, and emotional stress. It can be massaged for muscle relaxation. Lemon verbena can be used in most skin cleansers and conditioners because of its volatile oil. It can make a fine astringent for oily, sensitive, and irritated skin.

Medicinal uses: Lemon verbena has a strong lemon scent. Central and South Americans make tea with apple peel for flatulence and indigestion. Iranians make tea with lemon verbena, ginger, and clove to treat colds, flu, and upper respiratory problems.

Licorice (Glycyrrhiza glabra)

Parts used: Root.

Biochemical contents: Saponin, volatile oil, amino acid, sugar 30%, starch, flavonoids, glycyrrhizin.

Energy: Warm.

Country of origin: Iran and Afghanistan.

Harvest time: Licorice root is harvested in fall.

Properties: Licorice has antiseptic, antispasmodic, anti-inflammatory, astringent, emollient, and sedative properties.

Cosmetic uses: Licorice is highly antiseptic and antibacterial

and is wonderful for an acne problems

skin conditioner. Its saponin content makes it good for conditioning and cleansing skin, especially skin with acne or irritation.

Medicinal uses: Licorice root contains sugar. Iranians make a special non-alcoholic beverage with its root extract. Licorice root contains glycyrrhernic acid and has a pale yellow color. Licorice is powerful to cure stomach spasm, coughs, colds, sore throats, and muscle spasms. It is a strong anti-inflammatory and antispasmodic similar to cortisone. The glycyrrhernic acid reduces throat irritation and fever. Licorice is being investigated for anti-cancer properties.

This plant has been very popular within Iranians since ancient times. They cut the root by length, soak it in water with fennel for several hours and use it for treating flatulence, coughs, fever, and nervous tension, increasing the appetite, improving sexual desire, lowering stomach acid, decreasing stomach spasm, and reducing inflammation of the stomach. Licorice is widely grown in Iran, and most European countries (France, in particular) import much licorice from Iran. Iranians get an extract from the boiled root, and the syrup is very useful for chest pain and whooping coughs. Chinese remove the root clean and wash it, add honey, and warm it up for fifteen to twenty minutes. This is for treating throat infections and immune system problems. Ancient Egyptians used licorice to re-

duce muscles spasm and arthritis pain, since licorice supports hormonal glands. They combined it with other herbs, like borage and wild yam, for different skin disorders and hormonal imbalance. Licorice can cause water retention and bloating, therefore its use should be minimal in premenstrual women.

Caution: Avoid large doses with high blood pressure or during pregnancy.

Lily (Lilium candidum L.)

Parts used: Flowers, bulb.

Biochemical contents: Alkaloid, essential oil.

Energy: Warm.

Country of origin: Japan, China, Iran, Europe.

Harvest time: Early to late spring.

Properties: It has antispasmodic, antiseptic and aromatic properties

Cosmetic uses: It has antispasmodic, aromatic, and soothing properties. It is used in skin cleansers, conditioners, and creams for eczema and acne.

Medicinal uses: Its bulb is widely used for asthma, coughs, nervous tension, and urinary disorders. It is a strong sedative and useful for lung congestion. Chinese use its soaked leaves and stalks for gastrointestinal problems. Indians use its bulb to regulate heartbeat, for coughs, and for chest pain. Lily is great remedy for nervous tension, insomnia and depression.

Lily of the Valley (Canvallaria majalis)

Parts used: Leaves and whole plant.

Biochemical contents: Cardiac glycosides, essential oil, saponins, and flavonoids.

Energy: Neutral.

Country of origin: Iran, European countries.

Harvest time: Lily of the valley leaves are gathered when the plant is flowering in late spring to early summer.

*Properties:*It has diuretic,cardioactive, and tonic properties.

Cosmetic uses: It is an ingredient in many skin lotions and conditioners. This plant has a pleasant aroma, so its essential oil can be used in body lotions.

Medicinal uses: Lily of the valley is very valuable for treating heart diseases, including congestive heart failure. It contains cardiac glycosides which increase the strength of heartbeats while normalizing heart rate. Ira-

nians call this plant "lover's flower" as they believe its pleasant aroma bring cheers and affectionates.

Caution: It is categorized as poisonous and should only be taken with consultation.

Lobelia (Lobelia unflata)

Parts used: Aerial parts.

Biochemical contents: Bitter glycosides, alkaloids, volatile oil.

Energy: Cool.

Country of origin: Iran

Harvest time: Lobelia entire plant can be harvested from summer to early fall.

Properties: It has antispasmodic, emetic, and anti-asthmatic properties.

Principle uses: Lobelia is a good for treatment of coughs, asthma, and bronchial problems. Lobelia is a popular plant in Iran for treating arthritis, muscle pains, and for relaxation of the nerves. Its alkaloid and glycoside contents make it suitable for internal cleansing and respiratory problems. Iranians grind dry lobelia with peppermint and smoke it like tobacco.

Caution: Use only under medical supervision.

London Rocket (Descurainia Sophia (L) webb)

Parts used: Seeds.

Biochemical contents: Glycosides, fatty essential oils, alkaloids, linoleic acid, stearic acid.

Energy: Warm.

Country of origin: India, Iran, Pakistan.

Harvest time: London rocket seeds are harvested from late summer through fall.

Properties: It has antispasmodic, aromatic, and cleansing properties.

Main uses: This herb has been used since ancient times by Iranians. Ancient Iranian physicians believed that London rocket had a warm energy and was a great remedy for indigestion and upset stomach. They soaked London rocket in water and rosewater, boiled it for few minutes, and added organic honey for upset stomach due to food poisoning. London rocket is used for the female reproductive system and stimulates sexual and adrenal glands. Ancient Iranians used London rocket with honey and rosewater during labor pain to relax the muscles and reduce the labor pain. London rocket can be used for skin disorders, especially in the case of paleness as it gives color to the skin. Chinese use London rocket seeds to reduce fever, constipation, and skin inflammation and disorders. Indians use London rocket flowers and leaves for bloody diarrhea, bronchitis, and fever.

Lovage (Levisticum officinale)

Parts used: Leaves, stems, flowers, and seeds.

Biochemical contents: Volatile oil, angelic acid.

Energy: Cool.

Country of origin: Iran, India.

Harvest time: Lovage leaves can be gathered during the summer.

Properties: Lovage has astringent, tonic, antiseptic, diuretic, and antispasmodic properties.

Principle uses: Leaves are used in soups and stews and the seeds in breads and cakes. Lovage is an aromatic stimulant and warms the digestive system. Iranians use lovage to relieve flatulence. They also make a stew with a combination of celery and lovage. Ancient Iranians made an infusion with lovage, peppermint, and borage, then added organic honey and drank for menstrual pain or muscle tension.

Caution: Should not be taken during pregnancy or kidney problems.

Male Fern (Dryopteris filix-mas)

Parts used: Rhizome.

Biochemical contents: Essential oil, tannin.

Energy: Warm.

Country of origin: Worldwide.

Harvest time: Fern rhizomes are gathered in the fall. The roots are dug in the fall, cleaned, and dried at a temperature of seventy degrees Fahrenheit.

Properties: Fern has antibacterial properties.

Medicinal uses: Male fern has been used by Iranians for centuries. They use male fern rhizome to kill intestinal worms because its rhizome contains a substance that is deadly to intestinal worm. Male fern grows anywhere in the United States, Europe, and Iran.

Caution: Male fern is potentially poisonous in overdoses.

Marigold (Calendula officinalis)

Parts used: Flowers.

Biochemical contents: Volatile oil, calenduline, glycoside, tannin, saponin, mucilage, flavonoid, essential oil.

Energy: Warm.

Country of origin: Worldwide.

Harvest time: Marigold flowers are gathered from summer to early fall.

Properties: It has astringent, antimicrobial, tonic, and anti-inflammatory properties.

Cosmetic uses: Marigold is used in the cosmetic and skin care industries. Its anti-inflammatory and antiseptic properties qualify it for all skin type cleansers, toners, and moisturizers, especially for irritated, sensitive skin. Marigold can be used as an astringent and healer. It contains tannin which reacts with proteins and produces a tightening and soothing effect on skin tissue.

Medicinal uses: Marigold is valuable for healing cuts and burns. Its antibacterial and antiseptic properties promote wound healing. Its tannin and mucilage render it good for stomach ulcers. Marigold is very popular in Iran for its beauty and medicinal use. Marigold is used for upset stomach and removal of warts. Iranians use it to stop internal, gum, and hemorrhoidal bleeding. Marigold is a popular flower in Iran during spring and summer. Almost every housewife plants this flower in her backyard for its beauty as well as medicinal uses.

Marjoram (Origanum marjoram)

Parts used: Leaves and seeds.

Biochemical contents: Volatile oil, tannins, glycosides, vitamin C, essential oil.

Energy: Warm

Country of origin: Iran, N Africa, Asia

Harvest time: Marjoram leaves are picked from late spring and late fall.

Properties: It has antispasmodic, astringent, antimicrobial, stimulant, and expectorant properties.

Cosmetic uses: Its volatile oil can be used in general skin cleansers and conditioners. Tannin contained in marjoram makes it especially good for sensitive and irritated skin.

Medicinal uses: This is a very popular herb, and Iranians include it in their daily diet by serving it fresh with meals or using it in soups, salads, and variety of dishes. As an infusion with other herbs, such as peppermint and tarragon, it is a good cleanser and promotes digestive secretion. Some use marjoram to relieve emotional and muscle stress, release retained water before menstrual periods, and relieve painful periods. Ancient Iranians used marjoram with peppermint for tension headache and arthritic pain.

Marshmallow (Althea officinalis)

Parts used: Roots and leaves.

Biochemical contents: Mucilage, tannins, starch, flavonoid, and pectin.

Energy: Cool.

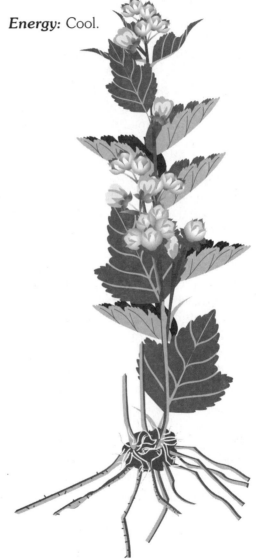

Marshmallow (Althea officinalis)

Country of origin: Iran.

Harvest time: Marshmallow leaves are gathered in summer and its roots in late fall.

Properties: It has anti-inflammatory, soothing, expectorant, diuretic, and emollient properties.

Cosmetic uses: Marshmallow is used generally in creams and cleansers for sensitive skin. Its high mucilage content is highly soothing and healing on sensitive and inflamed skin.

Medicinal uses: Marshmallow root is useful in treating urinary infections and stomach ulcers. High mucilage content makes it effective in treating stomach and intestinal inflammations. In Iran, marshmallow has been used over centuries for its medicinal values. People use it for different illnesses, particularly stomach and intestinal disorders. They combine marshmallow root powder with slippery elm powder and make a liquid pudding that is drunk on an empty stomach to protect the wound from gastric acid and inflammation. They also make an infusion with marshmallow root. It releases starch, which soothes sore throats and relieves coughs. Some mix marshmallow root with honey and ginger for women after childbirth to relieve muscle tension and regain energy.

Meadowsweet (Filipendula ulmaria)

Parts used: Leaves, flowers, and roots.

Biochemical contents: Mucilage, tannin, flavonoid, volatile oil, vitamin C, and salicylic acid.

Energy: Cool.

Country of origin: Iran, European countries.

Harvest time: Meadowsweet flowers and leaves are harvested in summer; roots are unearthed in fall.

Properties: Meadowsweet has soothing, anti-inflammatory, antiseptic, antispasmodic, and diuretic properties. It has a toning effect on skin tissues.

Cosmetic uses: Meadowsweet can be used in most skin conditioners and moisturizers, especially those made for sensitive skins and disorders, such as rosacea. The mucilage, tannin and volatile oil is powerful for treating inflammations of skin afflicted with acne or boils. The salicylic acid content qualifies it for skin exfoliation. Salicylic acid in this plant can be used along with other alpha-hydroxy acids for skin peeling.

Medicinal uses: Its salicylic acid is a major ingredient for aspirin, promotes excretion of uric acid and treats fever and arthritis. Iranians use meadowsweet with marigold for treatment of stomach ulcers, due to high content of mucilage and tannin in meadowsweet.

Milk Thistle (Silybum Marianum (L.)gaertn.

Parts used: Roots, leaves, flowers, and fruits.
Biochemical content: Tyramine, glycosides, alkaloids.

Energy: Warm.

Country of origin: N. Korea, Iran.

Harvest time: Leaves, flowers are harvested in summer and roots are collected in late fall.

Properties: It has antiseptic, antispasmodic, and antibacterial properties.

Medicinal uses: Tyramine content in this plant makes it very good for internal bleeding. Tyramine is a chemical substance which changes to Epinephrine in body. Tyramine substances exist in food such as beers, malt, grains, chicken and roosters, livers.

Indians use milk thistle leaves for fever reduction, and they also use the seeds for internal and external bleeding.

Milk thistle increases oxygenation in the brain and helps improve memory and concentration. Milk thistle roots, leaves and flowers are very bitter which make this plant very good for digestion as well as liver and gallbladder detoxification.

Ancient Iranians use extract of milk thistle for treating hepatitis, tuberculosis and gallstones, some people use milk thistle to cure headaches and to stop ocean sickness.

Caution: Milk thistle should not be taken with antidepressant drugs because tyramine content in milk thistle does not agree with antidepressant drugs. It may raise the blood pressure, causing headache, elevating heartbeats, and potentially cause brain stroke.

Mistletoe (Visum album)

Parts used: Leaves, berries, and branches.

Biochemical contents: Saponin, resin, mucilage, alkaloid. European mistletoe contains polysaccharides, lignin, flavonoid, caffeine, and other acids.

Energy: warm.

Country of origin: Iran, India, North Africa, Europe.

Harvest time: Mistletoe is harvested in fall. Both European and American species have similar properties.

Properties: It has stimulant antiseptic, cleansing, and anti-inflammatory properties.

Cosmetic uses: The large amount of saponin in mistletoe makes it a good skin cleanser and conditioner. It is an anti-inflammatory and can be used to reduce the inflammation and irritation of acne and other skin problems.

Medicinal uses: It has two chemical compounds, one affecting heartbeats and tensing intestinal muscles and the other lowering blood pressure. It is classified as a toxin due to its viscotoxene content. There are two kinds of saponins in mistletoe which are used in the adhesive industry. Indians use it internally as a laxative and for increasing sexual desire. Chinese use it from March to August. Soft green branches are used in an infusion to treat kidney problems, to increase milk supply in nursing mothers, to strengthen muscle and bone and to lower blood pressure. Ancient Chinese used it to cure liver inflammation and increase hair growth. Ancient Iranians used it to regulate circulation and cure cold energy diseases. Europeans use mistletoe to reduce high blood pressure and normalize heartbeats associated with tension and anxiety. Iranians use it for insomnia, depression, and in winter, to enhance the immune system.

Caution: European mistletoe berries are highly toxic; use under medical care.

Motherwort (Leanurus cardiaca)

Parts used: Aerial.

Biochemical contents: Alkaloids, volatile oil, bitter glycosides, tannin, flavonoids, vitamin A, and essential oil.

Energy: Cool.

Country of origin: Iran, Asia, Europe.

Harvest time: Motherwort can be gathered from early summer to late fall.

Properties: It has antispasmodic, anti-inflammatory, antibacterial and cardiotonic properties.

Cosmetic uses: This plant is highly antiseptic and anti-inflammatory. It is used for skin disorders and irritation.

Medicinal uses: The principle use of this plant is to regulate menstruation, relieve painful periods, and treat female disorders. Iranians make an infusion with the combination of motherwort, crampbark, and chamomile that is used for heartbeat regulation, especially when related to emotional stress and anxiety after childbirth. Its alkaloids lower blood pressure and fever. Chinese use motherwort for painful periods, insomnia, and emotional stress. Ancient Chinese used it on daily basis as a method of contraception.

Caution: Should not be taken during pregnancy.

Mugwort (Artemisia vulgaris)

Parts used: Aerial, leaves.

Biochemical contents: Volatile oil, tannin, flavonoids, bitter principal, and essential oils.

Energy: Warm.

Country of origin: Asia, Europe.

Harvest time: Mugwort leaves and flowers should be gathered from mid-summer to late fall.

Properties: It has stimulant, antibacterial, anti-inflammatory and bitter tonic properties.

Cosmetic uses: Its volatile oil is fine for skin toning and conditioning. It can be used in lotions for irritated, inflamed skin and for skin disorders, such as eczema and acne.

Medicinal uses: Since ancient times, mugwort has been used in Iran for missed periods, menstrual pain, nervous tension and insomnia. Europeans use mugwort to treat rheumatism and gout because it excretes uric acid. Chinese strongly believe this plant can help to prevent miscarriage. They get syrup from its green parts which is then used externally to reduce inflammation. Smashed green leaves are used to reduce tension headaches, muscle tensions, and labor tension. Its dried leaves are used like a tobacco to soothe asthma. Fresh leaves used as an infusion to regulate menstruation. Steamed fresh leaves are good for asthma and crush kidney stones. Bitter glycoside enables it to treat and detoxify the liver and gallbladder.

Caution: Avoid during pregnancy.

Mullein (Verbascum Thapsus)

Parts used: Leaves and flowers.

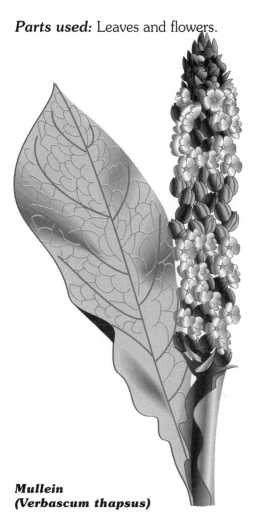

*Mullein
(Verbascum thapsus)*

Biochemical content: Volatile oil, saponin, mucilage, flavonoids, glycosides.

Energy: Warm.

Country of origin: Iran

Harvest time: Mullein leaves and flowers are gathered from July to September.

Properties: Mullein has antiseptic, anti-inflammatory, expectorant, diuretic, and antispasmodic properties.

Medicinal uses: Its saponin and mucilage are good for the treatment of bronchitis, coughs, asthma, and upper respiratory disorders. Mullein is an expectorant, helping to cough up excess secretions of phlegm that accumulate in the lungs. Iranians use mullein tea for insomnia, nervous tension, and bladder irritation. They also ground fresh leaves and flowers and then rubbed this into the rheumatic spot with olive oil to ease the pain. Ancient Iranians used an infusion of mullein with hyssops and peppermint to treat colds and upper respiratory problems.

Myrrh (Commiphora molmol)

Parts used: Dried gum resin.

Biochemical contents: Volatile oil, polysaccharides, resin, gum.

Energy: Warm.

Country of origin: Africa, Iran.

Harvest time: Myrrh resin is collected from cut branches of the trees and dried for use.

Properties: Myrrh has antiseptic, stimulant, anti-inflammatory, and antispasmodic properties.

Cosmetic uses: Myrrh contains large amounts of volatile oil. Being antiseptic, astringent and anti-inflammatory, it is highly qualified to treat acne, as well as problematic, sensitive, inflamed, and reddened skin. It can be used in skin cleansers, moisturizers and emulsifiers.

Medicinal uses: Because of its antiseptic and antibacterial properties, myrrh has been used traditionally in Egypt and Iran to treat sore throats, coughs, and painful periods. In Iran, it is believed to be gifted with the ability to kill negativity and bad energy. It is burned along with other herbs, such as wild rue, on a wedding eve, at the birth of a new baby, and on many other special occasions in order to kill bad energy. Thursday is believed to be holy for Iranians so they burn myrrh with wild rue at that time. Ancient Iranians also used myrrh for indigestion, gum infections, menstrual pain, and excess gas and water in the lower abdomen that cause menstrual pain. Iranians believe that using myrrh during pregnancy make the baby clever and open-minded.

Nasturtium (Tropaeolum majus)

Parts used: Flowers, leaves, and seeds.

Biochemical contents: Volatile oil, essential oils, tannin, vitamin C.

Energy: Warm.

Country of origin: Iran.

Harvest time: Nasturtium flowers are collected from early spring to late fall, leaves all year round, and seeds from midsummer to late fall.

Properties: It has anti-microbial, antiseptic, and soothing effects.

Principle uses: Nasturtium is a strong and powerful anti-microbial used for treating local bacterial infections and respiratory infections, such as bronchitis. Nasturtium also has antiseptic properties which are useful for liver detoxification. Nasturtium makes a delicious spring salad.

Nettle (Urtica dioica)

Parts used: Aerial parts, leaves, root.

Biochemical contents: Vitamins A, B complex and C, minerals (silica, potassium, sulfur, iron, zinc, copper).

Energy: Cool.

Country of origin: Iran.

Harvest time: Nettle leaves and stalks are gathered in May; the roots are unearthed in fall.

Properties: Nettle has astringent, antibacterial, antimicrobial, antiseptic, anti-allergies, and diuretic properties.

Cosmetic uses: Nettle is ideal for use in general skin care, cleansing, and shampoos. It is a good treatment for acne and skin blemishes and balances oily skin and hair. Nettle has the ability to purify the blood and to clear acne and most skin disorders, such as eczema and psoriasis.

Medicinal uses: Nettle is very rich in most Vitamins and minerals. It is an excellent blood cleanser, It cleanses the blood and tissue and help with many problems such as constipation, skin disorders, arthritis pain, and gout.

In Iran, nettle has been used since ancient time for constipation, and muscle tension. Ancient Iranians ate steamed nettle leaves every day for healthy skin, and hair. They used the extract of nettle root, with burdock root to treat boil and acne.

Some pregnant Iranian women use nettle for a few weeks before childbirth to ensure a plentiful supply of Vitamin K and iron in the blood and to release the uterus muscle tention.

Chinese, use nettle with sarsaparilla for arthritis and joint pain.

In India, nettle is used for tention headache, and weight control. Because nettle increases metabolism and also excrete uric acid. One research showed up to six glasses of nettle excrete uric acid. One research showed up to six glasses of nettle tea every day may possibly cure chronic headache, skin disorders, and cancer of stomach.

Oak (Quercus)

Parts used: Bark.

Biochemical contents: tannins, volatile oil, essential oil.

Energy: Warm.

Country of origin: Worldwide.

Harvest time: The bark of young oak trees is carefully pared from the trunk or branches from mid-spring to late spring.

Properties: It has astringent, anti-inflammatory, and antiseptic effects.

Cosmetic uses: Oak contains a high percentage of volatile oil and tannins which puts this plant in the cosmetic category. It can be used as an ingredients for all skin type cleansers and conditioners as well as creams for oily, sensitive skin.

Medicinal uses: Volatile oil content is valuable for the treatment of cuts, burns, bleeding hemorrhoids, and diarrhea. Oak bark is a powerful astringent because of its tannin content. Its therapeutic properties render it an excellent gargle for throat infections. Oak bark can be burned to kill germs and bacteria, especially during winter. Iranian burn oak bark and eucalyptus during wintertime to kill the bacteria and refresh the air.

Oat (Avena sativa)

Parts used: Whole plant, seeds, oatmeal.

Biochemical contents: Saponin, alkaloids, protein, starch, fiber, most minerals (silica, calcium, iron, magnesium, copper, zinc), vitamins B complex, and vitamins A, C, E and K.

Energy: Cool.

Country of origin: Iran

Harvest time: Oats are harvested in late summer.

Properties: They have antiemetic, antispasmodic, antidepressant, tonic, diuretic, expectorant, and sedative properties.

Cosmetic uses: Oat is used for cleansing and conditioning for all types of skin. It is superb for skin rejuvenation and for sensitive skin. Oatmeal can make a great skin scrub since it softens the skin tissue. Yogurt is added to oatmeal, and the mixture is massaged in and left on like a mask. It cleanses and removes dead skin, tones and softens the skin tissue. Oat can be used in soaps, or it can make a soothing bath for irritated skin.

Medicinal uses: Oat is a wonderful remedy for nervous tension, insomnia, tension headache, and depression. Since ancient times Iranians have used oat and oat straw to promote hair growth and reduce mental stress. Iranians make a variety of soups and dishes with oat. Oat is a protein-rich grain and is also high in minerals and vitamins, especially vitamin B complex. Iranians believe it balances the memory, promotes calmness, and provides the best remedy for the nervous system, depression and stress.

Anti-inflammatory and soothing properties make oat valuable for the treatment of urinary infections and stones as well as rheumatism. Infusion of oat bran is idea for people who are losing hair. Soak oat straw in water overnight, strain the mix with cooked grain, and drink in the morning before breakfast. This promotes the growth of hair. The alkaloid component of oats stimulates the central nervous system and may be used to alleviate fever. Oat bath soothes rheumatic joints and muscles, chronic pains, and bladder, pelvic and emotional stress. For chronic conditions, take oat bran bath twice a week and drink three cups of oat infusion a day for as many weeks as necessary.

Olive (Lea europaea)

Parts used: Fruit and leaves.

Biochemical contents: Vitamins A and E, bitter glycoside, tannin, magnesium, potassium, iron, copper, zinc, and fat.

Energy: Warm.

Country of origin: Iran, Europe, India.

Harvest time: Olives are harvested from late fall to winter.

Properties: Olive has soothing, purgative, antispasmodic and therapeutic properties.

Cosmetic uses: Olive can be used in most skin and body cleansers and moisturizer. It is highly therapeutic and may be used as a massage oil to reduce muscle tension.

Principle uses: Olives have been called the liver's best friend and the best cleansers for the digestive system. Olives are the fruit of a beautiful tree. They contain a large amount of fat, which keeps the body warm and gives it energy. Olives are helpful during the winter. Eating fresh olives with meals everyday ensures good health. Fresh olives are very popular in Iran for increasing immunity energy and cleansing the liver. They also massage the forehead and neck with olive oil to reduce headache and fever.

Onion (Allium cepa)

Parts used: The whole plant.

Biochemical contents: Vitamin C, volatile oil, minerals especially iodine.

Energy: Warm.

Country of origin: Egypt, Iran, Asia

Harvest time: Onions can be picked from early summer to late fall.

Properties: It has antiseptic, astringent, antimicrobial properties and antibacterial properties..

Principle uses: Onion is used as a part of the everyday diet, whether fresh or cooked. Onion is highly antibacterial; it prevents colds, coughs, sore throat, flu, sinusitis, and other upper respiratory infections. Onion is good for stimulating the digestive system and increases the appetite. Onion is bactericidal. If an onion cut in half is left on the kitchen counter, it will kill all the bacteria in range. Onion is also wonderful in removing warts. Onion is rich in vitamin C and iodine. Recent studies indicate that onion eaten regularly can prevent cancers of digestive system. When eating raw onion, try to remove the thin skin between the layers; it can cause indigestion. Onion is a part of the Iranian meal everyday. They use it fresh with salads, cooked, and sautÈed. They also use onion to tenderize meat and to cover any bad aroma from it.

Medical uses: Onion and garlic are among the oldest plants used by mankind. Onions were cultivated by the ancient Egyptians, who made them part of their diet.

Onion reduces cholesterol, therefore reduces the risk of cardiovascular diseases. In the last two decades, studies by Dr. Victor Gurewich professor of Tufts University proved that onion increases HDL (high density lipoprotein) which, a "good cholesterol". in the blood which combats "bad cholesterol". Dr. Gurewich emphasized there are 150 different chemical compounds in onion, and his experiments indicated that onion is best taken raw, when it is more effective in increasing the HDL. Experiments by Indians reserachers have also proven that onion reduces the risk of cardiovascular diseases because it dissolves and reduces the fat that cause clogged arteries.

In the Mid-Eighteen century, Louis Pasteur "the father of bacteriology", discovered the power of onions. In experiments, he observed that onion and onion extract destroyed bacteria, especially tuberculosis and E-coli (bacteria native to the colon).

A Russian scientist experimented with 150 plants to determine which ones were anti-bacterial. He observed that onion and garlic are the most powerful of all herbs Chewed for three to eight minutes, onion sterilized the mouth tissue.

Dr. Irwin Ziment, a specialist in pulmonary diseases confirmed that onion is a powerful anti-bacterial agent that can kills the bacteria that cause colds and coughs. He also emphasized that onion is also expectorant that serves to expel mucus from the throat, sinuses and lungs.

Opium Poppy (papaver somniferum var nigrum)

Parts used: Seeds, syrup, and oil.

Biochemical contents: Alkaloid, fatty acid, codeine, morphine, benzyl alcohol, dL-lactic acid, vanillin acid.

Energy: Cold.

Country of origin: Iran, India.

Harvest time: Late summer to fall.

Properties: Opium has sedative, anti-spasmodic, and soothing properties. Opium poppy is a capsule-shaped fruit, as big as an egg, that produces opium. As the fruit's surface is cut with a sharp blade, the syrup excretion is dried up and turns brown.

Medicinal uses: Opium is a drug that contains several alkaloids, such as morphine and codeine. Opium has been used since ancient times for coughs, whooping cough, insomnia,

and diarrhea. It is also a pain killer.

In Iran, opium is widely used in small dosages for insomnia, severe coughs, fever, stomach upset, and gastrointestinal problems. Opium reduces sexual activities, causes forgetfulness, and reduces the appetite. Some people in Iran smell opium for insomnia and nervous tension. Opium flowers can be boiled with cilantro extract for treating ear inflammation. It is best used for coughs. As a child in Iran, my grandmother used small dosages of opium which she would take it before bedtime for her coughs, bronchitis, and lungs problems. Usually children, infants, elderly, and young girls during adolescence show sensitivities to opium. Western physicians approve and prescribe opium as a soporific drug in very small dosages. Excess use of opium may cause emotional stress, anxiety, and sleepiness.

Consult with a physician before using this drug.

Orange Blossoms (Citru aurantium)

Parts used: Essential oil.

Biochemical contents: Volatile oil, vitamin C, flavonoids, essential oils.

Energy: Cool.

Country of origin: Worldwide

Harvest time: Orange blossoms can be gathered from mid to late spring.

Properties: They have antiseptic, aromatic, antispasmodic, and astringent properties.

Cosmetic uses: Orange blossoms can be used in most skin toners and conditioners for deep skin cleansing and balancing pH level.

Principle uses: Essential oil of orange blossom is used in aromatherapy to treat anxiety and nervous depression. It also has tonic properties good for promoting and cleansing the digestive tract. Orange blossom is mainly used for aromatherapy, perfumes, baking, and pastries. Orange blossom can be added to most fruit jams for aroma and flavor. Iranian make variety of jams and pastries with orange blossoms. They also add it into black tea and drink it after meals for its aroma and for better digestion.

Oregon Grape Root (Mahonia aguifolium)

Parts used: Roots and rhizomes.

Biochemical contents: Alkaloid, berberine, bitter principle, tannin, minerals such as manganese, copper, sodium, and zinc.

Energy: Cool.

Country of origin: Iran.

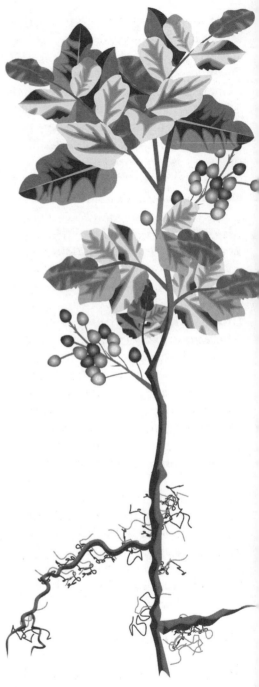

**Oregon Grape Root
(Mahonia aguifolium)**

Harvest time: Wild Oregon grape is a rocky mountain evergreen shrub with fruits resembling grapes. Its roots are gathered from late summer to fall.

Properties: Oregon grape roots have anti-inflammatory, soothing, and stimulating properties.

Cosmetic uses: Oregon grape root is excellent for all skin problems and disorders such as eczema, psoriasis, and acne. It has anti-inflammatory properties good for reducing the inflammation and irritation that results from acne and other skin disorders.

Medicinal uses: Oregon grape root contains bitter principle useful for liver and gallbladder detoxification and as a laxative for internal cleansing. Oregon grape root soothes, cools, and purifies blood, therefore, it can be prescribed for most skin disorders. Ancient Iranians used Oregon grape root with sarsaparilla and dandelion to cure skin disorders (such as eczema), constipation and arthritis pain as well as for liver detoxification.

Caution: Because of berberin, not to be taken during pregnancy.

Pansy (Viola tricolor)

Parts used: Flowers, leaves.

Biochemical contents: Volatile oil,

tannins, mucilage, and minerals.

Energy: Warm

Country of origin: Iran, Europe.

Harvest time: Pansy leaves and flowers are gathered from early spring to late fall.

Properties: Pansy has astringent, antispasmodic, soothing, anti-inflammatory, and tonic properties.

Cosmetic uses: Pansies are highly antiseptic and have strong healing and anti-inflammatory properties. They are used in general skin care creams, toners, and astringents, especially those made for sensitive skin.

Principle uses: Pansies have a strong flavor and are excellent for a variety of herbal salads, especially when mixed with dandelion, watercress, spinach, and nasturtiums. They are great sources of minerals, such as iron, potassium, zinc, and magnesium, and of vitamins, such as vitamins A, C, B complex, and K. Pansies are popular flowers in Iran especially during spring. They use pansies in backyards and also for garnishing foods and salads.

Papaya (Carica papya)

Parts used: Fruit, seeds, and leaves.

Biochemical contents: Enzymes, papain which helps in the digestion of protein.

Energy: Warm.

Country of origin: Hawaii.

Harvest time: Papaya leaves and fruits are collected mid-spring to late summer. The seeds are collected in winter.

Properties: Papaya has soothing, humectant, moisturizing, and toning properties on the skin.

Cosmetic uses: Papain is used for skin exfoliation, toning, and masks for all skin types.

Other uses: Papaya is a digestive fruit because of its papain content. Papain is used to tenderize meat and to contract blood during surgery. The seeds are taken to destroy parasites, and the leaves are a diuretic and slightly laxative. An infusion, for internal cleansing can be made with papaya, peach, and strawberry leaves, parsley, horsetail, and dandelion.

Parsley (Petroselinum Sativum)

Parts used: Leaves, stem, seeds.

Biochemical contents: Essential oil, glycosides, vitamins A, and C, minerals (calcium, iron, magnesium, and phosphorus).

Energy: Warm.

Country of origin: Worldwide.

Harvest time: Parsley leaves and stems can be gathered anytime during the growing season.

Properties: Parsley has astringent, antiseptic, antispasmodic, diuretic, and tonic qualities.

Cosmetic uses: Parsley is good for cosmetic, cooking, and medicinal use. It is an ingredient of general skin creams, toners, and conditioners. Being highly antiseptic, it soothes and moisturizes the skin, and in combination with other herbs such as fennel, creates a toning and anti-wrinkle effect on the skin.

Medicinal uses: Parsley is helpful for treating gout because it encourages uric acid elimination and is a strong diuretic suitable for treating urinary infections and stones. Parsley increases the flow of milk, tones the uterine muscles, purifies and cleanses blood, is slightly laxative, and stimulates the liver and flow of bile, especially in combination with other herbs such as dandelion, and gentian. Iranians use parsley in a variety of salads, dishes and medicines. They eat parsley everyday for cancer prevention as parsley may increase the production of white cells. They prescribe parsley for leukemia patients.

Parsley seeds are used to treat stomach gas and flatulence, bloody hemorrhoids, and kidney stones. Ancients used parsley to increases menstrual flow and used it as a suppository in uterus to induce miscarriage.

Ancient Iranians used parsely root to treat hepatitis, flatulence, painful periods, diarrhea, and kidney stones.

Fresh smashed parsely leave are used externally to reduce pain and inflammation on breast. Parsley leaves contain vitamins, minerals, and essential oils. Parsely can be chewed to fight bad breath.

Parsnip: (pastinaca secacul Russ).

Parts used: Leave, root

Bio-chemical content: Protein, carbohydrate, tannin, Vitamins (A, B1, B2, B3 and C), minerals (potassium, iron, calcium, phosphate).

Energy: Warm

Country of origin: Europe, Iran, N. America

Harvest time: The leaves are collected in summer and its roots are dug up in late fall.

Properties: Parsnip has soothing, and cleansing properties.

Cosmetics uses: Parsnip in very rich in most vitamins and minerals, so the plant may be used in skin creams and moisturizers for all skin type. Rich in protein, sugars and complex carbohydrates, it is an anti-wrinkle agent. Its tannin content makes it especially good fot dry sensitive skin.

Medicinal uses: European, especially French enjoy this pland in variety of dishes and salads. France's famed Pot-Au-Feu is made with parsnip root, beef and other herbs such as parsley, and chives.

Iranians make a delicious jam with parsnip root and eat it during winter time.

Parsnip root cleanses the liver, stomach, and kidneys, and it reduces the appetite.

Each 100 Grams of parsnip contains:

Water	79	gm
Protein	1/7	gm
Fat	0/5	gm
Carbohydrate	15	gm
Calcium	50	m.g
Phosphate	77	m.g
Iron	0/.7	m.g
Sodium	12	m.g
Potassium	541	m.g
Vitamin A	30	IU
Thiamin	0/08	m.g
Riboflavin	0/09	m.g
Niacin	0/02	m.g
Vitamin C	16	m.g

Pasque Flower (Anemone Pulsatilla Syn.)

Parts used: Aerial parts.

Biochemical contents: Glycoside, saponin, resin.

Energy: Cool.

Country of origin: Iran.

Harvest time: Flower and stalks are gathered in the spring.

Properties: It has antispasmodic, antimicrobial, and sedative properties.

Cosmetic uses: Saponin qualifies it for skin cleansers and toners and for pH balance.

Medicinal uses: Pasque flower is an excellent treatment to relieve earache. Being antispasmodic, it may be useful for tension headaches and menstrual periods. Iranians use this plant for anxiety, insomnia, and arthritis pain.

Caution: Fresh plant is poisonous. If dried, do not stored for more than a year.

Passion Flower (Passiflora incarnata).

Parts used: Flowers, fruits, and vine.

Biochemical contents: alkaloid, sugar, flavonoids.

Energy: Warm.

Country of origin: Iran, European countries.

Harvest time: Passionflower is gathered from mid-spring to late summer.

Properties: It has antidepressant, tranquilizing, and soothing properties.

Principle uses: Passionflower is a good tranquilizer, used for tension, anxiety, insomnia, and depression. It works directly on the central nervous system to relax mental and physical stress. It has a gentle sedative effective in relieving pains caused by neuralgia. Ancient Egyptians used it to treat asthma. To treat insomnia and depression, combine one tablespoon of each passion flower, skullcap, valerian, and peppermint, and one teaspoon licorice. Add thirty-two ounces of boiled water, and make a tea that is taken before bedtime. Ancient Iranians used passion flower, with chamomile and borage, to reduce menstrual pain, tension headache, muscle spasms, and anxiety attacks.

Pennyroyal (Hedeoma pulegioides)

Parts used: Leaves, flowers.

Biochemical contents: Bitter glycosides, tannins, and volatile oil.

Energy: Warm.

Country of origin: Europe, N. Africa, Asia, Iran.

Harvest time: Pennyroyal should be gathered in summer before flowering.

Properties: It has astringent, stimulant, anti-inflammatory, and aromatic properties.

Cosmetic uses: It can be used in skin toners and cleansers. The volatile oil gives it healing and anti-inflammatory properties to be used for disorders of the skin, including sensitivities and irritation .

Medicinal uses: The volatile oil in pennyroyal makes it very good to use for stomach flatulence and colic. Its anti-inflammatory property is good for muscle tension and arthritis pain. In Iran, pennyroyal, in combination with other herbs such as elder and marshmallow, is used to treat colds, sore throat, muscle pains, and tensions that result from colds and flu. Iranians use pennyroyal with dandelion and peppermint for internal cleansing. They also smoke the leaves for preventing bacteria entering home.

The Chinese use pennyroyal to treat whopping cough, coughs, chest pain, sinus pain, hepatitis, hiccups, stomach upset, and flatulence.

Ancient Iranians used pennyroyal to increase menstrual flow. They also made suppositories to induce miscarriage.

Caution: It promotes menstruation; not to be used by pregnant women.

Peppermint (Mentha piperita)

Parts used: Leaves, stems.

Biochemical contents: Alkaloid, volatile oil, tannins, mucilage, and mentho, essential oil.

Energy: Warm.

Country of origin: Iran, Europe.

Harvest time: Peppermint aerials are gathered from late spring to fall.

Properties: It has antispasmodic, astringent, anti-catarrh, stimulant, tonic, antimicrobial, antiemetic, and aromatic properties.

Cosmetic uses: Peppermint has antiseptic properties, so it is good for skin care masks and for conditioners made for oily and sensitive skin. It soothes and relaxes the skin tissue and stimulates circulation. Menthol, its active principle, has antiseptic properties which can soothe acne.

Medicinal uses: Peppermint stimulates the digestive system and reduces water retention, thus it is a fine remedy for menstrual pain related to water retention. Peppermint can be used in combination with other herbs such as dandelion, gentian, centaury, and parsley to cleanse the system and to stimulate and detoxify the liver and gallbladder. Iranians use peppermint for indigestion, stomach pain, headache, and upper respiratory problems, such as sinus, colds, and coughs. They use peppermint in variety of dishes, salads, and pastries. Peppermint is frequently used in aromatherapy for anxiety and depression.

Poke Root (Phytolacca americana)

Parts used: Berries and root.

Biochemical contents: Saponin, tannin, sugar, and resin.

Energy: Cold.

Country of origin: Iran, India, Asia.

Harvest time: Poke root should be collected late fall or spring.

Properties: Poke root has cleansing, anti-inflammatory, and antispasmodic properties.

Cosmetic uses: It is used in skin cleansers and conditioners. It is helpful for skin disorders and irritants, and it is also used to reduce pain and skin inflammation.

Medicinal uses: Poke root is used as an antibacterial and anti-inflammatory for arthritic and rheumatic complaints. The berries can be used to help weight loss. In Iran, in combination with herbs such as ginger and devil's claw, it is used to treat arthritis and tension headaches. Since poke root by itself may exhibit toxic properties, it had better be used in combination with other herbs. It is wise to begin with small doses and gradually increase.

Caution: To be taken under supervision.

Potato (Solanum tuberosum)

Parts used: Tubers.

Biochemical contents: Starch, vitamins A, B1, B6, and C, minerals (potassium, iron, and manganese).

Energy: Cool.

Country of origin: Worldwide.

Harvest time: Potatoes are harvested from late summer to late fall.

Properties: They have antispasmodic, soothing, and anti-diarrheal properties.

Cosmetic uses: Potato contains starch and potassium, which enables it to soothe burned and inflamed skin and tone large oily pores. Potatoes can be sliced thin or grated and applied on burned and inflamed areas to prevent blistering.

Principle uses: Potato is a very good food, especially in winter, when foods are heavy or greasy. The potassium content of potatoes helps the absorption of nutrients, and it changes consumed fats into saponins and dissolves them. Potatoes are wonderful for insomnia and nervous tension, especially if taken for dinner. They stop diarrhea and control overproduction of stomach acid. Potatoes are best when baked or boiled in their skins because they lose less vitamin C and potassium with the skin intact. Iranian bake potatoes, beets, and turnips for a winter afternoon snack. This combination provides all kinds of vitamins and minerals and helps the body increase the immune system.

Potato is not recommended for individuals with high blood sugar, because it contains high amount of glycemic index which raises the blood sugar quickly.

Potato's leaves and green parts can be used externally to treat rheumatic pain, and muscle tention.

Potato's skin is anti-oxidant and contains Chlorogenic acid, and it may prevent some cancers.

In 1960 Florida University discovered the power of potatoes by experimenting and observing potato's skin prevents oxidation of polyunsaturated fat, and it prevent cells damage by free radicals. This is due to of its antioxidant and antiviral content.

Caution: Green potatoes are poisonous.

Each 100 Grams of Potatoes Contain:

Raw Potatoes:

water	79.8	gm
Protein	2.1	gm
Fat	0.1	gm
Carbohydtates	17	gm
Calcium	7	gm
Phosphote	53	gm
Iron	0.6	gm
Potasium	407	gm
Thiamin	0.1	gm
Riboflavin	0.04	gm
Niacin	1.5	gm
Vitamin C	25	gm

Baked Potatoes:

water	75	gm
Protein	2.6	gm
Fat		
Carbohydtates	19.5	gm
Calcium	9	gm
Phosphote	65	gm
Iron	0.7	gm
Potasium	503	gm
Thiamin	0.1	gm
Riboflavin	0.04	gm
Niacin	1.7	gm
Vitamin C	20	gm

Prickly Ash (Zant hoxylam amerrcanum)

Parts used: Barks and berries.

Biochemical contents: Tannin, alkaloids, resin, and volatile oil.

Energy: warm.

Country of origin: Iran, India.

Harvest time: Prickly ash berries can be gathered in late summer; bark is collected in the spring.

Properties: It has tonic, stimulant, anti-inflammatory, and astringent qualities.

Cosmetic uses: Prickly ash can be used in most skin cleansers and conditioners. The tannin content makes it a good remedy for skin disorders. It is anti-inflammatory, reduces skin irritation, and relaxes irritated skin.

Medicinal uses: Prickly ash is used to treat arthritic and rheumatic complaints. Powdered prickly ash bark can be chewed to relieve toothache. The anti-inflammatory properties make it good for menstrual pain and muscle tension, especially arthritis and joint pain. In Iran, prickly ash is used with marjoram and ginger to relieve arthritis and rheumatic pains. They also massage the sore area with a powder of prickly ash bark and olive oil to reduce inflammation and pain.

Psyllium (Plantago psyllium)

Parts used: Seeds, leaves, and husk.

Biochemical contents: Tannins, mucilage, glycoside, silica, alkaloid, and fatty acids.

Energy: Cool.

Country of origin: Iran.

Harvest time: Psyllium seeds are harvested from late summer to early fall.

Properties: Psyllium has demulcent, laxative, and purgative properties.

Medicinal uses: Psyllium husks and seeds are considered excellent colon and intestinal cleansers. They lubricate stool and help to increase its bulk, ease the passage of feces, and relieve constipation. Some clinical research in Germany shows that psyllium has laxative and anti-diarrheal properties. Psyllium husks and seeds contain large amounts of fiber. When soaked in water, they expand and become a gel. Psyllium contains large amounts of tannins and silica which qualifies the plant as a treatment for hemorrhoids Iranian have used psyllium since ancient time for liver cleansing and to release warm energy from the blood and liver. They also mix psyllium with cilantro to cure skin disorders such as acne and eczema.

Caution: Inhaling psyllium powder may cause asthma and unsoaked seeds may cause gastrointestinal problems.

Pumpkin (Cucurbita pepo)

Parts used: Seeds and whole fruit.

Biochemical contents: Vitamins A (beta carotene) and C, sugar, starch, and minerals (zinc, potassium, magnesium).

Energy: Warm.

Country of origin: Worldwide.

Harvest time: Pumpkins are harvested from late summer to the end of fall.

Properties: Pumpkin has antispasmodic, anti-catarrh, and soothing properties on skin disorders such as boils.

Cosmetic uses: Pumpkin is good for skin disorders, especially acne and boils, due to its rich vitamins A, C, and zinc content. The seeds and oil are particularly helpful. If pumpkin has been steamed for a few minutes and applied to acne five to ten minutes daily, it dries up acne and gives elasticity to the skin as well.

Medicinal uses: Pumpkin is used to treat sore throats, coughs, and colds. In Iran and Mediterranean countries, one suffering from laryngitis will steam and cook the pumpkin, then try to eat it hot to soothe the larynx and relax the throat. Pumpkin is commonly used by singers or people who have to speak loudly. Pumpkin seeds are very rich in vitamin A and zinc, and they are valuable for treating skin disorders, such as acne and eczema, and for flushing intestinal worms.

Pumpkin and its seeds both are considered anti-cancer. Several year ago one scientist in Poland discovered that there is a chemical in pumpkin named Protease trypsin which can stop the growth of viruses in the intestine that cause cancer. Pumpkin has a strong source of carotenoids and beta-carotene which are both anti-oxidants and protect the body cells against free radicals.

One research study showed in New Jersey, a group of men who were addicted to tobacco after using pumpkin quit their habit, and some of them reduce the amount of tobacco they were using.

Another scientific research study proved those people who have lung cancer should eat substantial amount of pumpkin, carrot and sweat potatoes to fight the cancer.

Radish (Raphama sativus).

Parts used: Roots, leaves, and seeds.

Biochemical contents: Glycoside, volatile oil, saponin, sulfur, zinc, and vitamins A, B complex, and C.

Energy: Warm.

Country of origin: Iran, India, Asia.

Harvest time: Radishes can be harvested from late spring to late summer; black radishes are harvested during winter.

Properties: Radish has antibacterial, antiseptic, detoxifying, diuretic, and cleansing properties.

Cosmetic uses: The volatile oil of radish and its saponin content make this plant work as a cleanser and conditioner for all skin types, especially oily skin. The antiseptic and antibacterial properties in radish are ideal for oily skin masks and creams.

Medicinal uses: Radish is a fine remedy for coughs, colds, sore throat, and upper respiratory infections. The sulfur content of radish soothes the chest and throat. It is antibacterial and fights upper respiratory infections. Radish increases the circulation and appetite, promotes bile production, and is good for liver and gallbladder detoxification. Radish can also be a good remedy for kidney and bladder stones. There are many different kinds of radishes. Any kind of radish juice is good for expelling stones from the bladder and kidneys. Simply drink the juice in the morning before breakfast. It helps in crushing stones and discharging them in urine.

Radishes generate heat in the system and can dissolve fat. They give a special glow and color to the skin.

Iranians, eat radish leaves to clean the stomach and colon, and apply smashed radish externally to treat rheumatic pain, and backache.

They also drink radish juice to expel stones of bladder and kidney.

Chinese, and Indians use all parts of radish. They use radish seed to treat coughs, fever, cold, indigestion, stomach ache and to increase the flow of urine. They also include radish and cabbage in their daily diet to ensure stomach health, and to prevent cancer.

In Japan extract of radish roots is used to treat rheumatic pain, coughs, dirrhea, and back pain.

Raspberry (Rubus)

Parts used: Fruit and leaves.

Biochemical contents: Citric acid, vitamins A, B, C, and E, volatile oil, minerals (calcium, iron, and phosphorus), sugar.

Energy: Cool.

Country of origin: Most countries.

Harvest time: Raspberry leaves can be picked throughout the growing season; fruits are gathered from early summer to mid-fall.

Properties: Raspberries have astringent, tonic, and diuretic properties.

Principle uses: Fresh fruits are widely used in jams, cakes, and ice creams. Indians use raspberry leaf tea during the last few weeks of pregnancy to ease the childbirth and tone the uterine and pelvic muscles. They also use a leaves and fruit tea after childbirth to encourage the flow of milk. Iranians use raspberry to reduce high blood pressure and sugar. Raspberry leaves are a good remedy for diarrhea, and since they have cool energy and volatile oil, they help ease sore throat.

Red Clover (Trifolium pratense)

Parts used: Dried flower heads.

Biochemical contents: Flavonoids, glycosides, and phenolic acid.

Energy: Cool.

Country of origin: Iran, China, India.

Harvest time: Red clover flowers are gathered from late spring to fall.

Properties: Red clover has antispasmodic, astringent, expectorant, sedative, and tonic properties.

Cosmetic uses: Red clover is a prime remedy for skin disorders, such as

acne, eczema, and psoriasis. It is used in ointments or creams, toners and conditioners for all skin types.

Medicinal uses: Red clover has expectorant and antispasmodic properties for treating coughs, whooping cough, respiratory ailments, bronchitis, and all diseases associated with mucous congestion. Red clover is a very useful for skin diseases and conditions, such as acne, eczema, and psoriasis in children and adults. To treat skin disorders, make an infusion of red clover, dandelion, yellow dock, burdock, chickweed, and echinacea. Drink three

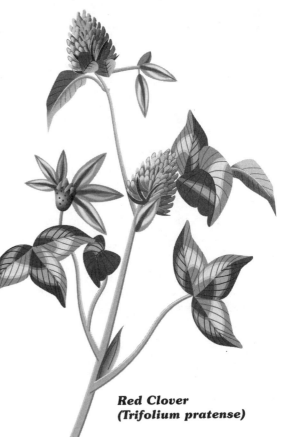

Red Clover
(Trifolium pratense)

to four cups a day for treatment of skin disorders and colds. Iranians drink red clover and yarrow tea for colds and flu. Recent studies show that red clover may be useful for the treatment of tumors and cancers of various kinds. Indians use dried flowers for bronchitis and whooping coughs. Chinese and Japanese use steamed flowers for blood purification, asthma, whooping cough, and throat and stomach cancers.

Rhubarb (Rheum palmatum)

Parts used: Rhizome.

Biochemical contents: Tannin, glycoside , gallic acid, starch, pectin.

Energy: Cold.

Country of origin: Iran, China, India, Europe.

Harvest time: Rhubarb root is dug up in China, Turkey, and Iran.

Properties: It has astringent, and laxative qualities.

Cosmetic uses: A variety of acids in rhubarb are used in skin creams or moisturizers. The properties of alpha hydroxy acids help tone skin tissues and increases exfoliation (sloughs of dead skin). It soothes and heals irritated skin.

Medicinal uses: Rhubarb is used for constipation, and in small doses, it helps diarrhea. It has digestive properties, increases the flow of bile, detoxifies liver and gallbladder; and stimulates blood circulation. Iranians make stews, soups, and jam with rhubarb. They also make syrup with rhubarb and take it before meals to increase the appetite, and also to regulate the bowl movement.

Rhubarb is a laxative which does not irritate the stomach.

Ancient Iranians used rhubarb to treat indigestion, bloody diarrhea, flatulence, gastrointestinal problems, kidney and bladder stones.

Chinese use rhubarb to treat constipation, female problems, whopping cough, and to produce red blood cells.

Rhubarb with rice many be used to treat upper respiratory problems.

Caution: Rhubarb is not recommended for individuals who have hemorrhoids.

Rose (Rosa)

Parts used: Hips, flowers, and leaves.

Biochemical contents: Tannins, pectin, and vitamins B, C, E, and K, essential oil.

Energy: Warm.

Country of origin: Iran, European countries .

Harvest time: Roses are gathered in spring, and rose hips and leaves are collected in fall.

Properties: Rose has diuretic, astringent, tonic, and laxative qualities.

Cosmetic uses: Its alpha hydroxy acid properties help balance the pH levels of the skin and exfoliate the dead layers. It also soothes sensitive skin. Aromatherapists use rose for anxiety and depression. It is also valuable in perfumery. Rose hips are a wonderful source of vitamin C. Rose hip tea is good for colds and flu, and rose leaves are cathartic, easing constipation and problems of gallbladder. Iranians use rose in jams and pastries, and use the extract of rose for skin cleansing.

Medicinal uses: Rose has been used since ancient times for food, perfume, cosmetics, and medicines. It cleanses the liver and gallbladder, detoxifies the system, and is a laxative. Its extract is used to increase circulation, ease stomach spasms, and relieve chest and lung inflammation. Dried rose buds stop diarrhea and reduce headache. Its infusion gives strength to gums and teeth and cures mouth wounds. Some people may show a reaction by sneezing, nasal block, or lung sensitivity. Iranians make rose jam for wintertime, as it is very high in Vitamin C and it also cleanses the system.

Rosemary (Rosmarinas officinalis)

Parts used: Leaves, oil, and flowers.

Biochemical contents: Volatile oil, phenolic acids, camphor, and flavonoids, essential oil.

Energy: Warm.

Country of origin: Iran, Mediterranean countries.

Harvest time: Rosemary leaves can be gathered throughout the year, and flowers are gathered in summer.

Properties: It has astringent, antimicrobial, antispasmodic, antidepressant, antibiotic, aromatic, and stimulating properties.

Cosmetic uses: Rosemary is an ingredient for any skin cream, especially those for skin with poor circulation. Rosemary is a fine skin toner and conditioner and a good addition to shampoo. Aromatherapists use the oil for energy, stimulating muscles, and circulation.

Medicinal uses: Rosemary is a very good remedy for tension headaches, rheumatic pains and arthritis pain when taken either as an infusion or used externally. The essential oil is applied directly to the head with massage. Rosemary is antibacterial and anti-fungal. It stimulates digestion, the liver and the gallbladder, increasing the flow of bile. It is also a useful internal cleanser. Since rosemary by itself is very strong and stimulating, as an infusion it is better to combine it with other herbs such as chamomile, passion flowers, and apple peel. Ancient Iranians used it to cleanse lungs, liver and colon. It is great for tension headaches, for rheumatic and arthritis pains, for increasing menstrual flow, and for stimulating uterine muscles. Filipinos use rosemary for indigestion and for steam baths after delivery. The French make its infusion to treat muscular spasms and indigestion.

Rue (Ruta graveolans)

Parts used: Dried aerial part.

Biochemical contents: Tannins, essential oil, alkaloid.

Energy: Warm.

Country of origin: Turkey, North Africa, Iran, Mediterranean countries.

Harvest time: Rue can be gathered before flowers open during summer.

Properties: It has antispasmodic, antimicrobial, and stimulant qualities.

Principle uses: Rue was first discovered in Greece and migrated from there. Since ancient times, this plant has been used in Iran and Mediterra-
nean countries to relieve menstrual pain, muscle spasms, and tension headache. Experiments show that rue reduces heartbeats on frogs. Its alkaloid content, when burned or boiled, is bactericidal. Rue increases menstruation and can be used for miscarriages and to stimulate sexual desire. Iranians use rue to reduce fever, stomach pain, and intestinal pain. There is also wild rue which is widely used in Iran to increase menstrual flow and stimulate milk production. Indians use it for miscarriage. Wild rue is very popular in Middle Eastern countries to treat fever and stomach spasm. Iranian use a wild rue leaves infusion for rheumatic and joint pain. Iranian strongly believe burning wild rue can kill negativity and bad energy. Usually most Iranians burn wild rue on Friday eve as they believe Thursday or Friday eve is a sacred day. They also burn wild rue in the first minute of the new year to kill negative energy for the entire year. They also burn it for sickness, weddings, and new born babies. Ancient Iranians prescribed an infusion of wild rue leaves for three consecutive months for women who cannot become pregnant. Wild rue increases circulation and lowers blood pressure.

Caution: Rue should not be used during pregnancy.

Saffron (Crocus satwus)

Parts used: Dried flowers.

Biochemical contents: Essential oil, bitter glycosides, natural dye.

Energy: Warm.

Country of origin: Iran.

Harvest time: Saffron flowers are harvested in the fall and very carefully dried in the shade.

Properties: Saffron has aromatic, antispasmodic, and dyeing properties.

Main uses: Iranians use saffron for garnishing and dyeing rice and a variety of foods, such as stews, puddings, cakes, and desserts. Saffron is a most expensive spice and very aromatic. Saffron is used as a powder mixed with warm water to release its orange-yellow color. Because it is water soluble, saffron can be used for painting, but not for fabric dyeing. In Iran, saffron is used in traditional ice cream for its color and aroma and saffronic ice cream is very popular within Iranians.

Sage (Salvia officinalis)

Parts used: Leaves.

Biochemical contents: Volatile oil, saponin, glycoside, alcohol, phenolic acid, tannins, camphor, essential oil.

Energy: Warm.

Country of origin: Asia, North Africa.

Harvest time: Sage leaves can be gathered in early summer.

Properties: Sage has astringent, antimicrobial, anti-catarrh, and stimulant properties.

Cosmetic uses: Sage is highly antiseptic, and its phenolic acid content is antibacterial. Sage is excellent for soothing and healing of acne and for problematic skin in form of masks, cleansers, and acne lotions. Aromatherapists use sage for elevating energy. The essential oil of sage can also be used in the bathtub for stimulating energy. If feeling negative and low, the best remedy is either smudging or boiling and steaming sage. Let its aroma linger in the house. It draws a lot of good energy into any home.

Medicinal uses: For centuries, sage has been esteemed for its healing power. As a hot infusion it is excellent for colds. Its phenolic acid is antibacterial and excellent for sore throats and laryngitis. Gargle with hot infusion of sage, salt, and fresh lemon juice three to five times daily to kill bacteria in throat and soothe the inflammation and coughs. Sage stimulates the digestive system and is useful for painful periods. Its estrogenic properties make it useful for treating menopausal hot flashes. Sage also has a reputation for drying up the flow of milk. It has become popular in China and Europe since the 9th century. Chinese use dried sage in beverages, such as herbal tea. In England, it is used as a non-alcoholic beverage. In the USA, it is used as an aromatic herb to tenderize meat. Ancient Iranians believed that extract of sage was good for wounds, burns, scratches, stopping milk production, sore throats, and coughs. Its small branches are used in steam baths and for inhalation. Sage mixed with honey, boiled in water, then soaked in a piece of cotton for 15 minutes and applied to wounds is good for fast healing. It stimulates sweat glands and increases perspiration.

Sandalwood Oil (Santalum album)

Parts used: Flower.

Biochemical contents: Essential oil, tannins.

Energy: Cool.

Country of origin: India.

Harvest time: Sandalwood can be gathered in the spring or early summer.

Properties: It has aromatic, anti-inflammatory, and soothing properties.

Cosmetic and principle uses: Sandalwood has a heavy, luxurious oil used in aromatherapy for tension, anxiety, and sexual stimulation. Sandalwood oil can be used for a massage and in a hot tub to relax and soothe the mind and release tension. Mix it with rosewater for massaging on the forehead to reduce tension headache. Iranians use its perfume. Its leaves resemble walnut leaves and are aromatic. In Indonesia, its trunk is powdered and its oil is used as a medicine. Chinese use its powder for upset stomach, vomiting, colic, and backache. They also mix it with rosewater and use it for skin disorders, headache, and fever.

Sarsaparilla (Smilax ornata).

Parts used: Root.

Biochemical contents: Saponin, glycoside, sarsaponin, sugar, and fat.

*Energy:*warm.

Country of origin: Japan, China.

Harvest time: Sarsaparilla roots and rhizomes can be dug up throughout the year.

Properties: Sarsaparilla has astringent, diuretic, anti-inflammatory, and anti-rheumatic properties.

Cosmetic uses: Sarsaparilla is used for skin diseases, such as psoriasis and eczema.

Medicinal uses: Sarsaparilla is a blood purifier, useful in treating rheumatism, and a good alternative for psoriasis, eczema, acne, and all other skin diseases. An infusion is made from a combination of equal parts of sarsaparilla, burdock root, yellow dock root, dandelion root, and red clove for skin disorders. One ounce of the combination is added to a pint of boiling water, and three cups are taken daily. This will purify and cleanse the blood and the results will appear in two to four weeks. Sarsaparilla has been used traditionally in Iran for arthritis and rheumatic pains. It makes a delicious tea to drink plain or with ginger. Chinese use the ground stalk as an antitoxin for food poisoning, for overflow of menstruation, and for body fluid reduction, especially around knees. They use it for sexual diseases, arthritis and joint pains, and backache. In the Philippines, it is used for internal cleansing and regulating menstruation. Its stalks are useful as a blood cleanser and detoxifier. A mixture of sarsaparilla and wine is good for toothache. Fifteen grams of sarsaparilla root with 450 ml. of boiling water drunk with sugar is good for muscle weakness, coughs, lung inflammation, joint pain, and some sexual diseases. Its ground root is great for wounds, acne, and eczema. Indians use ground root mixed with water and cow's milk to treat bloody diarrhea.

Caution: As medicine is taken a for long period of time, if it is taken by a warm energy person, he or she should be over age 40, and if cold energy, should be over 30.

Senna (Cassua)

Parts used: Leaves and pods.

Biochemical contents: Essential oil, tannin, and resin.

Energy: Cold.

Country of origin: Iran, India.

Harvest time: Senna pods are collected during the winter.

Properties: It has laxative and soothing properties.

Principle uses: Iranians have used it for constipation since ancient times. Senna leaf is bitter, and this bitter property makes it good for detoxifying the liver and gallbladder, for cleansing the system, and for relieving constipation. In evenings before sleeping, one should drink its infusion.

Caution: Should not be used during pregnancy.

Skullcap (Scutellaria lateriflora)

Parts used: Aerial part.

Biochemical contents: Volatile oil, tannin, flavonoid, glycosides, and sugar.

Energy: Cool.

Country of origin: Iran.

Harvest time: Skullcap aerial parts should be pick from late summer to early fall.

Properties: Skullcap has antispasmodic, tonic, anti-inflammatory, and sedative properties.

Medicinal uses: Skullcap is an excellent tonic for the nervous system, treating anxiety, depression, nervous headache, and insomnia. Anti-inflammatory and antispasmodic properties qualify it for stomach ulcer and urinary infections. It also has considerable detoxifying properties that are good for liver and internal cleansing. It is one of the most effective herbs for use in quitting alcohol, for insomnia and for mental depression.

Caution: Large doses may cause dizziness and confusion.

Skunk Cabbage (Symplocarpus foetidus)

Parts used: Root.

Biochemical contents: Volatile oil, silica, iron, manganese, and resin.

Energy: Warm.

Harvest time: The underground part of skunk cabbage should be unearthed in the fall and not be kept for more than one year because they deteriorate with drying.

Properties: Skunk cabbage has antispasmodic and expectorant properties.

Medicinal uses: Skunk cabbage has an unpleasant smell, but is a prime remedy for upper respiratory disorders. It is prescribed for tightness of chest and asthma. Iranians use this plant for muscle pain, muscle tension, and tension headaches.

Caution: Fresh plant can cause blisters.

Slippery Elm (Ulmus fulva).

Parts used: Bark.

Biochemical contents: Protein, iodine, and mucilage.

Energy: Neutral.

Country of origin: Iran

Harvet time: Slippery elm bark is stripped from the trunk in spring. The older the bark, the better the quality.

Properties: It has astringent, anti-inflammatory, demulcent, and emollient qualities.

Medicinal uses: The infusion (slippery elm powder in hot water) is used to soothe sore and irritated throats, coughs, and lung dryness. Iranians use slippery elm powder with comfrey root, marshmallow root, licorice and ginger to treat stomach ulcers and gastrointestinal problems. To make slippery elm gruel, mix four to six tablespoons of slippery elm root powder with warm water or warm milk and honey. Stir until desired consistency, and add ginger for flavoring. This liquid pudding is to be directly applied on the affected area. Slippery elm powdered with licorice is great for stomach ulcer.

Soapwort (Sapmaria officinalis)

Parts used: Rhizome.

Biochemical contents: Saponin.

Energy: Cool.

Country of origin: European countries especially France, it grow in China and Japan.

Harvest time: Root and rhizome are collected in fall.

Properties: Soapwort has expectorant and diuretic qualities.

Cosmetic uses: Excellent for treatment of eczema, psoriasis, boils, and acne.

Medicinal uses: Its medicinal properties are due to saponins which lower surface tension and produce a lather which eliminates uric acid and its anti-inflammatory properties for gout and rheumatic pain. Iranians use its steam inhalation for upper respiratory problems, such as asthma and coughs. In China, people soak soapwort root in water for sexual diseases. Powdered root gives a lather and is used for cleaning silk fabric.
Caution: Internal use may cause severe vomiting and dizziness.

St. John's Wort (Hypericum Perforatum)

Parts used: The whole plant.

Biochemical contents: Volatile oil, tannins, flavonoids, glycosides, chlorophyll, pseudohypericin, alkaloids, vitamins A and C, unstable fatty essential oil, and resin.

Energy: Warm.

Country of origin: Iran, and most countries.

Harvest time: The aerial parts of St. John's wort are gathered in the summer and dried in shade.

Properties: It has astringent, anti-inflammatory, and antispasmodic properties.

Cosmetic uses: It is useful in skin disorders, such as acne, inflamed skin, and skin with broken capillaries. It soothes and heals inflamed and irritated acne.

Medicinal uses: St. John's wort is good for lifting the immune system and energy level. Because of its antibacterial properties, it heals wounds and eases pain by lowering skin temperature. In Iran and Mediterranean countries, this plant is used for mental depression. The herb is very useful for treating problems of the nervous system and emotional stress, especially during menopause. It is diuretic, eliminates waste material, and is good for internal cleansing. Ointment of St. John's wort is good for healing burns, wounds, and cuts. St. John's wort leaves contain a red-colored syrup. This substance in France is used externally to treat burns, wounds, and cuts. In India, this plant is used to kill intestinal worms and to regulate menstruation. St. Johns wort increases the flow of menstruation, urine, and bile, and it cleanse the liver and gallbladder. St. John's wort is great for treating tension headaches and relieving nervous tension. Mix oil of St. John's wort flowers with olive oil; heat for a couple of hours, stir occasionally; and strain after twenty four hours. This oil can be used externally for wounds, cuts, and burns. Also massage joints and muscles with this to relieve rheumatic joint pain. An infusion of its leaves is used to increase appetite and to cure hepatitis, liver, and kidney disorders.

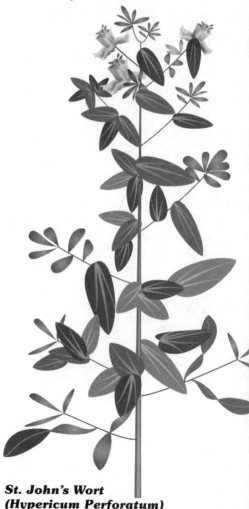

**St. John's Wort
(Hypericum Perforatum)**

St. John's wort has been known and used for two thousand years for external and internal cures. Scientific research about St. John's wort shows that this plant increases the body's immune system. The most exciting medicinal power in this plant was discovered in 1988 when scientists in New York discovered that St. John's wort increases the production of white cells and its antibacterial power helps to conquer HIV viruses. After that research, most patients who had AIDS started using St. John's wort. The results were positive and many improved. One of the most exciting and interesting effects of St. John's wort is its biochemical hypericine which weakens AIDS viruses. The result of one scientific animal research experiment in Proceedings of the National Academy of Sciences indicates that St. John's wort has activities against HIV viruses. They experimented on rats by injecting St. John's wort orally, and the results were one hundred percent positive. Research studies have shown that AIDS often attacks the brain. Extract of St. John's wort passes throughout brain cells and treats the disease. Its leaves and flowers contain an essential oil which can be expressed with finger pressure. The oil can be massaged in to reduce rheumatic pain and tension headache.

Pliny, a famous early Italian scientist soaked St. John's wort in red wine to cure snake bites. Greek physicians used the plant to heal burns and cuts. Abu Ali Cinna and other ancient Iranian physicians used St. John's wort for healing burns and cuts and for stimulating the flow of menstruation. Nicholas Culpepper, a British herbalist in the 17th century, indicated in his book that if St. John's wort is boiled in wine and drunk, it is a cure for skin disorders, diarrhea, fever, and liver detoxification. During the 16th century, John Gerard, a famous herbalist, categorized St. John's wort as a most valuable plant for wound healing and useful for curing disorders of liver and kidney stones.

Stillingia (Stillingia sylvatica)

Parts used: Root.

Biochemical contents: Tannin, glycoside, alkaloid, and resin.

Energy: Cool.

Harvest time: Stillingia roots can be dug up from late summer to fall.

Properties: Stillingia has astringent, anti-microbial, expectorant, anti-inflammatory, and antispasmodic properties.

Cosmetic uses: Stillingia reduces inflammation and irritation of skin disorders, such eczema, and psoriasis.

Medicinal uses: A blood purifier and cleanser, it is decreases arthritic and rheumatic pain, stomach ulcers, and intestinal inflammation because of its anti-inflammatory and antimicrobial properties. It is also used for menstrual pain and muscle tension. Iranians use an inusion of stillingia with sarsaparilla, burdock and blue flag for skin disoders such as acne and eczema as well as arthrities pain.

Stone Root (Callinsonia canadensis)

Parts used: Leaves and roots.

Biochemical contents: Saponin, tannins, volatile oil, and silica.

Energy: Cool.

Country of origin: Iran

Harvest time: Stone root is dug up in fall.

Properties: It has antiseptic, anti-inflammatory, antispasmodic, and soothing properties.

Medicinal uses: Stone root is principally used for the treatment of kidney and bladder stones, for the reduction of back pressure resulting from kidney stones, and for cuts and burns. Iranians apply fresh stone root with grated potatoes on burns to reduce pain and inflammation, and they also use an infusion of stone roots for hemorrhoidal

pain and bleeding. Since this plant is highly diuretic and antiseptic, it is helpful in treating problems of the digestive system.

Sugar Cane

Parts used: Branches, stalks.

Biochemical contents:
Polysaccharides 15%, oxalate calcium, pectin.

Energy: Warm.

Country of origin: Asia.

Harvest time: Sugar cane is harvested from early summer through fall.

Properties: It has soothing and calming actions

Cosmetic uses: It is used in creams for skin exfoliation and in toners. It has anti-wrinkle properties. Glycolic acid, derived from sugar cane, is a most important ingredient in beauty creams. It can reduce pH balance in the skin.

Medicinal uses: Chinese use it topically to cure acne, boils, burns, and wounds. They also burn the stalks and mix the ashes with olive oil for wounds and itches. Indians boil the stalks for measles, backache, liver detoxification, vomiting, and hemorrhoids. Polysaccharide in sugar cane is a preservative and produces energy. Ancient Iranians believed that sugar cane soothed nerves, regenerated blood circulation, and stopped internal bleeding. Sugar cane is great for coughs and lung irritation, if used warm. It cleanses the bladder and stimulates sexual desire. Excess use after meals causes stomach gas and indigestion. If mixed with fresh organic butter, it is good for wounds, itches, and skin irritation.

Ancients believed sugar as stimulant and energetic, but recent research shows that it is not only is stimulant, but is also soothing, antidepressant, and relaxing to those suffering from insomnia. Many scientific experiments have shown that the amount of sugar in blood is not related to physical and mental strength. Eating sugar causes physiological and chemical changes in brain, and those changes give energy to and relax the brain. Sugar cane's carbohydrates stimulate insulin in the blood, increasing tryptophan, which enters the brain immediately and produces serotonin. This soothes and relaxes the mind. Dr. Judith Wurtman has shown that the amount of tryptophan is directly related to the amount of serotonin. Dr. Norman states that some people suffer from seasonal affective disorder, which is related to the reduced production of serotonin in the brain, during winter. The result is insomnia and depression. Since in winter there is less daylight, the production of serotonin in the brain reduces and causes mental depression. During such periods, more carbohydrates are needed.

For better mental relaxation and concentration, about 2 1/2 tablespoons of carbohydrates a day is a must. People who are greater than 20% require 50% more. Experiments have shown that if the above dosage of carbohydrates is taken a day, it will reduce mental depression, anxiety, and nervous tension, therefore one can sleep better.

Caution: Overeating sugar cane may cause one to become overweight.

Summer Savory: (Satureja hortensis).

Parts used: Leaves.

Biochemical contents: Tannins, mucilage, essential oil, and phenolic acid.

Energy: Warm.

Country of origin: Iran, Meditteranean countries and Europe.

Harvest time: Summer savory leaves are collected from early summer to fall.

Properties: It has antispasmodic, astringent, anti-inflammatory, and antiseptic properties.

Principle uses: It is used to season meat and soups and is mixed with other herbs in salads. Summer savory stimulates the appetite and digestive system. It is very refreshing and cleansing. It may be used to ease menstrual pain. In Iran and

Mediterranean countries, summer savory is used in daily meals, salads, and summer soups. Italians make a sauce of this herb for a variety of dishes.

Sunflower (Helianthus annuns)

Parts used: Oil and seeds.

Biochemical contents: Vitamins A, C, E, and zinc.

Energy: Warm.

Country of origin: Iran.

Harvest time: Sunflower seeds are gathered from the flower from late summer to fall.

Properties: Sunflower seed oil has an emollient and toning properties on the skin.

Cosmetic uses: It can be used in skin cleansers and creams for all types of skin due to its emollient and moisturizing elements.

Principle uses: Sunflower seeds are very rich in vitamin A which is useful for treating eye problems. The oil is used in cooking. Sunflower seed oil is a laxative that increases the flow of bile. In Iran, sunflower seeds are used to reduce high blood cholesterol, and the oil is used in cooking.

Sweet Bay (Laurus nobilis)

Parts used: Leaves.

Biochemical contents: Essential oil, uric acid.

Energy: Warm.

Country of origin: Iran, India, Europe.

Harvest time: Sweet bay leaves are gathered throughout the summer and dried in the shade. The color fades from green to brown, and it will lose aromatic oil if dried in the sun.

Properties: It has aromatic, antispasmodic, and antiseptic properties.

Cosmetic uses: It is used in skin conditioners and cleansers. The essential oil can be used in aromatherapy for depression and muscle tension.

Medicinal uses: Leaves are traditionally used in Europe for menstrual flow and miscarriages. Ancient Europeans used its extract for treatment of nervous tension, stomach ulcers, muscle tension, and to increase blood circulation. The oil can be massaged over pain that is due to low blood circulation. Indians use the fruits for menstrual flow and to stop diarrhea. Sweet bay leaves are beneficial for toothache Leaves with vinegar reduce headache, stomach gas, liver pain, and colic. Its fruits are beneficial for liver disorders and gas. Ancient Iranians massaged the extract of sweet bay fruits with rose oil and vinegar for earache and headache.

Sweet Flag (Acorus calamus)

Parts used: Rhizome.

Biochemical contents: Volatile oil, azulene, tannins, mucilage, and camphor.

Energy: Cool.

Country of origin: Iran

Harvest time: Sweet flag rhizomes can be gathered in fall.

Properties: It has anti-inflammatory, antiseptic, antispasmodic, soothing, and antibacterial properties.

Cosmetic uses: Sweet flag is ideal for sensitive skin. Its azulene content soothes nervous and sensitive skin, tannins promote healing of irritated skins, and mucilage soothes inflamed tissue. This plant is also antiseptic and can make a great conditioner for all skin types, especially sensitive skin.

Medicinal uses: Its mucilage and tannins make sweet flag useful for gastrointestinal problems and upper respiratory inflammation. Europeans use it for stomach/ bowel problems as it stimulates the salivary glands and the

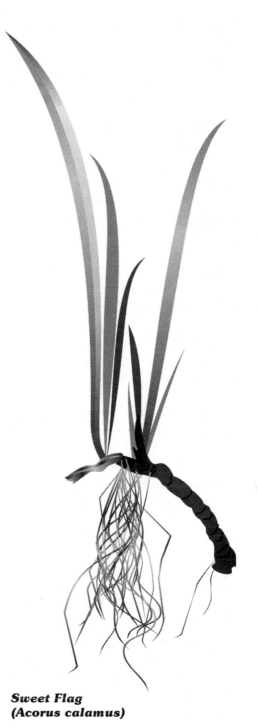

**Sweet Flag
(Acorus calamus)**

production of stomach juices. Iranians use sweet flag for coughs, colds, and asthma. Chinese use it for toothaches and headaches. European rhizomes have a lower concentration of aserone than those from Iran or India.

Caution: The Food and Drug Administration has classified it "Unsafe".

Sweet Violet (Viola odorata)

Parts used: Flowers and leaves.

Biochemical contents: Essential oil, volatile oil, mucilage, and glycoside.

Energy: Cool.

Country of origin: Iran, Europe.

Harvest time: Sweet violet flowers and leaves are gathered in the spring.

Properties: The herb has expectorant, antiseptic, demulcent, diuretic, emollient, antipyretic, and laxative properties.

Cosmetic uses: Being highly emollient, sweet violet soothes and lubricates the skin. It is ideal for use on both dry and sensitive skins and for disorders, such as eczema. It contains mucilage that forms a gel when mixed with water, making it easier to use on the skin.

Medicinal uses: Its mucilage and emollient contents are useful for stom-ach pain, coughs, asthma, and sore throat. Ancient Iranians used an infusion of sweet violet with red clover and sarsaparilla to cure skin disorders such as acne, eczema, and arthritis pain. Ancient Egyptians used it for skin inflammation and stomach ulcers. Sweet violet leaves are rich in salicylic acid, qualifying it to treat arthritis pain and bladder inflammation. Violet is soothing and cooling on the brain and nervous system, and it may be used for insomnia, tension headache, and mental depression. Sweet violet leaves are antiseptic; its roots are antipyretic and diuretic. Use of sweet violet dissolves, cools, and heals pimples and chronic skin diseases. It is also used for cold sores, coughs, sore red eyes, and for dissolving respiratory mucus. Fresh root can be used as a syrup to reduce coughs.

The cough syrup recipe is as follows:

1/2 cup of fresh violet blossoms
2 cups of water
2 cups of honey

Boil water, pour blossoms in, cover, and let steep overnight in a glass container. Strain. Bring the purple liquid to boil. Add honey. Pour in a clean jar, and use as needed. This syrup is very useful for coughs, asthma, whooping cough, and reducing inflammation in lungs. Infusion of fresh leaves is used for stomach, breast, bladder, lung, and kidney pain and inflammation.

Tarragon (Artemisia dracunculus)

Parts used: Fresh or dried leaves.

Biochemical contents: Essential oil, volatile oil, tannin, bitter glycosides.

Energy: Warm.

Country of origin: Iran, Russia, European and American mountains.

Harvest time: Tarragon leaves can be harvested from late spring to fall.

Properties: Tarragon has antispasmodic, antiseptic, and stimulant properties.

Principle uses: Tarragon contain bitter principle which is highly digestive; it increases the appetite and flow of bile. Tarragon leaves can be chewed to strengthen gums and to prevent them from bleeding.

This plant is found in most Mediterranean and Iranian cuisine. Tarragon is very refreshing and can be used fresh in salads or dried in different dishes. It is good for seasoning meatballs or meat loaf. Tarragon, along with other herbs such as oregano, thyme, marjoram, chives, parsley, basil, and mint, can make a great snack, cleanse the system, satisfy hunger, and stimulate the digestive tract. It has a peppery, spicy flavor and can be added to many dishes.

The herb should be washed, chopped, and served with feta cheese and fresh bread as a light meal or afternoon snack (see recipes on Cold Summer Soup and Meatballs).

Tea Tree (Melaleuca alternifolia)

Parts used: The essential oil.

Biochemical contents: Volatile oil, camphor, and phenolic acid.

Energy: Warm.

Country of origin: Asia.

Harvest time: This tree is an Australian native, and leaves are best collected and pressed in the summer.

Properties: Tea tree has antiseptic, anti-fungal, antibacterial, and antipyretic properties.

Cosmetic uses: It is excellent for skin cleansers, toners and acne lotions. Due to its anti-fungal and antiseptic properties, it is used as a bactericide and germicide on infected skins.

Medicinal uses: Primary clinical use of tea tree oil is as an antiseptic. Tea tree oil is highly fat soluble. Its antiseptic efficiency may be related to its antimicrobial activity and its ability to penetrate tissues. Tea tree oil is an excellent remedy for acne, boils, and eczema and is used in shampoos for oily hair and the treatment of head lice.

Thyme (Brassica rapa)

Parts used: Leaves and flowers.

Biochemical contents: Essential oil, tannin, glycosides, flavonoids, and bitter principal.

Energy: Warm.

Country of origin: Iran, Mediterranean countries.

Harvest time: Thyme flowers and leaves are best gathered in late spring to fall.

Properties: It has antiseptic, stimulating, soothing, and aromatic qualities.

Cosmetic uses: It can be incorporated in skin toners and conditioners to heal and soothe boils, irritated skin, and skin disorders.

Medicinal uses: Thyme is a great remedy for urinary infections. It increases flow of urine and menstruation. Infusion of thyme is good to treat uterine pain and to crush bladder stones. In Iran, some women use it as suppository or douche to cleanse the uterus after her period. In France, they use infusion of thyme for arthritis pain, and coughs. Infusion of thyme with honey is good for colds, flu, asthma, whooping coughs, migraine headaches, and stomach indigestion. Thyme is used for chronic respiratory problems and for gastrointestinal problems, indigestion and diarrhea. Thyme's fresh leaf infusion with salt may be used as a gargle for laryngitis or sore throat and is soothing to irritable coughs. Iranians use thyme for easing indigestion and internal cleansing. It is highly bitter and diuretic and therefore useful for liver and gallbladder detoxification. Iranians use this herb with herbs, such as oregano, basil, tarragon and peppermint in variety of salads and dishes.

Turnip (Brassican rapa)

Parts used: Roots, seeds.

Biochemical contents: Vitamins A and C, minerals (zinc, magnesium, potassium, iron, phosphorus), volatile oil, and tannins.

Energy: Warm.

Country of origin: Iran, and most countries.

Harvest time: Turnip leaves and roots are collected from late summer to late fall.

Properties: It has antibiotic, antibacterial, antimicrobial, and anti-inflammatory qualities.

Medicinal and other uses: Turnip is highly antiseptic and antibacterial, thus, one of the best remedies for colds and infections of the throat, sinus, and lungs. Turnip is best used in soups or steamed. If suffering from throat or sinus infection, steamed turnip can be a fine remedy for upper respiratory infections and colds. Turnip contains large amounts of phosphate that is good for nerve and brain relaxation. Turnip is one of the liver's best friends since it normalizes liver function and increases the flow of bile. It is also diuretic, increases appetite and sexual activity, and aids vision. Turnip is a popular winter vegetable in Iran and Mediterranean countries, used to protect against viruses and bacteria. Iranians eat steamed turnip during winter time to enhance the immune system.

They also make a soup with turnip to treat colds, sinus, and sore throat. (See chapter 19 recipe on turnip soup).

Turnip contain large amount of vitamins and minerals, especially potassium and calcium, which make this plant very good for individuals who suffer vitamin and mineral deficiencies, and for patients recovering from surgery, when most minerals and vitamins are depleted. Turnip extract is helpful in treating coughs, and bronchitis. Steamed turips increase the appetite, vision, flow of urine, and help crush bladder stones. New scientific research indicates that the roots and leaves of turnips may be very effective in preventing cancers.

Valerian (Valeriana officinalis)

Parts used: Root.

Biochemical contents: Volatile oil, alkaloids, tannins, fatty essential oils, glycosides. Valerian root contain valeric acids.

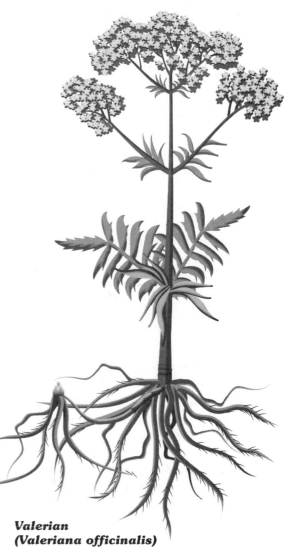

Valerian
(Valeriana officinalis)

Energy: Warm.

Country of origin: Iran, Asia and Europe.

Harvest time: Valerian roots dug up in fall and dried in shade.

Properties: Valerian has antispasmodic, sedative, astringent, and aromatic qualities.

Medicinal and other uses: Valerian is an excellent remedy for anxiety, nervous tension, and insomnia and is also good for treating headaches. Valerian root is dark brown in color and aromatic. Its aroma becomes stronger after drying. It has a bitter taste and as an antiseptic is useful for cleansing. In China and Japan, valerian root is used for muscle spasm, nervous tension, headache, insomnia, menstrual muscle pain, and fever. Indians use it for anxiety and most menstrual cramps. In Iran, valerian has been used since ancient times for muscle strengthening and liver cleansing, to reduce menstrual pain, nervous tension, and stomach pain, and to increase sexual desire. It increases urine, therefore is very useful for urinary and kidney infections. Valerian is also very useful for hemorrhoidal pain and for discomfort since it soothes muscle spasm. Another name for valerian is cat grass. Cats love its aroma. In Iran, they boil valerian root with borage, peppermint, cinnamon, fennel and honey for menstrual cramps, headache, and emotional stress. Valerian also has a strengthening property on the heart. Valerian root syrup with essential oil of valerian, mixed with vodka and white sugar, is used for emotional, mental, and nervous tension, for headache, and for insomnia.

Vervain (Verbena officinalis)

Parts used: Aerial parts.

Biochemical contents: Volatile oil, tannins, glycosides, alkaloids.

Energy: Cool.

Country of origin: Iran

Harvest time: Vervain should be gathered in the summer before the flower.

Properties: Vervain has tonic, sedative, expectorant, astringent, antispasmodic, and anti-inflammatory properties.

Medicinal uses: Vervain has been used traditionally to treat headaches, especially migraines, and nervous exhaustion. The glycoside in vervain increases flow of milk and is useful for liver and gallbladder cleansing. Tannins and volatile oil content make vervain very useful for stomach pain. Iranians make infusion of vervain with passion flowers and chamomile for nervous tension and insomina they also get oil form its leaves and massage over forehead and neck for tension headache.

Wahoo (Eucnymus atropurpureus)

Parts used: Root and bark.

Biochemical contents: Volatile oil, bitter glycoside, tannin, and gallic acid.

Energy: Warm.

Country of origin: Iran

Harvest time: Wahoo bark is stripped off the roots in fall.

Properties: It has astringent, anti-inflammatory, tonic, diuretic, anti-spasmodic, and anti-catarrh properties.

Medicinal Uses: Wahoo contains bitter glycoside. It is one of the best herbs known for liver disorders and detoxification. It removes liver congestion, allows flow of bile, and helps digestive processes. Its tannin content is useful in inflammation and stomach and intestinal pain reduction. Iranians use wahoo to relieve constipation and menstrual pain and for detoxification. Wahoo, in combination with other herbs like dandelion, gentian, and centaury, can normalize liver function and help skin disorders or problems.

Iranians make infusion with wahoo, senna leaves and ginger for internal cleansing and constipation.

Walnut (Luglans)

Parts used: Fruit and leaves.

Biochemical contents: Bitter principle in fresh walnuts, tannin, glycoside, vitamins A and B, minerals (iron, copper, calcium, and phosphorus).

Energy: Warm.

Country of origin: Iran, and then worldwide

Harvest time: Walnut are collecting from mid-fall to winter (they are usually fresher in early fall).

Properties: Walnut has soothing and antispasmodic qualities. The fresh hulls are used for coloring.

Principle uses: Walnuts are good for diabetics. It controls sugar and cholesterol levels, kills intestinal worms, is a bactericide, and is a good remedy for diarrhea. Fresh walnut leaves can be boiled and applied on eczema or can be gargled with salt for sore throat. Walnut prevents some female diseases and itching, especially during pregnancy, and prevents miscarriage and bleeding during pregnancy. Its copper content prevents cancer. Walnuts with raisins and figs are good for the memory, strengthen the stomach, soothe chest pain and sore throat, and are slightly laxative. Walnut jam with honey increases sexual activity. Ancient Iranians believed that sleeping under a walnut tree would cause nightmares.

Watercress (Nasturtium officinalis)

Parts used: Stems and leaves.

Biochemical contents: Volatile oil, vitamins A, C, and E, minerals (calcium, copper, iron, phosphorus, magnesium) and glycosides.

Energy: Warm.

Country of origin: Iran.

Harvest time: Watercress leaves and stems are picked in spring to late summer.

Properties: The herb has antispasmodic, astringent, stimulating, and cleansing properties.

Cosmetic uses: It is an ingredient in most skin cleansers and toners, useful for balancing the pH level of skin tissues, and is also antiseptic.

Medicinal and other uses: Watercress has been used as a therapeutic herb in most countries. In China, Indonesia, and India, people make soups with watercress and pork to treat coughs, colds, flu, and sore throat since it contains a substantial amount of vitamin C. Watercress has stimulating and nutritious qualities. It is used to treat coughs and bronchitis, to invigorate digestion, for blood or internal cleansing, and is diuretic, thereby helping detoxification. Iranians use it to ease indigestion and keep the blood pressure low. They use it in many dishes and salads. Eaten fresh or with bread, it strengthens the gums.

White Birch (Betula)

Parts used: Young leaves, sap, oil, and bark.

Biochemical contents: Saponins, volatile oil, tannins, vitamin C, bitter glycoside, and salicylic acid.

Energy: Cool.

Country of origin: Iran

Harvest time: Birch leaves are collected in late spring to summer. The bark is gathered from May to late September.

Properties: Birch has diuretic, tonic, antiseptic, and antispasmodic properties.

Cosmetic uses: Birch possesses cleansing, soothing, and anti-inflammatory properties that reduce irritation. It is relaxing and wound healing. It can be included in shampoos, skin care cleansers, and moisturizers. An infusion of this herb can be used for toning and conditioning the skin.

Medicinal Use: There are many different types of birch, i.e., white, black, and sweet birch. Salicylic acid is the major ingredient of aspirin, and the properties of birch oil are much the same as that of aspirin. The oil has an aromatic flavor and is used in the candy trade. The oil is also very helpful for the treatment of rheumatism. Indians use the sweet sap of the birch trees as source of sweetening and a basis for fermenting beer. They also use the dried bark as an astringent, antiseptic and antipyretic. An infusion is an excellent remedy for treating bladder infections, rheumatism, arthritis, and gout. Ancient Egyptians used the birch bark externally to ease the muscle pain and birch sap combined with cloves to treat the skin diseases such as acne.

Iranians make an infusion with white birch, devil's claws, borage, valerian, and marjoram to treat muscle pain and arthritic complications.

White Poplar (Popalus)

Parts used: Bark.

Biochemical contents: Glycoside, tannin, and essential oil.

Energy: Warm.

Country of origin: Iran

Harvest time: White poplar bark is collected from late spring to summer.

Properties: It has anti-inflammatory, soothing, and antispasmodic qualities.

Medicinal uses: White poplar has almost the same properties as white willow. Both are anti-inflammatory and used for treatment of arthritis, rheumatism, joint inflammation, and joint pain. Iranians use white poplar to reduce fever and tension headache. They make an infusion or decoction with white poplar bark combined with white willow bark, ginger root, and wild yam. Put one ounce with thirty ounces of boiling water, infuse for twenty minutes, and drink three to four cups daily to reduce tension headache, fever, and inflammation of arthritis.

Wild Cherry Tree (Prunus serotina)

Parts used: Bark.

Biochemical contents: Tannins, glycosides, and other organic acids.

Energy: Warm.

Country of origin: Iran

Harvest time: Wild cherry bark is collected in fall.

Properties: It has astringent, expectorant, and sedative properties.

Medicinal uses: It is sedative, great for the nervous system, insomnia, and mental depression. Its glycosides are very useful for internal and liver cleansing. Wild cherry syrup is very good for treating coughs and asthma. Iranians use the bark to treat diarrhea and stomach ulcers.

Wild Rue (Peganum Harmala)

Parts used: Seeds, leaves, aerials.

Biochemical contents: Four kinds of alkaloids, glycosides.

Energy: Warm.

Country of origin: Iran, Turkey, Syria.

Harvest time: Wild rue is harvested from early summer through fall.

Properties: It has antiseptic and stimulating properties.

Medicinal uses: Wild rue increases menstrual flow and stimulates milk production. It is useful in the case of miscarriages. Its seeds are sedative. Iranians use it to treat fever and stomach spasm. Men use it for intestinal worms. An infusion of its leaves is useful for rheumatism and joint pain. It reduces lung and chest inflammation. Iranians strongly believe that it kills negative energy. They regularly burn it to disinfect their houses. Ancient Iranians use its infusion for women who could not conceive for three consecutive years.

Wild Yam (Dioscorea villosa)

Parts used: Root and rhizome.

Biochemical contents: Saponins, alkaloids, tannins, starch, and sugar.

Energy: Warm.

Country of origin: S. America, Iran

Harvest time: Wild yam is a tropical plant and is uprooted in fall.

Properties: It has antispasmodic, anti-inflammatory, and anti-rheumatic properties.

Medicinal and other uses: Wild yam has traditionally been used for threatened miscarriage. It is good for menstrual pain. Iranians use wild yam for headache, muscle tension, and hormonal depression, such as menopause and PMS. Wild yam has antispasmodic properties and is anti-inflammatory making it excellent for arthritis, urinary, and uterine pain.

Willow (Salix)

Parts used: Bark.

Biochemical contents: Tannin, salicin.

Energy: Cold.

Country of origin: Iran, India

Harvest time: Willow bark is collected in spring.

Properties: It has anti-inflammatory, antiseptic, astringent, and anti-pyretic properties.

Medicinal uses: Willow has been used in European and Asian countries for thousands of years for reducing inflammation and joint pain. Iranians use it to treat arthritis, inflammation, the swelling of rheumatism, and back, knee, and joint pain due to its salicin content. Salicin is closely related to the active ingredient of aspirin. Iranians also massage willow bark powder with olive oil over sore muscles, joints, and temples to ease tension headaches. The following is a recipe to make a tincture for arthritis: Combine two ounces of equal parts of willow bark powder, poplar bark, licorice root, devil's claw, marjoram, and ginger root. Place the herbs in a glass container that can be tightly closed. Pour 16 ounces of vodka (35%) over the herbs, and close the container tightly. Keep the container in a warm place and shake it twice a day. After two weeks, pour the mixture through a cheesecloth, and squeeze it over a bowl to wring out all the liquid. Then pour the liquid into a brown glass container. Take one teaspoon of tincture every four hours as needed. As the strong bitter flavor can disturb the stomach, better add some honey.

Witch Hazel (Hamamelis virginiana)

Parts used: Leaves and bark.

Biochemical contents: Volatile oil, tannins, saponins, and flavonoids.

Energy: Cool.

Country of origin: Iran, India, Asia

Harvest time: Witch hazel leaves are picked in the summer.

Properties: It has astringent, antimicrobial, antiseptic, and anti-inflammatory properties.

Cosmetic uses: Witch hazel is one of the best natural healers and astringents. As an astringent, it is used for deep pore cleansing and toning the skin pores. Tannins in this plant reacts with proteins and produce a contracting and tightening effect on the skin tissue. Witch hazel is highly antiseptic which is best for skin toning, deep sanitation, and acne. It can be applied on bruises. Its compress is helpful for varicose veins and stops bleeding.

Wood Betony (Stachys officinalis)

Parts used: Dried aerial.

Biochemical contents: Tannins, alkaloid, betaine.

Energy: Cool.

Country of origin: Iran, Asia

Harvest time: Wood betony aerials should be collected in the summer. Wood betony has tonic, sedative, anti-inflammatory, and aromatic qualities.

Medicinal uses: Wood betony is good for nerves, chronic headaches, and anxiety. Iranians use it for muscle spasm, menstrual pain, and arthritis pain by combining it with rosemary, passion flower, and feverfew for migraine headache and anxiety.

Woodruff (Asperula odorata)

Parts used: Leaves, stems, and flowers.

Biochemical contents: Tannins, citric acid.

Energy: Neutral.

Country of origin: Europe, Asia.

Harvest time: Woodruff leaves and flowers are gathered in summer.

Properties: It is aromatic and soothing.

Principle uses: Woodruff is aromatic and used in air fresheners. Mediterraneans make a jam and tea with woodruff leaves and flower. Since it has sedative properties, it is a good tranquilizer. Europeans use an infusion with green leaves for tranquilization, detoxification, and to act as a pain killer. French take its infusion before bedtime for spasms and insomnia. In the USA, it is mixed with passion flower, skullcap, blackberry, rose and cinnamon for relaxation and the treatment of insomnia.

Wormwood (Artemisia absinthium)

Parts used: Aerial part.

Biochemical contents: Azulene, essential oil, phenol, and bitter principle.

Energy: Cold.

Country of origin: India, Afghanistan, Iran

Harvest time: Wormwood ntry of originleaves and flowers are collected in summer.

Properties: It has tonic, anti-inflammatory, stimulant, and antimicrobial properties.

Medicinal uses: Wormwood is traditionally used for the treatment of hepatitis and to expel worms. It has bitter principle which promotes the secretion of bile, detoxifies the liver and gallbladder, and internally cleanses. Wormwood can kill long intestinal worms Ascarde . Wormwood reduces the sugar in urine very rapidly. Two tablespoons of wormwood bud powdered, sifted for 3-4 days in the morning on an empty stomach.

Iranians use wormwood for the treatment of fever and intestinal parasites and they also use the ashes of burned leaves with olive oil to prevent hairloss.

In India wormwood is used to kill intestinal worms such as ascarid, and also to reduce blood sugar. Wormwood can be used with senna to help excrete worms.

The buds of wormwoods are like a tiny seeds, it has a grey color, and change to reddish brown with age. It is very bitter and it has a strong smell. To excrete long worms, use dried powdered wormwood buds soaked in honey, for three to four days then add milk and drink in the morning on an empty stomach. It is also good for asthma, gripe and hiccups.

Dried leaves with olive oil has also been used to treat baldness.

Wormwood should be taken with caution for individuals who have stomach problems, as it many induce nervousness.

Caution: Excess doses may damage the liver.

Yam (Sweet Potato) (Ipomoea Batatas (L.) Lamk.)

Parts used: Roots

Biochemical contents: Sugar, starch, calcium, protein, potassium, iron, Vitamins B1 and B6, and beta-carotene. Each 100 grams of raw yam contains 70 grams of protein, 1.70 grams of fat, 243 mg of Vitamin A (8800 I.U), .01 Vitamin B1, 6% Vitamin B6, 21 mg Vitamin C.

Energy: Neutral.

Country of origin: Spain, USA.

Harvest time: Yam is harvested from late summer throughout winter.

Properties: It has soothing and anti-depressant action.

Cosmetic uses: Because of the high percentage of beta-carotene, protein, and minerals in yam, this plant is highly qualified for all skin type creams, especially those for dry and mature skin. It has humectant properties which are great for wrinkle prevention.

Medicinal uses: Yam is very rich in most minerals and vitamins, especially vitamin A (beta-carotene), and it is highly nutritious. It is ideal to eat yam during mental depression and insomnia. Chinese use sweet potato to treat stomach and kidney pain. Yam is very high in potassium therefore it is ideal to use it for bladder and kidney infections. Iranians make syrup with yam to quench thirst and to treat fever and colds. Yam is also a good remedy for those who get ocean sickness. In Indonesia, people apply ground yam leaves externally on burns, cuts, and joint pain. Stalks and branches are used for arthritis and rheumatic pain. In India, people use sweet potato roots to treat constipation.

Yarrow (Achillea millefolium)

Parts used: Aerials and flowering heads.
Biochemical contents: Volatile oil, saponins, azulene, camphor, tannins, amino acids, salicylic acid, sugar, bitter glycosides, alkaloids, and flavonoids, and 47% fattt essential oil.

*Energy:*Warm.

Country of origin: Iran, Europe.

Harvest time: It should be gathered in early summer to fall.

Properties: It has astringent, antiseptic, anti-catarrhal, tonic, anti-inflammatory, soothing, antispasmodic, and stimulant properties.

Cosmetic uses: Because of its saponin content, yarrow is mainly used as a skin cleanser. Azulene in yarrow is anti-inflammatory for sensitive and sun-damaged skins. Yarrow can be applied on brown spots and blotchy skin to fade the pigmentation. Avoid using it in the sun.

Medicinal uses: The tannins in yarrow make it good for wound healing. The alkaloids lower blood pressure, stimulate digestion, tone the blood vessels, and reduce fever. One research in U.S.A showed because of its antipyretic property, yarrow reduces fever in rabbits in lab animal.

Yarrow contains proteins, carbohydrate complex, and azulene, which are anti-inflammatory. If used externally, yarrow helps in healing wounds.

Iranians use it to treat arthritis, muscle spasm, gout, cold, flu, rheumatism, and nerve tension due to its anti-inflammatory and salicylic acid content. They also use the extract of yarrow with lemon juice and egg

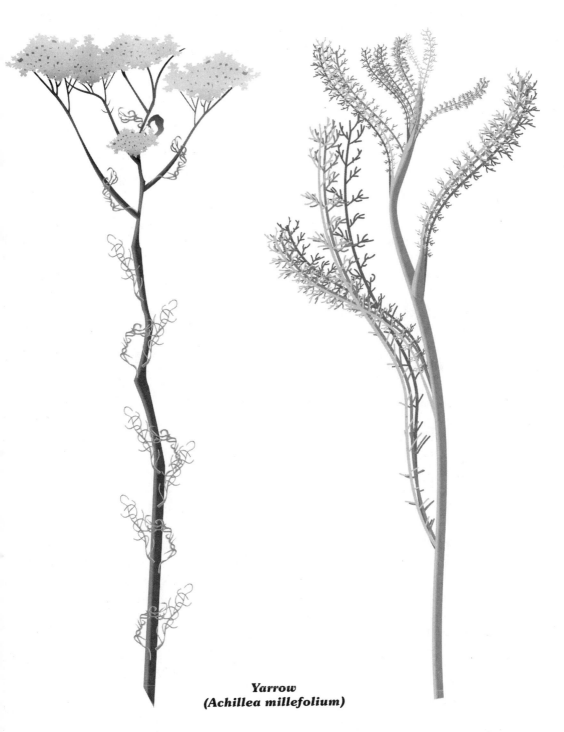

Yarrow
(Achillea millefolium)

white to reduce brown spots (pigmentation).

Chinese use fresh yarrow for stomach ulcers and wound healing. In Sweden, it is an ingredient of beer. They also mix it with arnica, sage, and rosemary to make a tea which is good for internal and stomach detoxification.

Indians use yarrow to increase menstruation. Recent research showed there are chemical properties in yarrow which help stop inernal and external bleeding.

Yellow Dock (Rumey crispus)

Parts used: Root.

Biochemical contents: Tannin, anthraquinone, glycosides, and iron.

Energy: Cool.

Country of origin: Iran, Afghanistan, India.

Harvest time: Yellow dock root is unearthed in summer.

Properties: It has tonic, laxative, and anti-inflammatory properties on skin disorders.

Cosmetic uses: Yellow dock is extensively used for a variety of chronic skin diseases and eruptions, such as eczema, psoriasis, and acne. Yellow dock has cleansing and anti-inflammatory properties to reduce skin irritation and infection.

Medicinal uses: Yellow dock is categorized as a blood cleanser and purifier, and one of the best remedies for skin disorders such as acne, eczema, psoriasis and boils.

Yellow dock is anti-inflammatory, and therefore useful for inflammation of stomach and gastrointestinal problems. It is mildly laxative, so it is good for treating constipation and congestion of liver and gallbladder.

A remedy is made by combining yellow dock with burdock root, red clover, sarsaparilla, borage, and skullcap. One ounce of this combination is simmered in a pint of water for twenty minutes. The dose is three cups daily.

Yellow Flag (Iris pseudacorusl)

Parts used: Dried rhizome.

Biochemical contents: Volatile oil, salicylic acid, starch, alkaloids.

Energy: Cool.

Country of origin: Iran, European countries.

Harvest time: Yello flag rhizomes are unearthed in fall.

Properties: It has anti-inflammatory, astringent, tonic, and diuretic properties.

Cosmetic uses: Because of its volatile oil content, it is very antiseptic and a useful ingredient of skin toners and cleansers for skin complaints, such as acne.

Medicinal uses: In Iran, this plant is widely used for its cleansing properties. It purifies blood and cleanses toxin from the system. Because of its salicylic acid content, it is useful for treating arthritis and rheumatic pain and eliminates uric acid.

Caution: Fresh root is poisonous.

Yucca (Yuccu)

Parts used: Root.

Biochemical contents: Saponin.

Energy: Cool.

Country of origin: Southeast India, Southwest Asia, tropics.

Harvest time: Yucca root is collected in fall.

Properties: It has astringent and antispasmodic properties.

Medicinal uses: Southwestern Americans use yucca as both a fruit and a medicine. Yucca is used to reduce arthritic and rheumatic pain. Its infusion is useful to prevent intestinal cramping and diarrhea. It is used in the paper industry, and it acts as a laxative due to its saponin content. Yucca is also used in soaps and shampoos. In the USA, it is used for arthritis. The extract is used in tablets and sold at health food stores. It has shown no side effects.

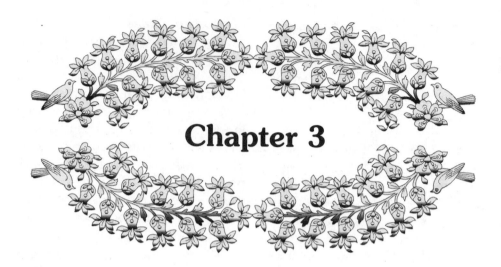

Chapter 3

Uses of Fruits

Apple

Parts used: Whole fruit, seeds, skin, leaves.

Energy: Neutral.

Harvest time: Apple fruits and leaves are gathered from spring to late summer.

Properties: Apple has soothing, antispasmodic, antibacterial and cleansing properties. Apples contains A, B, D, C, and E vitamins, potassium, selenium, manganese, magnesium, phosphoric acid, essential oil, and phosphorus.

Main uses: Apple is a superb remedy for diarrhea, bloody diarrhea, and gastrointestinal problems. Apple is a very precious fruit; if used everyday, it practically ensures health forever. Apple is one of the best remedies for arthritis, kidney and bladder stones, and infection. Steamed apple is great for indigestion and upper respiratory disorders. Try to eat apple with its skin because its peel contains manganese that helps digestion. Grated apple is best for children's diarrhea. If one has an upset stomach, vomiting, grips in stomach, or gets motion sickness, apple is the best remedy. Apple is excellent for pregnant women and for stomach ulcers. It controls stomach acid overproduction and also destroys harmful bacteria and toxins in the stomach.

Apricot

Parts used: Fruit, seeds.

Energy: Cool.

Properties: Apricot contains minerals, vitamins (especially A, C, D, and B), and sugar.

Uses: Apricot is considered to be an antioxidant that promotes white blood cells, fights free radicals, gives strength and energy, is great for indigestion, internal cleansing, and due to vitamin A, gives elasticity to the skin and promotes youthfulness.

Banana

Parts used: Fruit.

Energy: Warm.

Properties: Banana contains Vitamin A, B, and C, potassium, starch, and sugar. Banana has soothing and anti-spasmodic properties.

Uses: Potassium content makes bananas healthful for pregnant woman and babies. Use bananas to replace carbohydrates like cookies and cakes for children. Banana has to be picked and eaten ripe, otherwise it has no nutritive value. You can make banana bread and banana cake. Banana soothes the stomach and increases energy level.

Cherries

Parts used: Fruit, seeds, leaves.

Energy: Cold.

Properties: Cherries contain vitamins, especially vitamin C and A, potassium, sugar, and pectin. Cherry has diuretic, purgative, and detoxifying properties.

Uses: Cherry is a great fruit for nervous tension. It cleanses the stomach, purifies the blood, and is a great remedy for indigestion, especially the seeds and leaves. Cherry contains low starch, and its sugar content is not harmful. Its leaves and seeds are great for arthritis and joints. Its acid crushes and destroys stones in kidney, gallbladder, and bladder. Cherry gives glow and youthfulness to skin.

Figs

Parts used: Fruits, leaves and rhizome.

Energy: Warm.

Properties: Figs contain Vitamins A, B and D, potassium, and sugar. Fig has purgative, soothing, and laxative properties.

Main uses: Fig is a purgative fruit. If suffering from constipation, fig for breakfast is a wonderful remedy, and it helps to flatten the stomach. Sugar content in fig is very nutritive for children, especially fresh fig which is more cleansing and nutritious. Fig is a good remedy for people who have nervous tension. Include figs in your diet for at least a month, and you will see the benefits. Fig syrup is a great for sore throat and coughs. Fig makes delicious jam, which also reduces inflammation of gums. If you pick an unripe fig and cut the tail, the milk is the best remedy to dissolve and remove warts.

Grapes

Parts used: Fruits, leaves.

Energy: Warm, when ripe, and cool, when unripe.

Properties: Grape contains vitamins and minerals, especially vitamin A,C and D, pectin, sugar, tannin, organic acid, flavone glycoside. Grape has diuretic, astringent, tonic, and laxative properties.

Uses: Grape can be used to lose or gain weight, especially if used in the morning with empty stomach. If trying to lose weight, eat sour grapes for breakfast along with other fruits, like oranges and lemons, and if trying to gain weight, eat sweet grape with your breakfast. Grape stimulates liver function and metabolism, especially if taken in the morning. Grape can be used in many ways. It can be used in pastries and dishes, to make wine, and as raisins. Even leaves can make a delicious dish. Unripe grape is rich in vitamin C and can be used in many dishes.

Iranians harvest unripe grape and leaves late in spring, then extract the juice for a variety of dishes. Some people dry unripe grape and powder it to use it as a flavoring spice in baking chicken, fish and stews. The juice can be used in salads, soups, and different dishes. Grape leaves are very diuretic and make a delicious meal (stuffed grape leaves).

Lemon

Parts used: Fruit, skin, seeds.

Energy: Cold.

Properties: Lemon contains a large amount of vitamins C, A, and B, and minerals. Lemon has diuretic, antibacterial, and anti-spasmodic properties.

Uses: Lemon acts as a bactericide in the stomach and intestines and is great for pregnant women, people who want to lose fat, and those with arthritis, backache, or diabetes. Lemon helps to increase calcium and saliva; therefore, it improves digestion. It increases the flow of bile, and as such, it is helpful to lose fat. Lemon detoxifies liver and gallbladder. Eat whole lemon with skin and seeds, if you wish to have clean and purified blood.

Lemon is great for cleansing skin. Cut a lemon into halves and massage over the body. Sit in the sun for few minutes, and then wash. It helps open pores and soften skin. Lemon is good for pigmentation. If you have dark brown pigmentation, cut a lemon in half, beat with egg whites ,and massage this on dark spot for few minutes, then wash. Apply moisturizer. Repeat this 3 times a week. Fresh lemon is great for skin; apply directly on eczema areas for faster healing. Lemon peel can be used in perfumery or aromatherapy for antidepressant effects and release of nervous tension. Lemon skin can make a delicious jam and cake.

Orange

Parts used: Fruit, skin, blossom.

Energy: Cool.

Properties: Orange contains vitamins C, A, and D, citric acid, salicylic acid, pectin, potassium, and magnesium. Its skin contains alcohol and bitter principle. Orange is aromatic, antibacterial, purgative, antidepressant, anti-tension, and antioxidant.

Uses: Orange is anti-wrinkle and contains vitamin C which helps with the absorption of calcium and gives strength to bones and teeth. Orange is mildly laxative and increases the appetite. Fresh orange juice added to babies' foods gives vitamins C and B. Research shows that fruit acid increases calcium in body. Orange is great for colds, coughs, fever, gastrointestinal problems, and indigestion. Another research shows that,

taken daily, orange gives youthfulness and health, makes the skin soft and supple, and is great for nervous tensions and constipation. Orange is used in aromatherapy for depression and nervous tensions. Its blossoms are used in jam and cake.

Peach

Parts used: Fruit, leaves and seeds.

Energy: Cool.

Properties: Peach contains vitamin A, C, and D, and minerals. Peach is diuretic, and its leaves are laxative and antispasmodic.

Uses: Peach is a beautiful fruit that can be used as an antioxidant for breakfast, especially in order to lose weight. Peach is great for cleansing. It promotes bile production and is great for indigestion and stomach flatulence. Peach is best when washed and taken with its skin because most vitamins and mineral are stored under the skin.

Pear

Parts used: Fruit, seeds, and leaves.

Energy: Neutral.

Properties: Pear contains minerals, vitamins A, B, and C, and sugar. Pear is cathartic and has cleansing properties.

Uses: Pear is good for breakfast and

best taken with its skin. Pears have cleansing properties, increase saliva and the flow of bile, and ease nervous tensions, stomach pain, and fever. If suffering from a stomach ulcer, use steamed pear. Pear is good for diabetes.

Pineapple

Parts used: Fruit.

Energy: Warm.

Properties: Pineapple contains vitamins A, B, and C, potassium, sodium, sugar, magnesium, sulfur, phosphorous, and aroma. Pineapple has antibacterial and diuretic properties.

Uses: Pineapple is a tropical fruit that has warm energy. It is delicious, aromatic, diuretic, and in the stomach and intestines, bactericidal. Iranians use pineapple to delay periods.

Plums

Parts used: Fruit, leaves.

Energy: Cool.

Properties: Plums contains Vitamin C, A, and D, and minerals.

Uses: Plums are a great remedy for indigestion. Plums are in the category of those fruits that are good for rheumatism. It contains minerals and beneficial acids and is laxative, especially when used in the morning. It can make

great a remedy for nervous tension, memory, indigestion, and kidney function. Plum promotes the production of red cells. If dried, soak them in warm water for few hours, and they become like fresh fruit.

Strawberry

Parts used: Fruit, leaves.

Energy: Cold.

Properties: Strawberry contains Vitamin C, A, D salicylic acid, potassium and pectin.

Uses: The best use of strawberry is for kidney and bladder stones. Its salicylic acid helps to absorb body heat, can be good for arthritis and diabetes, balances pH, and, due to its alkalinity, is good for bladder infections. It can be used as breakfast along with citric fruits, if trying to lose weight. Strawberry promotes white cells and strengthens bones and joints. Strawberry might prevent some cancers. Strawberry leaves are laxative and diuretic, great for detoxification and internal cleansing.

Sweet Lime

Parts used: Fruit, skin.

Energy: Cool.

Properties: Sweet lime contains vitamins C, A, B, and D and minerals. Sweet lime has diuretic, antispasmodic, and antidepressant properties.

Uses: Sweet lime is used for sore throats, colds, coughs, and fever. Some think sweet lime has less vitamin C because it is not sour, however research shows that sweet lime grown in countries like Iran has twice as much vitamin C than sour lemon, and the vitamin can be preserved without citric acid. Other research shows that citrus fruits would contain more vitamin C if they were sweet. Ancient Iranians used sweet lime for fever and stomach upset.

Watermelon

Parts used: Fruit, seed.

Energy: Cool.

Properties: Watermelon contains vitamin A, C, B, and D and minerals. Watermelon has diuretic, purgative and antibacterial properties.

Uses: Watermelon is an antioxidant, helps to fight free radicals, and promotes white blood cells. Watermelon is diuretic and quenches thirst. It is a friend to the liver and gallbladder as it helps to cleanse and detoxify both organs. Watermelon treats sore throat, fever, colds, and high blood pressure and controls overproduction by the thyroid.

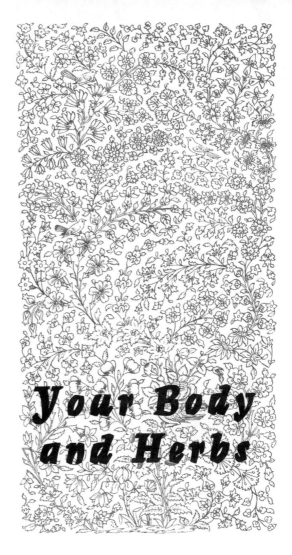

Your Body and Herbs

Your skin, that all-important first impression, tells it all.

It is said the eyes are the window to the mind. It could be said that the skin is "the window to the heart". Skin wrinkle lines reveal much about one's innermost feelings. Obviously, people don't like their deepest, heart-felt emotions constantly exposed, so they tint their window with various forms of cosmetics. Looking your best is a time-tested, sure-fire way of getting ahead in this world. So if you want to have a healthy and natural beauty, you better take good care of your skin with the all the oils nature provides.

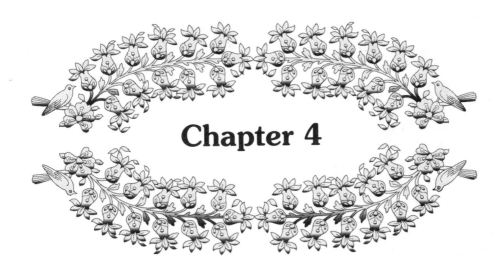

Chapter 4

The Structure of Skin

The skin is the largest organ of the human body. Healthy skin functions as a protective covering for our bodies in several ways. The elastic nature of the skin is designed to guard the sensitive underlying tissues and organs against physical and chemical damages. It prevents entrance of bacteria and harmful chemicals into the body. Firm and moist skin also protects underlying tissues from harmful rays of the sun. What is less obvious is that the skin is an active vital organ whose proper functioning is essential for our survival.

For example, if the body becomes cold, blood vessels in the dermis (deeper layer) will constrict and retain body heat, and if the body becomes hot, the blood vessels in the dermis will dilate, allowing blood to reach the surface to cool. Sense organs are also situated in the skin in the form of microscopic nerve endings which inform the brain about temperature, touch, pain, and pressure.

As we are constantly exposed to the outside world, if we fail to be in accord with our external surroundings, skin diseases may result. In fact, our skin is the mirror of our general health, thus it must be cautiously protected against damage.

Layers of the Skin

Skin has three layers known as Epidermis, Dermis, and Sub cutaneous Tissue, which are elaborated as follows:

Epidermis is the outermost layer of tissue and consists of dead skin cells. It is as thick as a sheet of paper and covers most parts of the visible body. It has four layers of cells which are from the outermost: the horny, granular, spinout, and basal layers. The horny layer consists of about 15 to 40 rows of dying cells. These cells are filled with a tough, waterproof protein called keratin. The granular layer consists of one or two rows of dying cells containing small grains of a substance called keratohyaline. The spinout layer is composed of 4 to 10 rows of living cells that have spine-like projections where the cells touch each other. The basal layer is made up of living cells consisting mainly of a single row of tall, narrow melanocytes. These cells produce a brown pigment called melanin.

Dermis, or true skin, consists of living skin cells that need nourishment to remain healthy. The dermis is the middle layer tissue and is from 15 to 40 times thicker than the epidermis. It primarily is made up of blood vessels, nerve endings, and connective tissues. The blood vessels nourish both the epidermis and the dermis. The surface of the dermis has many tiny elevations called papillae that help in connecting the dermis to the epidermis.

Subcutaneous Tissue consists mainly of connective tissue, blood vessels, and cells that store fat. It is much thicker than the epidermis and dermis. It consists mainly of connective tissues which help protect the body from blows and other injuries. It also helps retain body heat. The amount of fat in the subcutaneous tissue increases by overeating. If the body needs extra food energy, it will break down the stored fat.

In addition to these layers of tissue, structures associated with the skin include hair, nails, and certain glands, as follows:

Sebaceous Glands

Sebaceous glands are situated under dermis and empty into hair follicles. They secrete an oil called sebum which lubricates the surface of the skin and prevents dehydration.

Sweat Glands

Sweat glands assist the temperature control mechanism of the body. Adult skin contains several million sweat glands. Each day we secrete about a pint (0.5 liter) of sweat, but heavy exercise or hot surroundings increase the amount to one liter. Sweat glands also function like kidneys in that they excrete toxic substances, nitrogenous waste, and mineral salt. The skin can be called the third kidney of the body. If kidneys failed to function properly, the demand on sweat glands would be heavy.

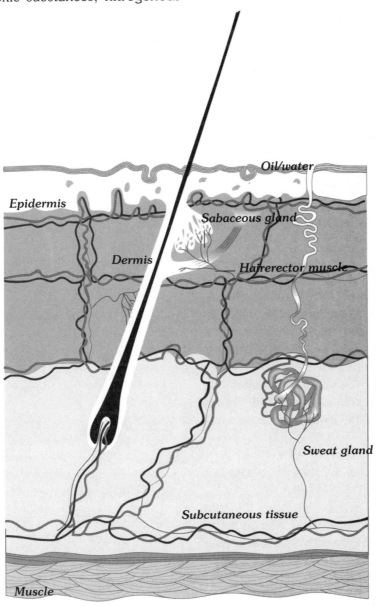

Epidermis

Oil/water

Dermis

Sabaceous gland

Hairerector muscle

Sweat gland

Subcutaneous tissue

Muscle

What Is Cross-linking?

Wrinkles in your skin are, in fact, an example of the aging process called cross-linking. As you age, many tissues are cross-linked, so your proteins lose their flexibility and some undesirable chemical bonds interconnect molecules in the skin. The result is loss of flexibility and an increased tendency for tear.

You can roughly measure the cross-linking in your skin this simple test: First, lay your hand flat on a table, then pinch the back of it. Hold the pinch for 5 seconds, and let it go. The skin in youngsters snaps back almost immediately. The skin of a person with much cross-linking present often keeps the pinched ridge visible for quite some time.

Preventing Cross-linking

There are many factors in life that cause cross-linking. Learning and knowing how to prevent cross-linking is a key to having a healthier, younger, and more beautiful complexion. Some examples of cross-linking prevention are as follows:

■ Avoid ultraviolet rays (sun).

■ Assist the skin's ability to bind and hold water.

■ Avoid smoking and alcohol.

Chapter 5

The Skin and Herbs

There are many environmental and internal factors that influence skin disorders. In this following chapter you will learn the cause of skin disorders and how to prevent and treat them.

Dehydration: Premature Aging (Wrinkles)

Harsh environmental influences can cause a loss of moisture and oil that can results in dehydration and wrinkles.

Cause: Lack of oil, moisture, and unbalanced diet are the major causes. As the body ages, the sebaceous glands become less active, consequently producing less oil. Poorly lubricated skin may not readily retain water. Loss of moisture in the skin can be caused by intense exposure to dry heat, cold, sun, and wind. As a result, skin becomes dry and loses its elasticity and the aging process sets in. Due to breakdown of the collagen and elastin fibers in the dermis, the skin loses its texture, and fine lines and wrinkles appear. Premature aging could begin from the age of twenty, if the skin is not treated well. Lack of sufficient water and liquids in daily diet can cause moisture loss in the skin too. Free radicals have also been found to be one of the major causes of skin aging. Polluted air, dust, dirt, and excess makeup must be removed from the skin every night, followed with a proper moisturizer to provide oxygen and better circulation.

Treatment: To prevent dehydration and premature aging, avoid exposure to sun, dry air, heat, cold and wind. Drink at least eight glasses of water each day, and eat a balanced diet. Extra vitamin A and C is very important as they increase the elasticity of the skin. Additional use of 15 mg of zinc a day helps the storage of vitamin A in the liver.

Eat fresh fruits, vegetables, and one tablespoon of yellow butter to get vitamin A and better skin lubrication. Herbs like dandelion, rich in vitamin A, also stimulate and cleanse the liver and blood. Get a good sleep every night, and exercise for better circulation of nutrients to the surface of the skin. Spend five minutes in the morning and evening to cleanse the surface of the skin with herbal skin care products, and for three to four minutes use acupressure massage on the skin tissues for better circulation and toning. Try to exfoliate the dead skin once a month. Refer to Minoo's hydro line along with acupressure massage techniques.

Herbs like fennel, chamomile, comfrey, and borage are great for moisturizing, softening, and toning the tissues. Jojoba oil is great for elasticity. Vitamin E is humectant.

I had a twenty year old customer whose skin was dry like a leather and quite wrinkled. She had olive, tanned skin, yet was unhappy because of her dehydration. When she came to me for a facial treatment, I found out she was sun worshiper and often basked in the sun, letting her skin bake without using any moisturizer. I put her under herbal treatment, proper diet, acupressure, and the Hydrating Facial Line. After a few weeks her skin started getting its elasticity and vitality. I am certain that it is never too late to take care of your skin by reducing and preventing both wrinkles and dehydration with the help of proper diet, acupressure, and alternative medicine.

Recommendation: To prevent premature aging, wrinkles, and dehydration, constant daily care that includes eight glasses of water, eight different kinds of vegetables and fruits, and eight hours of sleep is a must. Provide a healthy diet, exercise, and avoid the sun, dry air, and heat. Daily, cleanse and moisture balance the skin. If your skin feels dehydrated, keep your moisturizer along. Try using water-based skin care products to replenish the moisture. All the Minoo's products are hydrophilic (water-based), and they require acupressure massage and water. If you are using Minoo's line of herbal products, we suggest Hydro Line, as it is highly humectant (attracts moisture from the air and holds it longer in dry skins). Also try skin tissue acupressure massage every day, especially if you are using Minoo's herbal facial products.

Acne

Acne is a chronic inflammatory disorder of the sebaceous glands characterized by blackheads, pustules, and cysts. The affected areas are usually the face, back, and chest, areas where the sebaceous glands are naturally large.

Cause: The problem often appears during adolescence, usually from age 13 to 20, during a change of hormones, or during a change of lifestyle (eating disorder, emotional stress). Generally, acne is related to activity of the sex hormones and poor diet.

Sebaceous gland produces an oil called sebum that usually maintains the skin lubrication. During change of hormonal (adolescence), stress or wrong diet, the production of sebum oil increases and become thicker. In this case, excess sebum oils accumulate and can not reach to the surface of the skin resulting acne and inflammation. Diet that consists of greasy, spicy and hot energy foods may cause acne, as it may accumulate in the liver.

I had a particular customer who was suffering from acne who had tried different kinds of drugs for cure, but the results had been temporary. I immediately put her under alternative medicine and diet care, as well as proper facial massage techniques and products. Within a few weeks, she showed desired results and looked happier, healthier and more beautiful than ever.

Treatment: Skin cleansing is a most important part of the daily regime for all skin types in order to remove excess oil, especially during adolescence when sebaceous glands are more active. During this period, methods of skin treatment are important. If the skin is not treated properly, it will further damage the skin and tissues, causing scars, deep tissue depressions, and sensitivity. During this period some people become frustrated and mistreat their skin by using wrong products, over-scrubbing their skin with harsh alcohol-based solutions that could cause further skin disorders. They avoid using a moisturizer, wrongly thinking that a moisturizer may increase the oil on their skin. The best ways to cleanse acne skin are as follows:

Deep cleanse it with water-based cleansers containing eucalyptus, sage, burdock, peppermint, parsley. If the cleanser is not available, mix equal parts of fresh lemon juice with rosewater.

Steam the skin with eucalyptus and parsley at least three times a week for 10 minutes each time.

Make sure to apply moisturizer on your skin. No matter how oily your skin is, it still needs moisturizer.

Apply refreshing mask at least twice a week for circulation and refreshment.

Extract the blackheads and impurities to clean pores and allow oxygen flow. Lack of oxygen could also cause acne and impurities.

Never touch the cystic acne. Keep it clean, and apply an acne lotion of tea tree and burdock. Cystic acne is very nasty and takes a longer time to appear on the surface.

If you do not have an acne lotion, apply tea tree oil on the infected area for a few times daily. Hot compresses will help to make it ready for faster extraction.

Before extraction always check the surrounding area. If red, sore and inflamed, do not extract. Otherwise, extract and ensure full pus extraction. Clean with witch hazel, and wait a few days for healing and exfoliation.

Recommendation: Since blood nourishes your skin, it is very important to keep the blood clean and pure. Drinking eight glasses of water a day releases toxins from the blood and keeps it clean. Your diet should consist of fresh vegetables, fruits, carbohydrates such as steamed rice, potatoes, whole wheat bread, and fresh juices especially carrot juice, apple juice, and green vegetable juices. Try to provide in your diet at least 1500 mg a day extra vitamin C to prevent more acne, 15 mg of zinc to store vitamin A in your liver for a healthier skin, and vitamin E which helps to balance hormone production.

Mucopolysaccharides are very important for body function and protect cells against the invasion of bacteria, viruses, and fungi. The only foods that contain substantial amounts of muccopolysaccharides and mucoproteins are aloe vera and deep sea cold water fish.

Aloe vera juice provides a wide range of amino acids, minerals, vitamins, mucopolysaccharides, and mucoproteins. Black bilberry juice and pomegranate juice are very blood purifying and are recommended for acne cure. Herbs like Oregon grape, burdock, yellow dock, blue flag, dandelion roots, nettle and purple coneflower are also recommended for purification of blood. Burdock extract is highly recommended. The extract of this herb is very bitter, so add one tablespoon of extract to water or pure juice. Take at least four times a week to purify and cool the blood and nourish the skin.

Prevention:

Avoid refined carbohydrates, sugar, additives, and spicy foods containing hot chili pepper or cinnamon.

Avoid frozen and canned foods.

Avoid any type of caffeine, including coffee, chocolate, and cocoa.

It is wise to avoid shellfish (which are rich in iodine) and alcohol.

Avoid rich dairy products like cheese and creams.

Clean the skin daily, drink enough water, sleep well, and exercise.

Pimples:

Internal and external influences can cause over-activity of sebaceous glands and result in overproduction of sebum oil and pimples.

Cause: When the follicles become filled with oil, dead cells, and bacteria, they swell and rupture causing the debris to escape into the dermis. The debris is irritating and causes an inflammation called pimples.

Treatment: Pimples are easier to handle than cysts. They are superficial and less painful. They can be easily cleaned and extracted. Daily cleansing of the skin can prevent any kind of skin disorder like pimples. If pimples do appear on the skin, apply an acne lotion with tea tree oil. After 24 hours, the bacteria causing debris will be gone. Tea tree oil will also control sebum oil overproduction. Keep the area clean, and compress the infected area with hot water. Apply aloe vera gel, and steam with eucalyptus and lavender leaves.

Recommendation: Some people, and even some doctors, do not believe that diet affects skin disorders. It is quite the opposite; diet plays a major role in the health of your complexion. A balanced diet consisting of fresh and natural foods, vitamins, minerals, proteins, and fiber is very effective. As mentioned, blood nourishes the skin, so the cleaner the blood, the cleaner and healthier the skin. Consumption of green herbs and vegetables, fresh fruit, eight daily glasses of water, and non-additive foods is helpful to keep the blood clean. Avoid strong spicy and greasy foods (difficult to digest).

Encouraging normal liver functioning is also effective in maintaining a healthy complexion. Herbs that stimulate and cleanse the liver and internal systems, such as dandelion, gentian, centaury, and rosemary, can be added to the diet as salads or cooked foods. In general, a healthy diet, constant cleansing of the blood and internal systems, avoiding spicy and greasy foods, and avoiding emotional stress are recommended in this case.

Blackheads and Whiteheads

Technical names for blackheads and whiteheads are Comedones and Milia respectively. Blackheads and whiteheads on the skin are the result of a disorder in sebaceous glands caused by the accumulation of sebaceous matter.

Cause: Excess of sebum oil, generated by an overactive sebaceous gland, causes blackheads and whiteheads. The basic problem is a plug in certain pores or openings of the skin. The pores have an oil gland at the bottom of a tiny hair. For a number of reasons, microscopic cells and the oil from the gland plug the pores. If the pore's opening at the skin surface is clear the result is a blackhead, and if the opening is closed, the result is a whitehead. Whiteheads are the forerunner of pimples if the oil can't reach the surface of the skin.

Treatment: Treatment consists of daily cleansing of the skin to ensure removal of excess oil. As soon as blackheads or whiteheads are observed, remove them. If you are getting facials on a regular basis, ask your facialist to remove them. If not, you can give yourself a facial by removing impurities, blackheads and whiteheads. After cleansing your skin with milk cleanser, steam it for a few minutes. Pour a glass of water in a pot, boil it, and hold your face close to the steam for few minutes. Steaming opens your pores so blackheads and whiteheads become loose and surface. Extract them by wrapping a clean tissue around your index finger, placing it on the sides of the blackhead, and gently squeezing to let out the pus. Sanitize the area with a toner. The same method can be applied to whiteheads. As they are under the skin, their removal is harder. It is best to remove the whitehead as soon as it appears on the surface of the skin. So, get rid of whiteheads and blackheads as soon as they occur on the skin. Greasy and spicy foods, like cheese and cinnamon which irritate the sebaceous glands, must be avoided.

Recommendation: Avoid greasy food, daily cleanse the skin with Minoo's Products, and drink eight glasses of water daily.

Couperose (Broken Capillaries)

Couperose is characterized by broken capillaries and small blood vessels that can be seen beneath the surface of the skin.

Cause: Sensitive skins have strong adverse reactions to many environmental hazards. When blood vessels are not elastic enough to handle the flow of blood, smaller red vessels appear and the blood is forced through them, possibly stretching and breaking them.

Treatment: This reaction makes the capillaries lose elasticity. Usually fair skin has thin layers and a tendency to get sensitive faster. This skin type should avoid excessive exposure to sun and heat, cold and wind. The skin has to be kept moist all the time to prevent dehydration. Excessive use of alcohol and spicy foods should be avoided as well as exposure to drugs, household chemicals, and certain fumes. Avoid oil-based cosmetics and skin care products. It is better to use products with herbal ingredients, like chamomile, comfrey, cucumber, and marigold to soothe and relax the sensitive skin. Add carbohydrates like steamed rice, potatoes, fresh bread, fresh green vegetables and fruits to your diet. Take infusions including herbs like chamomile, comfrey root, evening primrose, burdock, or purple coneflower to nourish the skin and cool the blood. Skullcap can be used for the nervous system.

Recommendation:

Avoid sun and dry heat.

Keep the skin moist with herbal moisturizer.

Use Minoo's moisturizer for sensitive skin as it contains chamomile, calendula, cucumber, rosemary, and comfrey which soothe and relax the skin and decrease the redness.

Psoriasis

Psoriasis is characterized by dryness and redness, often afferscting the scalp, and elbow.

Cause: An excessive production of epithelial cells which constitute the surface layer of the skin causes psoriasis. The outer layer of skin sloughs off very fast. In some cases Psoriasis occurs after sudden shock, or long term stress which result in a disturbance of the adrenal glands.

Treatment: People suffering from psoriasis should take definite measures to reduce stress by regular exercise, relaxation techniques, or meditation. Herbs such as chamomile, skullcap, and vervain, which relax and strengthen the nervous system, can be

included in prescriptions to treat psoriasis. Licorice and borage may help to support the adrenal glands. To counteract the dryness of the skin, take infusions of herbs such as Oregon grape, burdock, and yellow dock roots, blue flag, nettle, red clover, and angelica that enrich the blood and help in balancing the hormones. In severe cases of psoriasis, because the skin exfoliates fast, the result may strain the circulatory system which eventually affects the heart. Herbs that support the heart and circulation, such as hawthorn, are helpful too. Spicy foods and beverages such as alcohol that stimulate the circulation and dilate the blood vessels should be avoided.

External application can help skin recover from dryness, so use of ointments or creams which contain lavender, comfrey, St. John's wort or mixture of lavender and olive oil for massaging dry parts are recommended. A herbal bath of yarrow and oatmeal soap is also beneficial. Additional herbal remedies to soothe and cool the blood are blue flag, cleavers, nettle, sarsaparilla, and Oregon grape.

Recommendation: Avoid stress.

Do regular exercise and meditation.

Avoid spicy foods and alcohol.

Take herbal baths, like yarrow bath.

Drink herbal teas like hawthorn,

chamomile, skullcap, and vervain to relax the nervous system.

Use herbs that balance the hormones and counteract the dryness like nettle, burdock, yellow dock, and red clover.

If you are suffering from psoriasis, a substantial amount of your nutrients are lost as the skin flakes constantly, and so, you should take extra vitamins and minerals through the skin to supplement the loss.

Take carrot juice, vitamin C, and vitamin B12.

Psoriatic skin contains an abnormal quantity of cholesterol; thus, include soy and sunflower oil, which contain lecithin, to help to clear fatty deposit.

Eczema

Eczema is characterized by rash, inflammation, and a sore, itchy feeling. It is a non-contagious skin disease. There are many causes for eczema. One of the most common causes is contact with irritants. Various types of eczema are as follows:

Dermatitis Eczema: This is caused as a result of contact with an irritant which damages the surface of the skin or penetrates deeper and causes allergic reactions.

Nutritional Deficiency Eczema: This kind of eczema is caused by lack of nutrition in the body, once deficiency is healed skin will quickly recover. Eczema in the case of pregnant woman, nursing mother or infant may be due to a lack of gamma linoleid acid. In this case plenty of herbal tea such as evening primrose, and borage is necessary for production of GLA in breast and to support the hormones.

Food Sensitivity Eczema: Some eczema is due to sensitivities to certain foods. First you should find out which food causes your sensitivity and try to avoid it in your diet for a few weeks to observe the result.

Arteries Stiffness Eczema : This kind of eczema causes stiffness of the arteries that prevents blood nourishes the skin, and often happens to old people.

Treatments: While preparing herbal remedies for any kind of eczema or skin disorders remember to use a mixture of different herb categories, i.e. primary herbs to work on a particular disease and secondary herbs for hormonal and third category herbs to support the nervous system.

Dermatitis Eczema: To prevent and treat this kind of eczema, avoid contact with strong household chemicals and biological detergents which can leave an irritating residue in clothes. Some creams and cosmetics may also inflame the skin.

Wool and nylon may irritate the skin in some people. In this case, the use of cotton is recommended. An infusion of herbs such as burdock, Oregon grape root, yellow dock, sarsaparilla, red clover, blue flag, purple coneflower, and cleavers helps to nourish and cool the blood and skin. Herbs like skullcap and vervain help the nervous system, and herbs such as borage, evening primrose, and licorice help in hormonal balancing.Include plenty of fresh fruits and vegetables to your diet. Drink plenty of mineral water and anti-oxidant juices such as carrot, orange and cantaloupe. Avoid junk foods and foods that have hot energy such as spices.

Use natural soaps and shampoos like oatmeal, and make your own skin cleanser with a mixture of jojoba and almond oils. Aloe vera and comfrey or a mixture of oatmeal, comfrey, and calendula help to soothe the inflammation.

Nutritional Deficiency Eczema: For treating this kind of eczema include vegetable oils, such as sunflower, corn, and olive, in the diet. Extra doses of vitamins C, A, B, and E are necessary to include in a diet for healthy skin. Drinking carrot juice everyday for a good dose of beta carotene (beta carotene is a precursor of vitamin A) and taking vitamin B6 can heal dry skin. Wholesome foods, plenty of fresh fruit, and vegetables are beneficial. Avoid junk foods, fried foods, and foods containing coloring, additives, and artificial flavoring. Avoid alcoholic beverages, and drink plenty of water and pure juices.

The main herbal treatment is an infusion of nettle, burdock, yellow dock, red clover, and purple coneflower which can help to nourish and cool the blood and skin. If you are under stress (which worsens the symptoms), take an infusion of skullcap, chamomile, vervain and oat. This soothes the nervous system and supports the adrenal gland (hormonal balancing). Internal treatment through an infusion of borage, evening primrose, and licorice can be helpful.

External herbal treatment consists of massaging essential oils of chamomile and lavender mixed with olive oil onto dry skin. Use skin care products that have a humectant agent in them like Minoo's Dry-Sensitive Nourishing Cream.

To reduce the inflammation, apply comfrey root or leaves mixed with fine oatmeal on inflamed area. You can make your own ointment with the above mentioned herbs, mixed with olive oil and vitamin E, to soothe and relax the eczema. I remember long ago, when in Iran, one of my aunts had eczema. Everyday she used to massage her skin with comfrey leaves and wheat germ oil to soothe inflammation. She also made nettle, oat, and wheat soup and tea to clean her blood and receive her vitamins B and A from it. After a few months of treatment, her eczema was cured. I used the same method of herbs on one of my customers who was suffering from eczema with the same results. Using herbs for different disorders might take longer for a cure, but the result is permanent as the root of the problem is attacked.

Food Sensitivity Eczema: This kind of eczema is noticed promptly. One may easily recognize the food that causes the sensitivity and resulting eczema. The most common foods that cause sensitivities leading to eczema are dairy products, spicy foods, chocolate, eggs, some seafood, acidic fruits, and vegetables such as oranges, tomatoes, egg plants, and peppers.

Internal treatment consists of infusions of herbs like nettle, purple coneflower, burdock, yellow dock, red clover, and sarsaparilla to nourish and cool the blood and skin. Also, combine these herbs with skullcap and wild oat to help the nervous system if you are under stress. Add herbs like licorice and borage to support the adrenal glands. Make an infusion with licorice, borage, skullcap, wild oat, vervain, one or two parts of blue flag, red clover, sarsaparilla, and burdock. Drink three to five cups everyday with plenty of carrot juice and an additional 15 mg of zinc.

Make an ointment with lavender and/or comfrey mixed with jojoba or olive oil, and massage it into the area. Avoid excessive hot energy and spicy foods as your liver can not tolerate it, especially during such an illness.

Arteries Stiffness Eczema: The main treatment for this kind of eczema is internal herbal remedy. The person should take herbs that soothe the nervous system and regulate blood circulation and hormonal glands.

Herbal teas, such as ginseng, and ginger, help to normalize blood circulation: teas with evening primrose, borage and licorice help to regulate adrenal glands; and skullcap, chamomile, and passion flower teas help to soothe the nervous system. Herbs such as burdock, Oregon grape root, dandelion bark, yellow dock, purple coneflower, chickweed, nettle, and cleavers help to nourish the skin and cool the blood. You can make an infusion or tea of each or any two of the above herbs, and drink three to five cups daily. External treatment of vegetable paste is recommend. To make a vegetable paste steam vegetables such as cabbage, cayenne, and garlic smash and apply them on the area with some warm fabric warp the area for several hours, repeat every day.

Aromatherapy is beneficial for any kind of eczema. To soothe and reduce inflammation topically, mix oil of jojoba, lavender, evening primrose, and marigold, and massage into skin. Use of sandalwood, lavender, and rose, by either steam inhalation or bath, is recommended.

Recommendation: In general, use of

herbs like blue flag, purple coneflower, burdock, yellow dock, sarsaparilla, cleaver, Oregon grape root, nettle, dandelion, and oat soothe and cool the blood; passion flower, skullcap, chamomile, melissa, wild oat, vervain, and valerian support the central nervous system; and licorice, borage, evening primrose, and wild yam support hormonal glands.

Warts

Warts are a contagious inflammatory skin disease characterized by an infection usually located on the hands, elbows, and soles of the feet.

Cause: Nutritional deficiencies, hormone imbalances, and stress are some of the common instigators of wart formation. If you are suffering from warts, strengthen your general vitality, immune system, and nervous system.

Treatment: To treat warts, correct nutritional deficiencies. Include vitamins A, B, C, and E in your diet for a healthy skin. Pure fresh fruit and vegetables, in forms such as carrot juice, and vitamin B6 also help for fast healing of the skin.

Avoid dairy products and fried, greasy, and spicy foods.

Take internal treatment with herbs. Use skullcap, vervain, and oat to relax the nervous system, especially if under stress; use burdock, yellow dock, nettles, red clover, and purple coneflower to nourish the skin and cool the blood; and use licorice, borage, and wild yam to balance the hormones.

For external remedy, apply fig and dandelion sap, from bottom fruit part, on infected areas. Rub the sap on the affected area, and leave it on for a few minutes. Repeat for seven to ten days. After ten days, the wart will fall off. Garlic is also beneficial. Crush a clove of garlic and tape it carefully on the wart. As a little girl, I often got warts over my hands or between my fingers. My mother would treat them with unripe fig sap. She would cut the fig and rub the sap or milk over my wart, repeating it after few hours. In few days, wart would fall off.

Rosacea

Rosacea is a disease associated with sebaceous gland function and is characterized by redness and dilation of blood vessels in the form of pustule.

Cause: The illness starts with overexposing sensitive oily skin to harsh environmental influences such as cold, wind, sun, household chemicals and fumes. Excessive use of alcohol, drugs, and spicy food can aggravate the sensitivity and cause redness, dilation of blood vessels, and formation of pustules, thus resulting in rosacea. Rosacea on the face is often in the form of a flushed appearance. Nose and cheeks are the most frequently affected parts. It is more common in woman after the age of 35. Imbalance in hormones, stress, nutritional deficiencies, and nervous tension can worsen the symptoms of rosacea.

Treatment:

To treat rosacea, sun, dry heat, chemical fumes, cosmetics and skin care products that contain chemicals, alcohol, perfumes, and mineral oils, and strong spicy foods should be avoided.

Include additional vitamins, such as vitamins B6, B12, and C, and minerals like zinc to help store vitamin A in the liver. Carrot and apple juices, fresh vegetables, and mineral water should be part of your daily diet.

Include internal infusions of herbs like skullcap, vervain and chamomile for the nervous system, burdock, yellow dock, and nettle to nourish the skin and cool the blood, and borage, licorice, or evening primrose to normalize hormone imbalances.

The cosmetics and skin care products should be free from perfumes and alcohol. Oil of lavender and chamomile mixed with cucumber paste and wheat germ oil, in the form of an ointment, soothes the skin.

Recommendations:

Avoid strong alcoholic beverages and spicy and artificially flavored foods.

Avoid inhaling fumes and chemicals.

Avoid using oil-, alcohol-, and perfume-based cosmetic products.

I have dealt with many cases of rosacea. When put under proper diet and herbal remedies, in a short period of time these people get good result.

Usually people with rosacea are those who have had large oily pores since an early age and have mistreated the skin. For example, they were overexposed to harsh environmental influences, such as free radicals, pollution, dry heat, dry cold, and sun. They had a poor diet, and in order to get rid of excess oil, they over-scrubbed their skin with wrong products in a wrong way. Those skin types later become oily, sensitive, and prone to different skin disorders, like rosacea. Make sure to follow the advice offered in this section, if you are suffering from rosacea.

Seborrhea

Seborrhea is a functional disease of the sebaceous gland, characterized by an excessive secretion of sebum which collects upon the skin.

Cause: Seborrhea, like rosacea, also starts with sensitive oily skin, strongly reacting to adverse environmental hazards such as exposure to sun, excessive heat, excessive use of alcoholic beverages, strong spicy food, fumes, and household chemicals. Reaction of the skin is in the form of an itchy and burning sensation. Skin affected by seborrhea has enlarged pores and appears coarse and shiny from the excess oil.

Treatment: To treat seborrhea, the following exposures and diets should be avoided:

Avoid overexposure to sun, dry heat, cold, household chemicals, fumes, and cosmetics and skin care products containing mineral oil, perfumes, and alcohol. Strong spicy food, milk products (especially cheese), alcoholic beverages, artificially flavored foods, and certain drugs should also be eliminated or greatly decreased in use.

Include additional amounts of vitamins like B6, A, and C and minerals like zinc and potassium in your daily diet.

Drink fresh carrot juice twice daily for extra vitamin A.

Include fresh fruits and green vegetables, eight glasses of water, and carbohydrates like steamed rice, potatoes, and fresh bread in your daily diet.

Take herbal infusions of borage and evening primrose for hormonal balance. Skullcap, chamomile passion flower, and vervain are for the nervous system. Nettle, burdock, lavender, cleavers, purple coneflower, Oregon grape root, yellow dock, and dandelion nourish the skin and cool the blood.

Use aloe vera gel with chamomile and lavender essential oils to soothe the skin.

Use oatmeal with lavender oil as a mask twice a week.

Use skin care products which contain soothing herbs like Minoo's Sensitive Skin Line.

Recommendation: Use herbal remedy and proper nutritional diet. Avoid spicy and artificially flavored foods, chemical fumes, and alcohol.

Asteatosis

Asteatosis is the condition of dry, scaly skin.

Cause: Asteatosis is referred to as dry, scaly skin characterized by absolute or partial deficiency of sebum, usually due to aging or bodily disorder. As the body ages, the sebaceous glands become less and less active, and the body does not retain water as much as when young. Moisture loss of the skin could be caused by intense exposure to sun, dry heat, cold, wind, nutritional deficiency, and lack of natural moisture.

Treatment:

Avoid overexposure to dry heat and sun.

Each day, add extra vitamins and mineral to your diet, drink enough water, take juices of fresh fruits and vegetables, like carrot, beet, and apple, and take enough minerals ,like zinc and potassium, to hold the vitamins in the body.

Infusions of herbs like red clover, rosemary, nettle, and yellow dock help to nourish the skin, while borage, licorice, and evening primrose are for hormone balancing.

Use herbal skin care products with ingredients like chamomile, jojoba, fennel (which contains hyaluronic acid), and vitamin E. Apply them with few drops of water on the skin. Minoo's nourishing creams are recommended.

Steatoma

Also known as sebaceous cyst, steatoma is a tumor of the sebaceous glands. Its size can vary from that of a pea to an orange, and it contains sebum oil.

Cause: Steatomas are caused by excess excretion of sebum oil, generated by overactive or disordered sebaceous glands. If sebaceous glands are larger than natural, the sebum oil produced cannot reach the surface, thus, thickening. Production of more oil by sebaceous glands leads to its accumulation, resulting in steatoma.

Treatment: If you observe symptoms of a steatoma, compress it with hot water at least five to seven times a day. Apply witch hazel or marigold extract to disinfect the area, reduce the inflammation, and make the sebum thinner.

Apply tea tree oil, burdock, or sage to the area as a germicide. Once inflammation is reduced, extract the area, and remove all the pus trapped beneath the skin. Sanitize the area with witch hazel.

Drink hot infusions of sage, burdock, and nettle to keep the blood clean. Bilberry and pomegranate juices also purify the blood. Extra intake of vitamin C that helps keep the skin from infection, zinc 15 mg a day along with carrot juice which help store vitamin A in the liver, herbs such as dandelion, centaury, and rosemary that stimulate the liver and gallbladder, and herbs such as wild indigo, dandelion, burdock, and garlic that fight infection are necessary and need to be added to the diet.

External herbal use of eucalyptus, witch hazel, and lavender oils is very antibacterial. Apply on the infected area at least three to five times daily until complete drying of disease.

Shingles

Shingles, technically known as herpes, is an acute exacerbation of a central nervous system infection caused by a virus.

Cause: Cases of shingles are characterized by skin blisters and pain in the nerve endings of the skin. The shingles virus is almost the same as the one that causes chickenpox. When the virus enters the body, it infects various parts of the nerves causing a few days of fever, after which skin erupts and rashes appear. These can run from under a rib to the back (dermatome) or be present on the face.

Shingles usually can be treated with injection or oral consumption of vitamin C which aids in the fast drying of blisters. If the face gets afflicted with blisters, the result can be permanent scarring.

Treatment: Herbs like echinacea, ginseng root, and St. John's wort that support the nervous and immune systems are important remedies. Take a tincture of 1/2 tablespoon of echinacea or echinacea tablet or capsule and make an infusion of echinacea, ginseng root, chickweed, and St. John's wort everyday. To soothe irritated areas of skin, apply infusion of rose, lime, or lavender twice a day. Mix one teaspoon of wheat germ oil with two teaspoons of grapeseed oil, and add 3 drops of each rosemary, geranium, and lavender. Apply like an ointment twice a day.

Wear comfortable clothing.

Do not use soap, especially if you have blisters on the face.

Use natural cleansers or cosmetic products. Minoo's herbal skin care products are recommended.

Do not eat spicy or acidic foods.

Take extra vitamin C, vitamin E, and zinc.

Drink carrot juice, and eat green leafy vegetables or cool energy foods like celery, dandelion, and cilantro.

Take a warm bath with essential oils of chamomile, marigold, and lavender.

Get enough sleep, and drink plenty mineral water.

In the case of shingles, it is advisable to consult your doctor too.

Cold Sores

Cold sores usually occur when the body has an infection or high temperature (fever) and are caused by herpes or chickenpox virus. In Iran, it is believed that emotional and mental stresses influence cold sores and that waking up with shock or fear from a nightmare while feverish and infected can also cause cold sores. They treat cold sores with the help of cold metals, putting the cold metal over the cold sores every morning and then applying eucalyptus and camphor ointment to disinfect them.

Two to four cups daily of an herbal

infusion of St. John's wort and echinacea, plenty of rest, and liquids are recommended in treating the problem.

Sunburns

Characterized by inflammation, redness, and dehydration and accompanied with pain and discomfort.

Cause: This is inflammation of the skin caused by exposure to ultra violet rays. Usually, fair skin damages more and faster than darker skin, as fair skin has little protective pigments. Damage to fair skin causes redness, discomfort, broken capillaries or sensitivities, and wrinkles. Damage to darker skin starts with redness and further oily pigments are increased.

Treatment: Usually sensitive skin has more reaction to U.V.R and it may lead to broken capillaries. If sunburn is deep and painful:

Apply fresh grated potatoes for 15-20 minutes to the burn area to reduce discomfort and burning sensation.

Apply herbal ointment or cream which contain Vitamin E, lavender, comfrey, and melissa to the burned area and massage it to be absorbed.

Drink plenty of mineral water and carrot juice to prevent dehydration.

Drink herbal tea such as chickweed,

dandelion, and blue flag the health of your skin.

Recommendation:

Avoid sun, and dry heat

Drink plenty of water and natural juices

Add plenty of fresh fruits and vegetable to your diet

Add one tablespoon of natural yellow butter, as Vitamin A in butter helps with skin lubrication and elasticity

Apply herbal cream every few hours to prevent skin surface dehydration and wrinkles

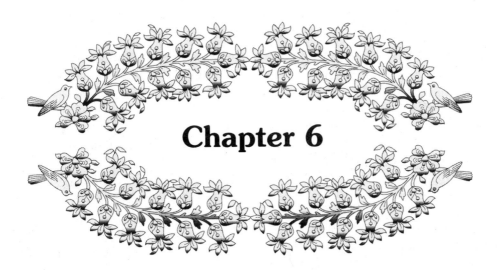

Chapter 6

The Digestive System and Herbs

The constant energy supply obtained from foods keeps the body alive and functional. The digestive process starts as soon as food is taken into the mouth, where it begins to be broken down. As it passes through the body, it continues to be broken down further at various stages so that the energy-rich nutrients can be properly absorbed. These changes take place in the digestive tract.

People can have a miserable life as the result of poor digestion. Poor digestion usually results from insufficient or excessive digestive secretion, emotional stress, and mental stress. If suffering from indigestion, certain types of foods, such as fatty and fried foods, need to be avoided. Sometimes fasting for a short time might be useful. Eat only simple wholesome foods, and avoid drinking water during a meal or immediately after the meal. Do not eat very late at night because the digestive tract will be overworked, causing indigestion and insomnia. Do not eat very fast. Drink water early in the morning or warm water with fresh squeezed lemon juice all day to clean up the system and rest your overtaxed body. Herbal medicines can improve the digestive organs and help to relieve acidity.

What Is the Digestive Tract?:

Throughout the middle of the body runs the digestive tract which secrets the digestive juices required to break down the food we eat into small molecules. Vital digestive secretions are supplied by the liver, gallbladder, and pancreas.

The active components of those digestive juices which cause the chemical breakdown of food are called enzymes. Enzymes are complex proteins capable of inducing chemical changes in other substances without themselves being changed.

When we eat a meal, the food is first broken down by both chewing and the action of saliva. It then passes down through the esophagus to the stomach, where it is further broken down by gastric juices. Then passing down to the small intestines, it mixes with digestive enzymes and bile from the gallbladder. Nutrients are absorbed into the bloodstream and transported by vessels to the liver. Indigestible remnants move on into the large intestine where the remaining water and sodium is extracted. Any remaining waste passes down to the rectum for excretion.

Elimination is a vital function of the digestive tract. In addition to voiding the residue of food and fluid, the intestine must also get rid of other metabolic waste products. If this process is impaired, a build-up of toxins will result. The health of the colon and its regular movement and evacuation are dependent on the amount of fiber and liquid taken daily in the diet.

Factors That Disturb Digestive Systems:

Nervousness and anxiety can interfere with the function of the digestive system. When one is worried or fatigued, eating may cause gastrointestinal disturbances. When we eat a meal, the circulatory system is automatically modified by the nervous system so that more blood is sent to the digestive tract in order to aid its functions. This process lowers the amount of blood reaching the muscles and brain. In the case of stress, however, a reverse process carries the blood away from the digestive tract to feed the brain and muscles, thus digestive functioning is reduced. During periods of stress, more acid is secreted by the stomach, which can cause indigestion and chronic ulcer.

Abdominal pain, constipation, diarrhea, flatulence, indigestion, nausea, and weight gain or loss are the common symptoms of digestive disorders. More serious problems include liver disease, stomach or colon cancer, and ulcer. Most digestive problems are caused by dietary factors such as too little fiber, lack of exercise, and emotional and mental stress.

Herbs for Better Digestion

In Iran, country people often eat bitter herbs to cleanse the liver and digestive system, especially after the holidays when lots of heavy, greasy food has been consumed. The liver needs to be cleansed and evacuated so that bitter herbs such as dandelion, agrimony and bilberry juice help cleanse the blood, liver, and digestive tract.

Iranian strongly believe in taking bilberry juice during holidays. Bilberry is a great source of vitamin C and purifies, soothes and cleanses the blood and liver. It is also good for high blood pressure, blood sugar, and cholesterol levels as well as for acne and boils.

Many of the early spring herbs are reputed as blood cleansers or purifiers. They contain glycoside, and often are very bitter in taste. They increase the secretion of digestive juices and restore the appetite. This is especially valuable after a winter diet of highly salted, heavy foods. Herbs such as gentian, dandelion, centaury, and peppermint strengthen the whole system and have a cleansing and antiseptic action.

Herbs to Cleanse the Colon

Cascara sagrada, psyllium husk, and peach leaves are considered to be excellent colon and intestinal cleansers. They lubricate the intestine and help to increase the bulk of the stool. Cascara sagrada bark also helps restore natural tone to the colon and painless evacuation. In Iran, this plant is known as "colon cleanser." Gentian and peppermint can be used for cleansing and digestion as follows:

1 tablespoon of dried gentian root
1 teaspoon of peppermint
16 oz of boiling water

Bring the water to a boil, add gentian, and simmer for 20 minutes. Add peppermint, and infuse for 10 minutes. Add a teaspoon of honey and fresh-squeezed lemon to taste. You can replace gentian with centaury or dandelion root.

Herbs for Appetite

Most herbs and spices are good for digestion and appetite. Their strongly aromatic or bitter scents and flavors increase saliva and stimulate secretion of gastric juices. Bitter herbs or spices taken before meals or aromatic seeds and leaves taken with meals are great for digestive system.

In the Middle East, spices are taken with drinks to increase appetite. For example, cold ginger or warm ginger tea is taken to increase the appetite and stimulate digestion. Spices are also added to foods for better flavor and better digestion. For example, meat and poultry do not digest as fast as carbohydrate and vegetables. Therefore meat is soaked with different spices for to deodorize and tenderize.

As another example, saffron, rosemary, tarragon, garlic, chili pepper, and dried lemon are also used for meat and poultry.

Spices with strong, warming volatile oils and antiseptic plants, such as ginger, caraway, cayenne, saffron, nutmeg, and fennel seeds are digestive, cleansing, antiseptic, stimulating, and have soothing effects on guts. Some appetizer recipes follow.

Brandy with Gentian Root
3 cups of brandy
3 tablespoons of gentian root, sliced
1 teaspoon of cardamom seed, powdered
3 tablespoons of dried orange peel

Combine the ingredients in a bottle. Cover for 3 days, strain, and keep in a glass bottle. Take two tablespoons before meals to increase the appetite.

Herbal Syrup:

1 cup of dandelion root, chopped
1 cup of centaury leaf, chopped
1 cup of sage leaf, chopped
1 cup of agrimony leaf, chopped
1 cup of peppermint and marjoram, chopped.
1/2 cup of honey
4 cups of water
1 teaspoon of crushed cardamom pods

Bring the water to a boil, add the herbs, and simmer for 25 minutes. Strain, add

cardamom pod and honey, and boil for 15 more minutes until slightly thickened. Take one teaspoon before and after meals for better digestion.

The application of aromatherapy can help prevent many digestive problems. Many plants contain essential oils that stimulate the digestive system. The fragrance of herbs and spices while cooking food can start the process, i.e., production of saliva. Later these herbs help break down food in the guts. The essential oil of aromatic herbs, spices, fruits, and vegetables should be incorporated into cooking and diet whenever possible. Warm energy and stimulating herbs like basil, marjoram, oregano, pepper, savory, thyme, ginger, and mint help create better and faster digestion.

Herbs to Relax the Digestive System

Normal function of digestive system depends on nervous control. To relax the digestive system, a relaxing herbal tea of hop and chamomile, skullcap and passion flower, and comfrey can be taken before meals.

Herbs to Reduce Stomach Inflammation

Inflammation of the stomach has the same feeling as that of ulcer. The same elements that cause indigestion may cause inflammation, stress being one of them.

In Iran, a variety of different herbs are used for stomach inflammation and flatulence, specially licorice.

Licorice has been very popular and widely used within Iranians since ancient times. It is a strong anti-inflammatory similar to cortisone, and is being investigated for anti-cancer properties. Iranian cut the root by lenght, soak it in water with fennel for several hours and use it for lowering stomach acid, decreasing stomach spasm, and reducing inflammation of the stomach, and flatulence. This plant is widely grown in Iran and most European countries import licorice from Iran to use it for the same purpose. People who live and work in cities frequently have this problem, the main reason being daily stress, which reflects on their stomach and causes indigestion, flatulence, or gastric discomfort. Many people have a variety of herbs at home which they use to soothe the stomach. They mix licorice with slippery elm bark and marshmallow root pudding with honey to heal inflammation. Warm herbal teas consisting of a mixtures of various herbs are also widely used.

Almost any disease and disorder, whether internal or external, can be the result of nervous system and hormonal disorder. Therefore, you should always take secondary herbs for central nervous system and hormonal disorder along with the primary herbs that are taken directly for the disorder. A vital part of treatment consists of changing diet, eating regularly, and ensuring less stress.

For stomach inflammation or gastritis, herbs like comfrey, slippery elm bark, licorice, marshmallow root, and chamomile are recommended. You can make pudding with slippery elm bark powder and marshmallow root powder. Add 2 tablespoons of these herbs in 3 cups of water or low fat milk. Stir until it thickens. Add honey and drink. This pudding not only soothes the stomach ulcer, but it also controls overproduction of acid and prevents further damage.

Make an infusion of marigold and comfrey for pain. Add licorice to support the hormonal glands, and add passion flower and chamomile to support the central nervous system. Infuse one part of licorice, marigold, and chamomile and two parts of comfrey and marshmallow root each. Drink everyday until the pain and inflammation are healed. Avoid spicy, greasy foods, caffeine, and acidic foods.

Herbs for Better Liver Function

The liver plays a central role in the cleansing of the body. It also plays a vital role in maintaining and regulating health and in overcoming diseases, thus, its proper functioning is very important. The liver's regular cleansing and detoxification of the body can be enhanced with the help of certain herbs. The liver is richly supplied with blood which helps in its filtering action and its regulating the sugar and amino acid levels.

There are two vessels in the liver, known as the hepatic artery and the portal vein. The hepatic artery brings fresh blood to the liver cells, providing oxygen; portal vein brings all the products of digestion to the liver so that it can filter and store glucose and fructose.

Bitter herbs like dandelion, centaury, and gentian have important effects on the liver, promoting the secretion of bile and helping in the detoxification of the liver cells.

The liver does not tolerate greasy and spicy hot energy foods well, as the storing of them causes skin disorders and internal problems. So it is very important not to take in a great deal of hot energy foods. If you do, try to cleanse and detoxify the liver by using bitter herbs, vitamin C, beta carotene, and zinc. A few of these herbs can be taken after heavy meals to help clear the residue. Infusion of golden seal root, gentian, rosemary, and barberry bark is a good liver regulating remedy.

Herbs for Gallbladder Inflammation and Gallstones

Gallstones are formed as a result of an excess concentration of bile. If you cleanse your liver and gallbladder at least once a week by including herbs that increase the secretion of bile from the gallbladder, you should never face any problem with gallstones.

Bitter herbs, like dandelion, gentian,

centaury, marjoram, rosemary, and peppermint, and also bilberry juice, barberry, and pomegranate juices can increase the secretion of bile and cleanse, detoxify and evacuate waste. Gallstones and inflammation of the gallbladder can be treated by using the bitter herbs dandelion, gentian, Oregon grape root, cleaver, and wahoo, which can be combined with soothing herbs like chamomile, lavender, marshmallow, and slippery elm. Golden seal root helps to regulate function of the liver.

Try daily additions of fresh dandelion leaves, peppermint, and rosemary to your salad and make an infusion of one part each gentian, Oregon grape root, golden seal, and lavender. Drink two to three cups at least three times a month.

Herbal Remedy to Reduce Indigestion

Indigestion is the result of eating inappropriately, like eating too much and too fast during stress or eating wrong foods. Dull stomach pain or heartburn after a meal are the sensations of indigestion.

To prevent indigestion, if under stress or tension, take an infusion of chamomile, lemon balm, or hops before your meal, to ease the tension. If you need to stimulate your appetite and regulate the digestive system, take bitter herbs like dandelion root or gentian before meals. To neutralize the stomach acid and prevent heartburn or indigestion, take herbs like mint, fennel, chamomile, lemon balm, and golden seal to relieve flatulence. These herbs are better than antacids. Avoid acidic and spicy foods.

Herbs to Stop Diarrhea

Frequent liquid bowel movements, often caused by infection and bacteria, irritate the digestive tract. Stress, fear, or taking laxatives can also cause diarrhea. Diarrhea and vomiting help to cleanse bacteria and poison away from the digestive system.

Iranians cure any kind of diarrhea by taking soft steamed rice with plain yogurt and hot peppermint tea with ginger. As the body loses a substantial amount of liquid and minerals during diarrhea, this loss can be replaced with warm water and honey and hot peppermint tea and ginger. They avoid cold energy foods and keep the stomach warm until all bacteria exit the system. If the diarrhea causes lots of flatulence and pain, they use a warm energy herbal tea like thyme, rosemary, sage, oregano and marjoram with honey and ginger, then they massage the stomach area with castor oil and marjoram and wrap it with a warm towel. Especially in the case of babies and old people, diarrhea may cause dehydration. Iranians make sure that their bodies receive extra warm liquid and antiseptic herbal tea blended with honey and ginger, and also keep the feet and stomach warm.

In any case of diarrhea, try to avoid foods for couple of days, especially most fresh fruit and dairy products (except yogurt). Take steamed rice with yogurt, garlic, and ginger. Herbs with warm energy like agrimony, ginger, cinnamon, rosemary, and gentian are recommended. Try warm infusion of agrimony with cinnamon and ginger. Do not take cold drinks during diarrhea, since digestive activity is aided by warmth.

Herbal Laxatives for Constipation

Constipation is usually the result of bad diet, stress, or lack of exercise. During stress, muscular tension can inhibit bowel activities, hence constipation. Toxic matter is released into the system during constipation, which can be relieved by regular exercise, abdominal massage, and adding plenty of liquid and fiber to our diet. Drinking eight glasses of water a day, fresh fruit like plums and watermelon, and fresh vegetables like corn and carrot juice are necessary for cleansing and regulating the bowel.

In Iran, fresh fruits, vegetables, and fresh herbs served with meals (like marjoram, peppermint, parsley, tarragon, dill, chives, cilantro and green onion) almost constitute the entire daily diet. These herbs cleanse and detoxify the digestive system, and as they contain fiber, constipation will not occur. Most people drink fresh fruits juices everyday and black bilberry juice twice a month to get rid of excess sugar, salt, cholesterol, and waste.

Herbal teas like dandelion root, rhubarb root, and yellow dock are mildly cathartic and help to relieve the constipation. Cascara sagarda, buckthorn bark, and psyllium husk restore natural tone to the colonic muscles, increasing colon activity and evacuation. Chamomile, valerian, wild yam, and licorice alleviate the tension. Infusions made of herbs like senna, fennel, peach leaves, papaya leaves, strawberry leaves, dandelion root, gentian, peppermint, rosemary, caraway, centaury, and anise are wonderful to relieve constipation. If you are constipated, take one tablespoon of these herbs with your favorite juice or herbal tea before you go to bed. By the next day, it will cleanse and release all the trapped toxin from your system giving a natural glow to your skin.

Flatulence

Flatulence is excess gas formed in intestine by the action of bacteria or ingested oxygen. We all swallow a certain amount of oxygen and nitrogen from the air each day which has to be dispelled. That air, during nervous tension, stress or anxiety can be formed into flatulence.

Certain foods can cause flatulence due to a lack of the enzyme necessary to digest that food (like lactose in milk or gluten in wheat) or by producing a gas in intestine. Some foods like beans, radishes, bell peppers, and cabbage encourage flatulence due to their sugar content which is converted to gas.

In Iran, beans are soaked, and they release the sugar which is trapped under the skin before cooking. Sometime beans, especially garbanzo beans and pinto beans, are peeled before boiling. They cook beans and other vegetables which contain a fair amount of sugar with herbs that contain volatile oils, like oregano, marjoram, peppermint, and garlic, in order to reduce the gas and make the food easier to digest.

After eating foods that can cause flatulence, they drink heavy peppermint and marjoram tea to reduce the gas. Nursing mothers should avoid eating vegetables like radishes, onions, cabbages, and bell peppers as the baby might get gastric distress or flatulence. These mothers are recommended to drink peppermint, marjoram, fennel, and mistletoe tea to increase their milk.

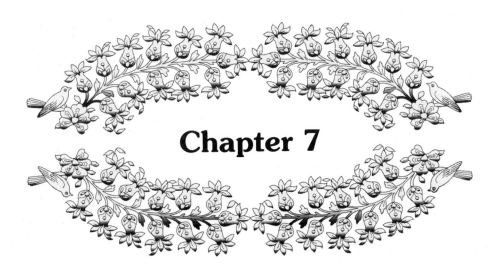

Chapter 7

The Circulatory System and Herbs

Herbs for Blood Purification and Circulation

Every minute, the heart beats about seventy times, pumping blood throughout the body. This process is known as circulation, which can increase during excitement and exercise. The circulatory system of the body mainly consists of the heart, veins, and arteries through which blood is carried to organs and tissues. Arteries, which carry the blood away from the heart, are responsible for bringing tissues the nutrients necessary for growth and maintenance. Arteries divide into many tiny capillaries, which link arteries and veins.

When blood leaves the heart, it flow through arteries and goes through tissues and organs. Deoxygenated blood, carrying waste carbon dioxide, returns through the veins to reach the heart. This blood is then pumped to the lungs where carbon dioxide is exchanged for oxygen. After the blood is oxygenated, it flows through the pulmonary veins back to the heart.

During circulation, the blood collects nutrients from the liver and intestines. The blood is filtered in kidneys. If the heart and blood vessels are in good health, circulation and transportation of oxygen and carbon dioxide by the blood should be normal.

Blood consists of red and white cells which float in a fluid called plasma. Plasma consists of salt, proteins, sugars, and other substances dissolved in water. Red cells carry oxygen from the lungs to the tissues, and white cells defend the body against bacterial or viral attacks and multiply during an infection.

Make an infusion of herbs such as burdock, yellow dock, blue flag, dandelion, bilberry, nettle, sarsaparilla, and coneflower and drink two to three cups daily as needed for blood purification and circulation.

Prevention of Cardiovascular Diseases

There are three groups of cholesterol: triglycerides, phospholipids, and sterols.

Cholesterol is produced in liver. Part of it enters the body through eating meals and is changed into lipoprotein molecules. Lipoproteins entering the blood are LDL (low density lipoprotein), VLDL (very low density lipoprotein), and HDL (high density lipoprotein). A healthy body produces an amount of cholesterol that can be burned and consumed. If LDL (bad cholesterol) is overproduced, then HDL will not be able to return it to the liver, so the excess will cause disorders by settling in arteries, thus impeding the normal circulation and causing cardiovascular disorders.

According to recent recommendations published in the USA, the total amount of either cholesterol should not exceed 200 ml/dl.

Very serious problems of the circulatory system are those that involve the heart. High blood pressure, heart diseases, and strokes are responsible for more than fifty percent of the deaths in western countries. Research shows that Great Britain has the highest number of cases of heart diseases in the world. The majority of these cases are due to inadequate exercise and diets rich in fat and sugar.

Exercise: You should take regular exercises at least 3 times a week. Regular exercise strengthens heart muscles and vessels.

Diet: You should have a diet high in fiber and low in both sugar and animal fat. Saturated animal fats can form fatty deposits in arteries and prevent smooth blood flow which can result in stroke. Drink at least eight to ten glasses of water a day. Drinking water and herbal teas, three to four cups a day, helps to get rid of fat, sugar, and salt deposits in the blood and makes the blood circulate easier. Try to have a diet consisting of fruits, vegetables, and herbs that contain saponin and glycoside for better circulation and cleansing.

Suggestions: Followings are some main suggestions to prevent digestive disorders.

Avoid Excess Meat: The results of a research study have shown that people in Kenya and Tanzania live exclusively on meat and milk provided by their cattle. Scientists call this regime as "the world's worst diet". An average person of these countries ingest up to 2000 milligrams of cholesterol a day, well over the maximum recommended daily intake of 300 milligrams. Yet their blood cholesterol level is remarkably low, about 1/3 of average cholesterol levels.

American researchers have long argued that these people must have specialized genes that prevent high cholesterol and cardiac diseases. The supposition of a genetic response to a high cholesterol diet does not, however, account for low cholesterol level found in these people. However, the study also showed that there exists a variety of wild tree barks that are added to their meat. They boil the meat slowly in milk, stirring the bark of acacia goetzei and other trees into the broth. They do not use these barks as flavorings in other foods. The study showed that these barks might play a sophisticated role in lowering blood cholesterol. Possibly they contain unique saponins and organic compounds with a sugar, like a core, that forms soapy foam when dissolved in water. If new cholesterol lowering substances can be isolated from these wild plants, millions of people could reduce their risk of cardiovascular illness, the gravest health threat in the west.

It has been scientifically proven that as soon as meat enters the stomach an increase of stomach acid secretion takes place for lengthy digestion. The waste of meat is a main cause of gastrointestinal and heart problems. Science has proven that meat contributes to diseases and disorders of the heart, and perhaps, to appendicitis, diarrhea, tuberculosis, different kinds of intestinal worms, liver diseases, and cancer. One research study shows that gastrointestinal problems and appendicitis in France, England, Belgium, and Romania are more than everywhere else in the world. It is because their diet consists mainly of eggs and meat that may not be well-cooked. Medium rare cooking of meat can cause growth of bacteria in stomach and lead to infectious diseases. Not only do diets that consist mainly of meat not give us vitality, but they may also cause heart and gastrointestinal diseases and even cancers.

Avoid Alcohol and Smoking: Avoid drinking alcoholic beverages and stop smoking. Nicotine constricts the arteries and reduces blood flow. Carbon monoxide in tobacco reduces the amount of oxygen in the blood and traps carbon dioxide in the lungs. Excessive use of alcohol also contributes to an accumulation of body fat.

Relaxation: Learn to relax at least 20 minutes a day. Lay on your back, relax, and meditate to reduce mental and emotional depression. Take a hot herbal bath of lavender, melissa, rose, sandalwood, orange and chamomile, ten to twenty minutes a day for physical and mental relaxation.

Aromatherapy: Aromatherapeutic oil can boost the circulation of the blood, thereby preventing less serious circulatory problems such as cellulite and varicose veins on the legs. Stimulating blood circulation is also extremely good for the skin, and strengthening the blood vessels can prevent broken capillaries. Massaging the tissue with essential oils like neroli, cypress, and lemon can stimulate the tissue and deliver fresh blood to the cells. Massaging also facilitates the entry of essential oils and boosts the circulation.

Herbal remedies: Herbs play an important role in circulation. For normal detoxification, circulation, and pressure of blood take herbs like horsetail, hawthorn, angelica, cayenne, and juniper. Horsetail contains silica, which strengthens the walls of veins. It has astringent action which helps to tighten up varicose veins. Silica encourages the absorption of calcium by the body and helps to guard against fatty depositions in the arteries. Angelica, juniper, and cayenne stimulate arterial circulation, and they could also be applied to areas of poor circulation. You can make a cabbage paste with ginger, cayenne, and garlic to stimulate the circulation to the area where it is applied.

Blood purification: Ingesting water is the best way to purify the blood. Next in importance are herbs. They can keep the blood clean from impurities that contribute to poor circulation and clogging arteries which result in cardiovascular diseases.

Include bilberry and pomegranate juice in your diet if suffering from high blood pressure and you need to release toxins from blood. These juices are especially helpful after a heavy meals, like the heavy, sweet and greasy foods we frequently partake in during the month of December. Drink one glass of bilberry or pomegranate juice for purification and cleansing. Herbs like dandelion root, centaury, and licorice are also blood purifying. Use alternative herbs like burdock, nettle, yellow dock, and blue flag to cleanse the tissue, nourish the blood, eliminate toxins, and ensure waste material evacuation from the body. Use alternative herb infusions with plenty of pure water.

High Blood Pressure

The major cause of high blood pressure is stress. To reduce high blood pressure, you should exercise, meditate 3 times a week, and learn to relax. Diet can play a major role in reducing blood pressure. If you are suffering from high blood pressure, adopt a meat-free diet, especially eliminating red meat that is rich in fat. Your diet should consist largely of fresh fruit and vegetables, especially garlic. You can add garlic either to your salad or take

1 clove a day by itself or with fresh bread.

It is also important to get rid of excess fluid from your body. Avoid taking much salt, as it causes water retention and increases the blood pressure. Avoid caffeine, which contributes to stress and tension. Drink fresh pure juices like carrot, grape and grapefruit juices, instead of tea or coffee. Fresh vegetables like lettuce, celery, cucumber, and all the cabbage family lower blood pressure. Herbs like hawthorn, yarrow, borage, valerian, mistletoe, berries, and lime flower also help in lowering blood pressure.

Low Blood Pressure

Low blood pressure usually occurs with poor diet and not eating regularly throughout the day. It is usually associated with dizziness, fainting, poor circulation, and headache, and it can cause insomnia. To increase the blood pressure level, the fastest way is to stimulate the circulation. Herbs like ginger, cayenne, pepper, and angelica stimulate the circulation and appetite at the same time. Infusion of honey, hot water, and ginger can help, and hawthorn and yarrow also level out the blood pressure if it is high or low. Four balanced meals a day are very important. Avoid acidic foods like lemon, orange, and grapefruit. Try not to have fruit and vegetables on an empty stomach. Always take your salad after your meal. Include grains and beans, like soybean, black beans, and lentils, in your diet as they are rich in protein and iron.

Low blood pressure causes headache. For rapid recovery, take a cup of hot low fat milk, one egg yolk, and 2 tablespoons of honey. Beat the yolk in honey until smooth, add hot milk, and drink it. Hot infusion of hawthorn, valerian or vervain with honey and ginger can normalize the blood pressure. Headaches are also associated with low iron. Include extra iron in your diet. Do not overdose the iron as it can be trapped in your liver and cause disorders. Take iron tablets, especially during menstruation. Include fresh red meat or beef liver to your diet twice a month as it helps to normalize the iron level. This is especially useful if you are suffering from dizziness or low iron.

Poor Blood Circulation

In Iran, people suffering from poor circulation or those with very pale skin are considered to be of a cool nature, and they should not eat much cool energy foods. Their diet should consist of warm energy foods to increase the circulation and bring back the color and vitality. For example, yogurt and cool energy herbs and vegetables should be avoided, or at least, they need to be mixed with hot energy foods to be balanced.

Honey with angelica and ginger is a good combination as a tea everyday.

When making salads, make sure radish, onion, cayenne, cabbage, and garlic are added. They all have warm energy and also stimulate blood circulation. If there is any area of the body that has low blood circulation, apply cabbage paste and cayenne and wrap the area with a warm towel. Within a short time, the blood circulation in that area is increased. Herbs like yarrow and hawthorn strengthen and dilate blood vessels.

In Iran, people suffering from localized low blood circulation use hot baths with cinnamon and ginger on that particular area and massage the oil of eucalyptus and rosemary with olive oil for stimulation. Aromatherapy also stimulates poor circulation. A massage of the essential oils of rosemary, sage, neroli, and lemon indirectly stimulates and increases the circulation.

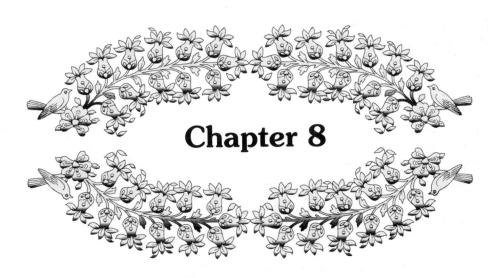

Chapter 8

The Urinary System and Herbs

Urinary System Disorders

The urinary system's main function is to produce and excrete urine, thereby controlling the body's water and chemical composition. Kidneys are the most important organs in this system. Without their constant work, the body would be poisoned by waste products. Therefore, kidneys also are responsible for the maintenance of overall health. Blood enters the kidneys and arteries and is then filtered out. The resulting fluid is conveyed to the ure-thra as urine.

The important material passing through the kidneys is reabsorbed and waste material excreted as urine. Valuable substances, like glucose and amino acids, are reabsorbed back into the bloodstream. About 98% percent of the water and nutrients are reabsorbed, and waste products, such as urea which is formed from the breakdown of protein, are passed into the urine and flushed out from the body. A healthy adult loses about 2 1/2 liters of water a day, 1 1/2 liters of which passes as urine. The remainder consists of moisture loss through bowel, perspiration, and breathing. Therefore, the kidneys' main responsibilities are regulation of water and salt, control of the acid/alkaline balance, and monitoring and increasing blood pressure.

Herbs for Urinary Disorders:

Herbs are not only beneficial for urinary disorders, but can also cleanse it. If kidneys function properly, the use of strong herbs is not necessary because they might stimulate and sloughs off the waste material throughout tissues and damage the kidneys. It is always wise to start by using gentle diuretic remedies which strengthen the kidneys and encourage effective debris excretion in the urine.

Herbs like prickly ash bark, rosemary, cough grass, and juniper are antiseptic and increase the flow of urine. If you suffer from kidney and urinary infections, herbs such as rosemary, couch grass, and juniper which contain volatile oils might be irritating. Therefore, do not take them during infections of kidneys or bladder. Drink plenty of water and herbal infusions of corn silk, horsetail, parsley, and goldenrod.

Bladder Infections

A bladder infection is caused by bacteria entering the bladder via the urethra. Inflammation is usually accompanied by a dull pain in the lower abdomen, the frequent urge to pass, a change of color in the urine to cloudy and reddish/orange due to pus or blood, and an unpleasant smell.

Cause: Cystitis (another word for bladder infection) is more common in women, especially pregnant women because the enlarged womb can press on the bladder. Because the urethra is shorter in women than men, access of bacteria to the bladder is easier. If bladder infections often happen to you, avoid using pantyhose as it stops the circulation of air, creating a moist environment that allows for the growth of bacteria.

These infections usually start with discomfort at the urethral opening and spread upward. They frequently happen in newly married women, and indeed, frequent sex can instigate the entrance of bacteria into the urethra of some women. These infections are usually caused by a bacterium called Escherichia coli, normally found in the bowel. Some people seem to have more Escherichia coli (bacteria native to colon) in their bowels than others, and because of bowel movements, these bacteria can potentially enter the urethral opening.

Treatment: If suffering from cystitis, take the following precautions:

After each bowel movement, make sure to wash the area with warm water.

Never use perfumed soap or deodorants. They can irritate the tissue of your urinary tract.

Always wear cotton underwear. Avoid pantyhose as it prevents air circulation and thereby dampens the area. Bacteria grow in dark, damp, and warm areas. Change your underwear everyday, and wash them with antibacterial soap instead of biological powders.

■ Avoid using internal tampons.

■ To fight cystitis, make your urine more acidic by drinking pure cranberry juice, two to three cups a day. Drink at least eight to ten glasses of water daily to help to clean the bladder. Avoid acidic and spicy foods, citrus fruit, peppers, and pickles which make the urine more alkaline.

■ Drink herbal infusions of boldo, buchu, bearberry, couch grass, horsetail, parsley, and marshmallow root, three to four cups a day.

■ Use comfrey and lavender ointments to soothe and prevent bruising of the vagina after intercourse.

■ Urinate within 15 minutes after each intercourse, and wash the area with warm water mixed with marigold. Urination flushes out germs which have passed into the urethra during sex.

■ During discomfort, heating packs of herbs like eucalyptus and rosemary can relieve and soothe the discomfort by disinfecting the area.

■ Make a massage oil of rosemary and eucalyptus, ten drops each, and add two tablespoons of olive or wheat germ oil, then massage the lower abdomen and back. In Iran, this technique is used to soothe menstrual and bladder pain and discomfort. They believe that massaging the essential of herbs containing volatile oil releases the pain and discomfort.

■ Diuretic herbal teas, like corn silk tea, are very useful. Drink five glasses a day, and eat the corn as well to release constipation and relieve the pain.

■ Other foods and herbs useful for cystitis sufferers are celery, fennel, and parsley. Take plenty of them fresh in a salad or use them in soup.

■ Infusions of barley and bargur, due to their cool energy and large amount of vitamin B complex, soothe and relax the area. Boil 4 oz of barley and bargur in 2 cups of water until cooked and tender. Strain, add a little honey, and drink several cups a day.

Herbal Remedy for Bladder Stones

Bladder stones are caused by increasing alkalinity in urine which results in crystallizing deposits that form into stones.

Cause: In an infection of the urinary tract, there can be trapped cellular debris, the presence of bacteria, and an increased alkalinity of the urine resulting in the deposition of phosphate, which forms a phosphate stone. The urine is more concentrated, causing formation of stones from urinary salts. Excessive uric acid can cause calcium excretion from kidneys into the urine which can also form into stones.

Treatment: The bladder has to flush excess salt out by the help of enough water.

■If suffering from bladder stone, drink at least ten glasses of water during the day and one before going to bed.

■To dissolve the stone, eat an alkaline vegetable and fruit diet.

■Do not eat citrus fruits as they make the environment acidic and irritated.

■Reduce protein from your diet since it tends to increase uric acid.

■The best remedy for bladder stone is RADISH JUICE. If you could drink at least 3 big glasses of radish juice every day, the stone and gravel would be crushed and released from bladder.

■Infusion of parsley, nettle, stone root, horsetail, agrimony, goldenrod, white birch, and gravel root, taken 5 cups a day, discharge stones through urine.

Herbal Remedy for Kidney Stone:

Lack of drinking enough water, thereby causing salt and materials to accumulate, can form stones in the kidneys.

Cause: Lack of water, unwashed fruits and vegetables, and tap water in some areas lead to the trapping of minerals, salts, and metals in the kidneys, especially if the kidneys do not have normal functioning.

Treatment: There are three different kind of kidney stones, i.e. uric acid stones, calcium oxalate stones, and calcium phosphate stones. If you have kidney stones, find out the type, then take the proper treatment for that particular stone.

Uric Acid Stones: As the urine is acidic, to dissolve these stones eat an alkaline diet of vegetables and potatoes (carbohydrate). Avoid eating any kind of meat especially liver, red meat, kidneys, fish, and sardines. Drink plenty of water everyday for better cleansing. Make sure to wash fruits and vegetables very well before eating. Take three to five cups of an infusion of at least 3 of herbs like parsley, fennel, horsetail, goldenrod, centaury, agrimony, nettle, marshmallow root, and gravel root everyday until the stone is gone.

Calcium Oxalate Stones: Those who have a tendency to form oxalate stones often secrete too much calcium in their urine which reacts with oxalic acid to form stones. To treat this kind of stone, avoid dairy products (which are rich in calcium), drink plenty of water, and drink mineral water rich in magnesium to increase the solubility of calcium. Avoid vegetables containing oxalates, such as parsley, spinach, beets, and rhubarb. Drink three to five cups of infusion made of at least 4 different kinds of herbs like agrimony, goldenrod, white birch, gravel root, marshmallow root, nettle and horsetail daily until the stone is dissolved.

Calcium Phosphate Stones: Calcium phosphate usually forms when there is an infection in the urine and the urine is alkaline. Eat foods such as red meat, liver, fish, eggs, and soybeans to acidify the urine. Drink plenty of water, and avoid dairy products. Drink three to five cups of an infusion consisting of at least two to three kinds of herbs like parsley, cough grass, corn silk, cleaver, marshmallow root, and gravel root everyday until the stone is dissolved.

To dissolve and flush all kinds of stones, take herbs like marshmallow root, gravel root, stone root, nettle, corn silk, cough grass, parsley piert, goldenrod, fennel, and horsetail. Goldenrod also helps to ease backache caused by kidney stones.

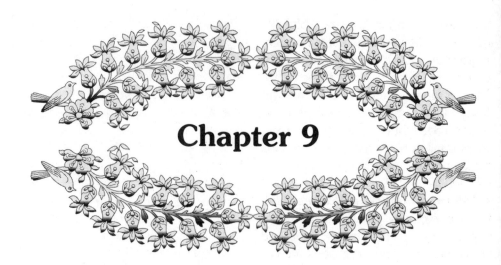

Chapter 9

The Reproductive System and Herbs

Herbal Remedies for Female Reproductive System

Since females have a complex and sensitive reproductive system, gentle herbal remedies are required. In Iran and Mediterranean countries, ever since the beginning of history, plant medicines have been used to reduce and prevent menstrual pains, prevent miscarriages, and delay menopause. Iranian use borage and valerian for menstrual pain. They make an infusion with rock candy and dried lemon peel and drink it as soon as the pain starts. They also massage warm olive oil, eucalyptus, rosemary, liquid rice pudding with butter and saffron to the low abdomen and low back to release excess gas and water. Ancient Egyptian and American Indian women used wild yam for its effects of easing menstrual pains and preventing miscarriages.

The female system operates on a 28 day cycle. The uterus prepares for pregnancy about two weeks after menstruation. That is the time when women ovulate and the uterus makes itself ready to receive the egg from the ovaries. If the egg is fertilized on its way to the womb after ovulation, pregnancy will occur. If fertilization of the egg does not occur, the cells which proliferated to thickly line the womb are sloughed off and menstruation occurs.

Chances of pregnancy depend on female body temperature and stability. If you want to increase the chances of pregnancy, have sexual intercourse from between the 11th day and the 14th day after the first day of your last period. Make sure that your body temperature is not low, that you are mentally relaxed, and that you and your partner take foods containing vitamins E (like peanuts), B6, and B12 as well as foods such as dates, nuts, wild yam, garlic, ginger and cinnamon that have warm energy. Wild yam and infusion of borage are also helpful.

Herbs to Reduce Menstrual Cramps and PMS

Many women experience excruciating pain during their menstrual period. This is common in young girls who have just begun to menstruate. Most women experience emotional and physical tensions like swollen legs and stomach, tender breasts, weight gain, pale skin, headaches, and insomnia a week before the period starts.

Scientists believe that hormonal imbalance between estrogen and progesterone (possibly high estrogen and low progesterone levels in the blood) a week before the period begins is the cause. The secretion of these ovarian hormones is under the control of the pituitary gland. Deficiency upsets the balance.

Herbal teas of marjoram, peppermint,

melissa, and thyme and warm energy infusions of ginger, cardamom, and honey can help to release excess gas and water which cause pain and discomfort. Iranians drink a very sweet warm liquid rice pudding, saffron, ginger, and honey, also adding egg yolk to it, three to four cups daily, with hot herbal infusion of peppermint and marjoram to release the pain and gas.

For PMS which can be related to emotional and mental stress syndromes, take substances which contain GLA (gamma linoleic acid), a precursor of a hormone called prostaglandin. Borage and evening primrose have been outstandingly successful in easing PMS. The body may produce the hormone when evening primrose and borage is taken.

Taking vitamin E, vitamin B6, calcium, and zinc is necessary for hormonal balancing before one's period.

Cramp Reduction: Painful periods or heavy cramps may possibly be the result of water retention, excess gas, heavy blood clots, or deficient flow. For painful periods associated with headaches, the following are some of the herbal remedies:

To treat painful cramps, take a herbal infusion like marjoram, peppermint, lemon verbena, tarragon, and juniper. Add plenty of honey with warm energy substances that contain alkaloid to release excess gas and water. Ginger and cardamom can be added too, since these two spices also have warm energy. If suffering from cramps, especially menstrual cramps, better take warm energy herbs and spices and warm energy foods to soothe the pain and discomfort and release the excess gas and swelling which cause pain.

■ Massage the lower abdomen and back with essential oils of eucalyptus, rosemary, and cypress to release the cramp tension, indirectly stimulate the hormonal glands, and normalize the secretion. There are certain essences in some plants that resemble female hormone. Herbs like cypress and tarragon have a chemical structure resembling that of ovarian hormones. They can also be used in baths, aromatherapy, and massaging the stomach. Herbal infusions or teas of sage, juniper, oregano, borage, and valerian with honey reduce menstrual tensions.

■ Avoid eating cold energy foods, fruits, and vegetables, especially onion, cabbage, pepper, radish, and spicy foods, during and a couple of days before your period starts in order to prevent more pain as these vegetables themselves can cause excess gas and water retention.

During the pain, try to lay on your stomach with a heating pad, and try to get a low back massage with essential oil of juniper, rosemary, and olive. This method can ease the flow of blood. Drink warm herbal teas of chamomile and crampbark.

Try to drink two to three cups of liquid rice pudding a day instead of solid food or vegetables. The recipe for liquid rice pudding is as follows:

1 cup of rice flour
1 cup of sugar or honey
4 cups of water
1/2 cup of olive oil or butter.
2 tablespoons of rosewater, or orange blossoms water.
2 eggs
1/8 teaspoon of grounded saffron and cardamom powder

In a large frying pan, roast the rice flour with butter or olive oil on a low fire for 15 to 20 minutes or until yellowish. In a separate dish, dissolve the sugar in water, and add saffron, cardamom powder and rosewater. Add this liquid to the fried flour. Now add the rest of the ingredients, and let it boil. If the pudding gets very thick, add more water. Before taking it off the stove, beat the eggs and add them to it. This pudding soothes and relieves menstrual cramps. The vitamin B6 in rice should give you energy and soothe the nerves that cause pain. Try two to four cups a day until the pain is eased.

To treat excessive or deficient flow related to menstrual cramps, make sure to use the above recipe and rest laying on your stomach. To treat a crampy period with excessive flow, take an infusion of a mixture of chamomile, lady's slipper, wild yam, and motherwort.

For treating the deficient flow type of menstrual cramps, use an infusion of a mixture of borage, valerian, motherwort, Chinese angelica, and false unicorn root.

If experiencing headache, try herbal infusions of valerian and vervain.

If your period is delayed, you may be pregnant, or if over forty, possibility menopausal. If neither, utilize an infusion of Chinese angelica, motherwort, and false unicorn, add ginger and honey, and drink three to five cups daily.

Pregnancy and Herbal Diet

During pregnancy you have a great responsibility to keep yourself physically, emotionally, and mentally in good shape for your baby's health and your health too. Remember that your baby eats just what you eat. Your treatment of yourself will affect your baby. You should relax mentally, emotionally and physically as much as possible. Smoking cigarettes, drinking alcohol, or using drugs that affect your baby's health must be stopped Four balanced meals and strolls must be included in each day, and you should get enough rest and sleep. Poor diet and lack of minerals or vitamins affects your baby's health as well.

During pregnancy, try to take addi-
tional dairy products and calcium everyday, as your child needs calcium for healthy bones and teeth.

Fish, protein, fruits, vegetables, fruit juices (like carrot, orange, and apple juice), grains (especially oats which are rich in vitamin B and minerals like calcium, iron, copper, zinc, magnesium, and silica), rice, and soybeans are very important ingredients to be included in daily diets.

Infusion of horsetail ,being a storehouse of minerals like silica, which helps the absorption and use of calcium, is very good for pregnant women. It helps in active bone and cartilage formation. Horsetail is also good for broken nails, white spots on nails, and lifeless hair, which are symptoms indicating calcium imbalance.

During the last three months of pregnancy, take raspberry tea to tone up the uterus muscles and ease childbirth. During the contractions, drink infusion of blue or black cohosh to strengthen contractions. Always consult your doctor before taking any herbal remedy during pregnancy.

Herbs for Miscarriages: No herbal medicine can be effective if you are in danger of a miscarriage because of the fetus being poorly developed. Consult your doctor. But if you are physically weak and think you might not be able to keep the pregnancy, take a rest, lift up your legs at least 2 hours a day, and take warm energy and relaxing herbs like skullcap, chamomile, peppermint, and melissa to relax your mind and body. Also, take infusions of wild yam, false unicorn, black haw, and evening primrose to strengthen the weakness and prevent miscarriage. Vitamins E and B6 are also helpful.

Herbs for Childbirth Pain: Take a 30 minute stroll everyday, especially during the last three months of pregnancy. Eight weeks before birth, take raspberry tea everyday, to help tone up the uterus muscles and ease childbirth.

Avoid eating too many sweets and fat foods. Drink enough water and chamomile tea during the contractions to help dilation. Try sipping a cold infusion of black cohosh or blue cohosh.

Consult your doctor before using these herbs.

Herbs for Breast Feeding: Many mothers seem to prefer to bottle feed their babies, often because their breasts do not produce enough milk, their nipples are cracked and wounded, or they work full-time and there is no opportunity to breast feed

Breast feeding is very beneficial for your baby's health, tones the uterine muscle faster, and puts the body back in shape faster. If your breasts do not produce enough milk, you should add a lot of green leafy vegetables, fresh fruit juices, milk, and dairy products to your diet. Take herbal drinks of fennel, goat's rue, blessed thistle, and parsley to increase the flow of milk and tone the uterine muscles. If your nipples are cracked and sore, apply fresh grated cucumber for 10 minutes, then apply comfrey or marigold ointment and massage to soothe and relax the nipple. Try to include parsley and fennel in your salads, or drink an infusion or tea of the above herbs everyday to increase the flow of milk. If you wish to dry your milk, try an infusion of sage.

In Iran, after childbirth, women try to breast feed the baby for at least nine months. They believe that breast feeding makes the baby physically, emotionally, and mentally stronger and healthier. Ancient Iranians believed that babies who were breast fed would have a healthy mind and be successful in their life. Nursing mothers should try to have a healthy diet by including herbs and foods that increase the flow and quality of their milk in order that their babies gets the best nutrition possible.

Herbs for Menopause: Menopause is a natural process that every woman must undergo at some time. It is a new phase of the life cycle. It generally occurs between the ages of 45 to 50, when women acquire new maturity, beauty, and self-awareness between their emotions and themselves. Some women experience this change with physical and emotional discomforts which usually lasts for a couple of years. They go through mental and emotional depression, hot flashes, skin dehydration, and insomnia.

In Iran, women start preparing themselves for menopause after the age of 50. They take extra vitamin B for mental and emotional depression and to prevent insomnia. As beets, barley, bargur, and oats are rich in vitamin B complex, they include barley soup with beet leaves in their daily diet. They take hot infusions of borage and valerian with honey and have full body massages with essential oils of sage, rosemary, and chamomile everyday, and drink sage and jasmine tea, if having hot flashes.

You can minimize the discomfort of menopause by doing regular exercise, eating four balanced meals, and getting plenty of water daily. Some women experience health problems, related to the drop of estrogen and progesterone, in the form of hot flashes, chills, depression, and skin dehydration. These symptoms are due to hormonal imbalance. To balance the hormones, take infusions of wild yam, false unicorn root, black and blue cohosh, and licorice. Vitamin E can also help in balancing the hormones.

■ If you have hot flashes, drink sage and nettle tea. Sage has an estrogen property that makes it useful treatment.

■ If your skin is dry, try vitamin E oil mixed with lavender and jojoba oil to moisturize the skin.

■ If you have depression during menopause, drink tea of borage, lemon balm, and rosemary, and add these herbs to your cooking along with wild oats. Borage contains a high percentage of gamma linoleic acid (GLA) that helps depression. Borage also brings the feelings of cheer and courage.

■ If you have physical tension, try rosemary and lavender oil in your bathtub with a tablespoon of baking soda to release all the physical tension and stimulate the muscles.

■ If you are emotionally depressed, boil sage in hot water and let the steam linger in your home. Sage can cheer the spirit and provide positive energy around you. You can also burn it in the fire place or on the stove.

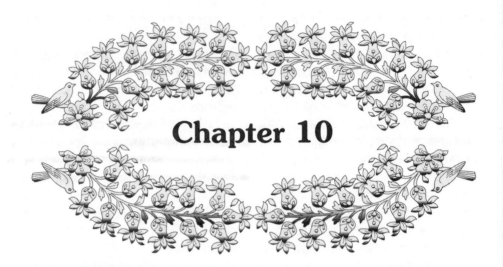

Chapter 10

The Nervous System and Herbs

Herbs for Nervous Systems:

The nervous tension of today's life with its pressures and stresses is manifested in mental, emotional, and psychological problems. There is a relationship between the human mind and body evident in the nervous system.

The human nervous system is made up of nerve cells called neurons. Neurons consist of a long fiber called an axon. The nerves are bundles of axons, which transmit messages, enabling the processing of information received from outside. The two main parts of the nervous system are called the central nervous system (the brain and spinal cord) and the peripheral nervous system, consisting of voluntary and involuntary systems.

There are two kinds of peripheral nerves, i.e., sensory and motor nerves. Sensory nerves send the sensory information to the spinal cord and brain, and motor nerves send the information from the brain to the body. Therefore, the spinal cord and brain process the information received from the peripheral system.

There are also sympathetic and parasympathetic nervous systems. The sympathetic nervous system prepares us to react to danger. As we sense danger, the sympathetic nervous system sends messages to the digestive system that reduce digestive activities and stop saliva flow. The mouth dries, the heart beats faster, skin becomes pale and cold as blood is withdrawn to feed the muscles, and sweat glands start secretion. In contrast, the parasympathetic nervous system acts to redress the balance by slowing the heartbeat, relaxing the muscles, and normalizing the body temperature.

Today, the tensions and stresses of modern life with the damaging effects of food processing and medication have caused more complications and sicknesses in the human body and nervous system. Fortunately, there are many herbal remedies, that stand as symbols of a natural and healthy way of life. Many herbs directly act on the nervous system to relieve the stress of life.

Make an infusion with at least 3 herbs like chamomile, passion flower, valerian, crampbark, and mugwort before going to bed to relax central nervous system. Herbs containing volatile oil can directly affect the limbic system of the brain via the olfactory organs.

Aromatherapy is another alternative to relax the nervous system. Essential oil of chamomile and rose calm the nerves. You can also take hot baths with essential oil of melissa, orange, and rose and burn candles made with essential oils of rose and lavender to relax your nerves. Full body massage with essential oils of lavender, rose, and

orange can help to relieve the nerves.

Restorative herbs such as vervain, skullcap, wild oat, ginseng, and echinacea are useful when your nervous system is down, for example, after a long illness. Echinacea not only helps to restore your relaxation, but also enhances the immune system, by increasing white cells against certain bacteria. Make a herbal infusion with echinacea root, ginseng root, and skullcap. Add honey, and drink 2 cups before sleeping. Avoid spicy foods, coffee, cola, and tea as these foods stimulate nervous tension.

Herbs for Migraines and Headaches: Migraines are one of the most common diseases of the nervous system. They are more common in women than men. They are usually in the form of a one-sided headache caused by sudden vascular changes in the brain. Sometimes swollen arteries on the face and head can be seen. Severe migraines are often accompanied by vomiting and nausea.

Migraine headaches can be due to hormonal imbalance (in which case it happens during or before periods), heredity, or stress. Sometimes accidents, trauma, or certain allergies to foods (like cheese, chocolate, egg, vinegar, and wine) cause migraine headaches.

In Iran, people who suffer from migraines get a massage of vinegar, salt, and olive oil on their temples and neck to reduce the tension. A hot infusion of skullcap and peppermint with rock candy is also helpful. Feverfew has always been used for migraine. People who suffer from migraines should eat substantial amounts of carbohydrates like potatoes, steamed rice, bread, and beans. Carbohydrate is converted to sugar, which feeds the brain.

If suffering from migraines, take fresh leaves of feverfew with other leaves like nettle and dandelion in your salad or sandwich to control the severity of the attacks. As soon as the first symptoms appear, infuse basil in hot water and drink. If your migraine is due to a hormonal imbalance, drink infusion of skullcap, passion flower, peppermint and chamomile with honey. Also take an infusion of feverfew, rosemary, vervain, and valerian. Add honey. Drink three to five cups until the pain is gone.

Avoid taking any kind of cola, coffee, tea, chocolate, hard cheese, alcohol, fruits (like orange and banana), and egg. Try to eat a large variety of vegetables and carbohydrates, and exercise regularly.

Herbs for Depression: Depression is a condition that may affect people at times, but it can become a serious illness. There are many causes (like job loss, loss of lover, death of a family member, etc.) for depression. Physical tension can increase depression.

If you are suffering from depression, find out the causes. If due to physical tension, upper body massage with essential oil of lavender or citric herbs can help to cheer the spirit, counter physical exhaustion, and strengthen and support the nervous system. Orange, neroli, marjoram, lavender, and melissa oils can help balance the nervous system. You can also eat these herbs with your salad or take as hot tea, drinking three to five cups daily. A hot bath with lavender and melissa helps in relieving physical and mental stress. A stuffed pillow with lavender helps relaxation.

Herbs like wild oats, ginseng, vervain, and skullcap are other herbal remedies for physical nervousness or physical depression. If your spirit is down, take herbs like sage, borage, St. John's wort, and lemon balm to cheer you.

Regular exercise and balanced diet are needed to help depression. Sometimes chemical or hormonal imbalances can cause depression. In the case of chemical imbalance, check with your doctor to find the problem. In the case of hormonal imbalance, try infusion of false unicorn root, sage, motherwort, borage, and evening primrose.

Aromatherapy with essential oils of orange, bergamot, sage, jasmine, and rose taken as a massage or in a bath are other alternatives.

Herbs for Anxiety: Anxiety can be

called "fears spread thin," in that, there is the experience of a lack of well being and a feeling of powerlessness. Anxiety is becoming increasingly common in today's lifestyles and society. It can also be the result of excessive demand of physical and mental energy that can lead to illness if the body's tolerance is low. Everybody differs in their reaction to physical and mental stresses. Some can cope with the high demands of life, while others reach their limits and react right away. It all depends on their physical resistance. Those who react right away get stress headaches, insomnia, digestive problems, and eating disorders. Take vitamin B complex everyday to increase physical and mental resistance to the pressures of life.

Since stress reduces the body's general resistance to infection, people under stress are susceptible to different illnesses, like colds, flu, and bronchitis. This, in turn, affects the health of the skin by interfering with levels and interactions of hormones. Taking extra vitamin C and antioxidants is very necessary to resist the attacks of bacteria and viruses.

Herbal Treatment: Herbs such as chamomile, valerian, hop, lime flower, lady slipper, passion, and skullcap restore and relax both the central and sympathetic nervous systems. Herbs like wild oat, skullcap, and vervain strengthen and support the nervous system. Massages of essential oils of lavender, rose, and orange reduce the stress. Take a warm bath with few drops of relaxing essences like lavender, basil, marjoram, ylang ylang, and sage.

To avoid insomnia, drink hot milk with honey or a hot herbal tea of skullcap, chamomile and mint to tranquilize and induce sleep. Regular exercise and meditation can help in relieving anxiety.

Herbs for Insomnia: Insomnia means not being able to sleep. There are many causes for insomnia, such as mental stress, depression, and anxiety. Other causes may be lifestyle, high tension, or lack of physical activity. Therefore, while the body is still full of energy, stimulants like smoking, alcohol or eating late in the evening can cause insomnia. Taking a nap during the day can shorten sleep at night. If your life is happy, regular exercise and meditation can help to calm a stressed nervous system. Avoid eating spicy foods, heavy meals, or caffeine before bedtime. Better avoid taking drugs, alcohol, tranquilizers, and sleeping pills for insomnia as they can undermine your general health.

Herbal remedies are safe with no side effects. Sedative herbs, like ginseng root and oats, are effective for sleep, especially for people suffering from nervous tension and fatigue. Herbal infusions of passion flower, skullcap, hops, lavender, and chamomile are effective against insomnia. Lavender bath helps to relax physical stress and overcome insomnia. Fill up your bathtub with fresh lavender, let it sit for few minutes and soak your body in it for at least 20 minutes. Listen to soft music or visualize a waterfall or ocean sound. Massage your body, especially the upper body and feet with essential oil of lavender, olive oil, or wheat germ oil to treat the physical and mental depression and exhaustion. Stop taking stimulants like tea, coffee, cigarettes, cola, and alcohol after five o'clock in the evening.

Fatigue

Most of the time, fatigue results from muscular pain after exercise, insomnia, or heavy sessions of mental work and emotional stress. Hormonal changes can also cause fatigue. Usually pregnant and menopausal women as well as children undergoing puberty suffer from fatigue.

In Iran, people who work hard for long hours everyday get upper body massages and foot baths with essential oils of rose and rosemary together with steam to release physical tension for a good night's sleep. When physically and emotionally fatigued, full body massage is also very popular. They usually stay in a steamed sauna and get full body massage with essential oils of lemon, orange, and orange blossom. Or they can drink a hot infusion of skullcap, peppermint, chamomile, fennel and rose, get a massage, wrap

themselves with warm towel, and go to bed. In case of fatigue due to hormonal changes, they drink an infusion or hot herbal tea of chamomile, lavender, sage, evening primrose, and borage, If fatigue is due to puberty, evening primrose and borage herbal tea is very effective. Usually substantial amounts of mucopolysaccharides and mucoproteins are added to the diet. These herbs protect cells against the invasion of bacteria, viruses, and fungi. The body slows down production of mucopolysaccharides at puberty, therefore, mucopolysaccharides from foods such as deep sea cold water fish, seaweed, and aloe vera juice must be supplemented during puberty.

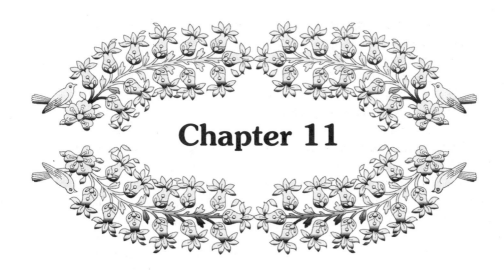

Chapter 11

Herbs for the Head and Neck

Herbs for Common Cold:

Common colds are caused by contagious viral infections normally affecting the nose and throat, causing coughs and sneezes. Its general symptoms are sneezing, mild fever, muscle pain, heavy eyes, sore throat, and headache. Colds are common during the winter or extreme changes of temperature. If bacteria invades vulnerable parts, colds can lead to sinusitis or bronchitis.

In Iran, during the coldest months of October through February, eucalyptus and sage are steamed in homes to keep the air clean and disinfected. Every afternoon steamed turnip, beets, and carrots are taken as antioxidants. Turnips contain antibiotic properties. They also drink hot herbal teas of echinacea, lavender, and marjoram after each meal to enhance their immune systems. For breakfast, banana shake with milk, honey, banana, almonds, walnuts, peanuts, dates, egg yolk and carrot juice is taken to give them energy, strength, and mental relaxation all day.

If suffering from a cold, herbal and natural remedies not only help in regaining your health but also have no side effects. Drugs or antibiotics can destroy bacteria outside cells, but they cannot touch the cold virus. Usually bacteria or viruses attack at the time when the body has a low vitality and immune system and cannot fight back. Chemical imbalance, vitamin deficiency during stress, depression, and fatigue also lower the immune system.

Colds run their course. Herbal infusions of echinacea and ginseng can help to restore vitality and deficiencies and also prevent infection. Aromatherapeutic oils can help keep cold germs at bay, prevent infection, and ease symptoms. Foods containing vitamin C are also useful.

As soon as you see the signs of cold, try an infusion of one half teaspoon of fresh or dried ginger, 2 lemons, 5 cloves, and 16 oz of water. Boil the water, add the ingredients, and simmer for 15 minutes. Add one tablespoon of honey, and drink it frequently. Echinacea tea also has a stimulating effect on immune defenses.

Try to have antioxidant fruits and vegetables, like carrot juice or orange juice, and lots of liquids especially if you have a viral cold. Get enough rest, and drink at least ten glasses of water, fruit juices, and liquid food, like chicken soup, each day. Drink at least three bowls of chicken soup containing lots of vegetables like onion, turnip, garlic, potatoes, carrots, celery, and tomatoes. Add lemon juice to taste.

Herbs for Sinus Headaches:

Headaches can have many causes such as flu, cold, neck tension and eyestrain. You should be able to know the exact cause and act accordingly. Some women suffer headaches during or before their menstrual periods. Sometimes headache is the result of sinusitis.

There are air-containing cavities in the skull called sinuses, which are lined with mucous membranes. When we have a cold, the nasal passages, lined with mucous membrane, react to the virus by producing mucus. This is the time when inflammation or chronic pain occurs. Overproduction of mucus causes pain and pressure across the face, temples, and around the eyes. Chronic sinusitis is usually accompanied with headache.

Keep your head and sinus area warm, and drink herbal infusions of bayberry, ephedra, eyebright, and echinacea to soothe the sinuses and release the excess mucus. Herbs like rosemary, pine, and marjoram with lemon reduce the production of mucus.

If sinus pressure comes from a virus, you should have a diet of vitamin C, garlic, onion, and turnip. Turnip contains natural antibiotics. The best remedy is to make a soup of 32 oz of chicken broth, two large onions, five cloves of garlic, five large turnips, two potatoes, and one cup of chopped cabbage. Boil all the ingredients in chicken broth for 30 minutes. Make sure to add fresh lemon juice. Before having the soup, do inhalations to clear the catarrh in the sinus. In a pot, pour two cups of boiling water and five fresh eucalyptus leaves or 10 drops of euca-lyptus oil, and let it boil. Inhale the steam, and massage your sinuses with eucalyptus oil for about seven to ten minutes after you have finished with vapor steaming. Cover your head and sinuses with a big towel to keep it warm, then eat your prepared soup and go to bed. Repeat this until the pain is gone. Otherwise, drink an in-fusion of hot lemon, peppermint, and fresh ginger, three to five cups a day to reduce the mucus production.

Onion is another remedy. Either eat raw onions to make you tear and help clear the mucus, or get onion juice and pour 1-2 drops in your nasal area. It might be discomforting, but it clears the sinuses and reduces inflammation.

Avoid eating dairy products, especially milk and cheese, chocolate, caffeine, eggs, and greasy foods that cause over-production of mucus.

For aromatherapeutic treatment, mas-sage essential oil of melissa, sage, rose-mary, and lavender with acupressure around the back of the neck, temples, and around the eyes. Also make a heat-producing ointment of a few drops of juniper or eucalyptus essen-tial oil to two tablespoons of grapeseed oil and massage it.

Herbs like ephedra, elder, rosemary, lavender, sage, thyme, and mint con-tain volatile oil and antibiotics and are ideal to treat sinus or upper body com-plications. Make an infusion of these herbs, add fresh lemon juice, and drink it hot ,three to four cups a day. Herbs like bayberry, mullein leaf, eyebright, ephedra, and agrimony contain tannins, which tone the mucous mem-branes. Herbs like fenugreek seed or leaf contain lecithin, which softens and dissolves hardened masses of accumu-lated mucus and disinfects the lungs. Herbs like marshmallow root relieve irritation of mucous membranes. All above recommendations would un-block nasal congestion caused by colds and reduce inflammation and discom-fort from sinus.

Herbs for Earache:

Since the ear is a very delicate organ, it may cause problems in many differ-ent ways. Earache is very common in young children and often due to colds, sinusitis, or flu.

If suffering from earache, strengthen immunity to infections by eating a wholesome diet with plenty of fruits and vegetables, such as hot turnip soup with plenty of garlic, onion, thyme, and lemon juice. Include extra vitamins and minerals (especially vitamin C and zinc). Avoid foods that produce mu-cus, such as milk products, chocolate, and artificial sweets.

Gargle with an infusion of sage, salt, and fresh lemon juice three or four times a day, and drink warm lemon drink. Take herbal infusions of echinacea, St. John's wort, and ginseng everyday to enhance the immune system. Take infusions of pasque flower, hyssop, chamomile, and mint.

Have your doctor ensure the integrity of the eardrums and the diagnosis. Be sure to check with your doctor about the use of herbal drops like the one made of 10 drops of tincture of eucalyptus oil, 20 drops of tincture of pasque flower, 5 drops of sage, and 1 oz of pure almond oil. If allowed, shake it well, and use 2 drops in the ear three to four times a day. You can also massage the side, front, and back of ears and neck with eucalyptus oil.

In Iran, they use cigarette smoking in the ear to reduce the inflammation and release the pain. They make cigarettes with colftsfoot, lavender, and eucalyptus and smoke it into ears. Coltsfoot contains tannin that reduces inflammation, and eucalyptus and lavender are antibacterial and antiseptic, which reduces the pain.

Herbs for Coughs:

Coughs can be symptoms of a variety of diseases. They can be associated with asthma, bronchitis, hay fever, flu, sore throat, and sinusitis, Coughs are commonly caused by colds. After finding out the type of cough, herbal remedies can then be chosen to clear and ease the cough. Coughs from the chest may produce white, yellow, or green phlegm.

An infusion of herbs like quince seed, slippery elm bark, and starch soothes the throat and coughs. Simmer two tablespoons of quince seed with 16 oz. of hot water for 15 minutes until water becomes starchy. Drink the water and seeds together. Marshmallow root powder and slippery elm also have the same effects on coughs. Add one cup of slippery elm root and marshmallow root with 3 cups of boiling water or low fat milk. Stir until thick. Add honey, and drink two to four cups daily. Herbal gargles help in killing the bacteria in the throat and reducing the inflammation. Add 1/2 cup of sage to 3 cups of boiling water, and let it simmer. Add salt and lemon, and gargle four to six times daily. Sage, which is antibacterial and antiseptic, soothes the discomfort.

Herbal infusions of sage, coltsfoot, lobelia, horehound, and licorice also expel the phlegm. Turnip (contains natural penicillin), garlic, and onion are antibiotics and recommended. Make a turnip soup by adding onion, garlic, rosemary, and cilantro. Take three to four cups daily with lemon to soothe the irritation. Another remedy is hot starch pudding. Dissolve two tablespoons of rice starch in 16 oz. of cold water. Heat, and stir until starchy. Add some honey and drink it hot to soothe the irritated throat and cough. If the coughs continue for more than a week, consult a physician.

Herbs for Sore Throat:

Sore throat can be caused by cold, flu, bronchitis, tonsillitis, or other viral or bacterial infections and by allergies to certain foods, dust, and pollens.

If sore throat is the result of bacterial infection and cold, do the following:

Gargle with infusion of sage, salt, and lemon juice, three to five times daily to kill the bacteria and soothe the inflammation. A recipe to make sage gargle is as follows:

I teaspoon of sage
1 teaspoon of rosemary
1 cup of boiling water
1 tablespoon of salt
2 tablespoon of fresh lemon juice

Bring the water to a boil, and add herbs make an infusion. Gargle four to six times daily to soothe sore throats.

Steam a turnip, salt it, and have it hot. Turnip contains antibiotics that fight infections and reduce inflammation and discomfort.

To disinfect the throat, take raw onion and garlic either with bread or plain. Chew the onion and let the juice spray in your throat. Also take onion soup made from chicken broth, onion, garlic, and turnip. Drink it hot with fresh lemon juice.

Take herbal infusions, including three or four of horehound, balm mint, ephedra, lobelia, mullein, elder flower, golden seal, coltsfoot, and blood root, to stop sore throat and release the tension and inflammation. Flax seed and slippery elm are also great remedies for sore throat.

Herbs for Laryngitis:

Laryngitis is an inflammation of the voice box, or larynx, that can be the result of a viral or bacterial infection. It causes a painful and dry throat, often with mucus, which usually is associated with a loss of voice. Laryngitis can happen to those who work in a dry, dusty atmosphere.

In this case, you need to gargle three to five times a day, and take steam inhalation of eucalyptus and sage leaves. Place a few leaves of each in 2 cups of water, and let it boil. Place a large towel over your head, and do steam inhalation for at least 10 minutes, twice a day. For gargle, place two teaspoons of salt in two cups of water. Add a few leaves of sage and simmer for 10 minutes. Drain, add salt, and gargle three to five times a day.

Herbal infusions of horehound, balm mint, elder flower, and rice starch drink three cups a day, soothe the irritation. To make rice starch drink, dissolve two tablespoons of rice starch in 16 oz. of cold water, heat, and stir until starchy. Add some honey and drink hot to soothe the irritated throat. Vitamin B contained in rice starch soothes the throat.

Herbs for Tonsillitis:

Tonsils are glands of lymph tissue located on each side of the back of the throat. Tonsillitis is an inflammation of the tonsils. It can be the result of viral or bacterial infections when the body has low resistance after a cold or flu or has a diet that is less nutritional and low in protein. The symptoms are fever, redness and swelling in the back of mouth, headache, and difficulty in swallowing due to enlarged lymph glands. Tonsillitis usually happens during childhood, and tonsils can be removed.

To prevent tonsillitis infection, especially in winter, gargle with a hot infusion of sage and horehound, four to five times a day. Rice starch is to be taken four to five times a day, and flax seeds soaked in hot water taken as a drink two times a day. To make the infusion, simmer sage in 2 cups of water for 20 minutes, strain, and add salt.

Fever

Fever is an abnormally high body temperature and can occur in both adults and children. A high temperature can be due to physical overexertion, but in adults, fever usually is associated with bacterial or viral infections, such as bronchitis, colds, flu, sinus infections, or tonsillitis.

Symptoms of fever, other than high temperature, are shivering and chills. All these symptoms mean that the body is fighting the infection.

In the case of fever, do not take solid foods for a couple of days. Avoid sour or citrus fruits; instead, replace these solid foods with pure cool water and pure fresh juices (especially watermelon juice). Get cold water and peppermint foot wash every two to three hours until the body temperature returns to normal.

After a couple of days, drink plenty of chicken soup with carrot juice for extra minerals. The body loses a substantial amount of minerals and vitamins during fever. Take steamed rice with fresh rosemary or more carbohydrates. Drink plenty of herbal tea made of chamomile, rosemary, yarrow, lavender, and lemon grass, and sweeten it with honey. Drink five to six cups a day. Massage wheat germ and rosemary oil on the temples and soles of feet.

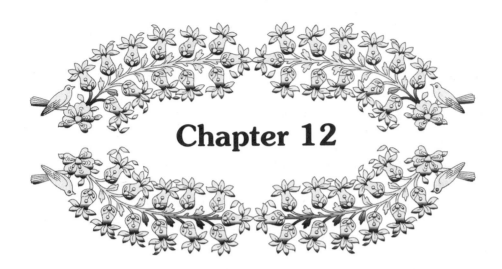

Chapter 12

The Respiratory System and Herbs

Herbs for Asthma:

Temporary constriction of small bronchial airways causes asthma, which is usually associated with shortness of breath, choking , and coughing. Many asthmatics are allergic to various foods, plants, feathers, pollens, dust, animal hair, fur, perfumes or chemical fumes, etc. They should avoid using essential oils, if allergic to them. Inhalation of essential oils may worsen an asthma attack. Try to discover the cause of the allergy. Avoid pets, if possible. Remove dust harboring curtains and carpets, feathers in pillows, and vacuum clean daily. Avoid household chemicals and perfumes.

Avoid stimulants such as coffee and chocolate. Replace them with an herbal tea of marjoram, rosemary and sage, made by adding one ounce of fresh or dried herbs to 16 oz. of boiling water. Infuse for twenty minutes, and drink two or three cups per day, especially during times of asthmatic exacerbation. Herbs like horehound, ephedra, lobelia, mullein, red clover, and coltsfoot relax the bronchi and expel the mucus; chamomile, lime flower, hops, and skullcap support the nervous system; licorice soothes the expectoration, supports adrenal glands, and provides natural cortisone against stress; and infusion of borage or evening primrose soothes respiration and strengthens the function of the adrenal glands.

If asthmatic, avoid smoking and drinking alcohol. Try to get daily exercise like walking, swimming, and yoga. Check whether you are sensitive to any food; it is wise to exclude eggs, dairy products, greasy foods, and preserved fruits containing sulfur dioxide. Carry your emergency inhalers.

Herbs for Bronchitis: Bronchitis is an inflammation of the larger air passages. There are two kinds of bronchitis: one can occur acutely after viral or bacterial infections such as colds, and the other, i.e., chronic bronchitis, is caused by long standing irritation of lining of the bronchi through smoking or living in dusty or fumed environments. Bronchitis is accompanied with constant coughing to dislodge the bacteria and by mucus blocking swollen bronchi, phlegm production, fever, and chest pain.

To treat bronchitis, drink plenty of fluids, especially fresh lemon and pineapple juices and hot herbal tea. Herbal healing of the illness is comprised of two parts.

Part One:
Use herbal infusions of eucalyptus leaves, hyssop, ephedra, elder, horehound, lobelia, mullein, mint, pine bud, and rosemary. Eucalyptus, hyssop, and bay are expectorant and soothe the lungs.

To make a good tea for bronchitis, boil 16 oz of water, add 1/2 cup of eucalyptus, clover and horehound. Leave it to steep for at least five minutes, then strain, add fresh lemon juice, and drink it hot. Tea made from marshmallow root and leaves and lavender is also beneficial.

Massage the chest with 1 tablespoon of wheat germ oil, 10 drops of eucalyptus oil, and 5 drops of oregano oil.

Part Two:
Take a herbal inhalation of eucalyptus and pine. Boil fresh eucalyptus and pine leaves in 3 cups of water, and inhale the steam for at least 15 minutes. Repeat three to four times a day.

Make an infusion with three to four kinds of herbs like hyssop, horehound, red clover, mullein, ephedra, comfrey, elder flower, bladder wrack, and skunk cabbage, which causes sweating.

Pour soothing herbs like comfrey and marshmallow root in boiling water. Simmer for 15 minutes, strain, add cardamom powder or ginger, and drink three to four cups daily. Licorice also soothes the bronchi.

Turnip soup is also a great remedy for bronchi. To 3 cups of chicken broth, add fresh turnip, onion, garlic, potatoes, thyme, and barley flakes. Cook for 30 minutes. Add lemon juice to taste, and drink it hot three to four times daily.

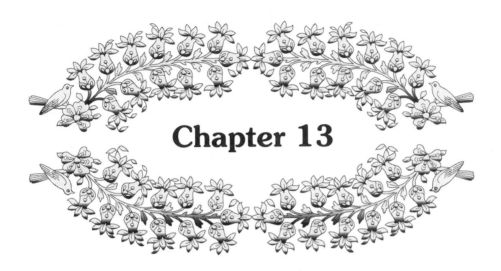

Chapter 13

The Musculoskeletal System and Herbs

Herbs for Arthritis:

Arthritis is an inflammation and stiffness of the joints, accompanied by pain, and discomfort.

There are many causes to arthritis. In woman, it usually occurs after the menopause, when her estrogen level drops causing a calcium decline in the bone.

There are different kind of arthritis. The most common ones are as follows:

Osteoarthritis:
Is a disease that causes the breakdown of joint tissue called cartilage, leading to joint pain and stiffness. Osteoarthritis is chronic, which means it lasts a long time and won't go away, and it usually begins after age 40. Osteoarthritis can affect any joint but often occur in finger, knees, feet, spine, and hips. Dietary measures are important in treating this kind of arthritis to repair the bone and cartilage.

Treatment: Exercise, Meditation, weight loss, heat massage, and herbal remedy.

Rheumatoid arthritis: Involves inflammation in the lining of the joints and/or other internal organs. Typically affects many different joints. It can wear away at the bone and cause loss of the synovial fluid, which lubricates the joints. This inflammation of the joints can cause intense pain and restrict movement. The symptoms are swelling and pain in the joints, fatigue, and weight loss.

Treatment: Exercise, rest, hot herbal compress, and herbal remedy.

Gouty arthritis:
This kind of arthritis is caused by accumulation of uric acid crystallized in the joints and is accompanied by pain. Typically affects many different joints.

Treatment: Exercise, herbal massage, herbal tea that contain salicylic acid such as devil's claw, and white birch. Salicylic acid eliminate uric acid deposit from the joints.

Dietary Recommendation:
Proper diet for all kind of arthritis is recommended.

1- (Exclude red meat, citrus, and sour fruits, foods containing oxalic acid like rhubarb that can cause painful joints, and coffee.)

2- Plenty of drinking water, especially mineral water. Maintain high level of calcium intake, especially if you are post menopausal woman.

3- Herbal remedy: The best herbal remedy for all kind of arthritis is devil's claw, which have anti-inflammatory properties compared to cortisone and a great reputation for treating arthritis. Take infusion of devil's claw, blue cohosh, black cohosh sarsaparilla, dandelion, nettle, white willow, ginger, and cardamon 3-4 cups daily for 6-8 weeks. If you are under stress add herbs such as skullcap, borage, and valerian to

release tention.

Herbal massage for all kinds of arthritis is recommended. Herbs that are stimulating and contain essential oil such as eucalyptus, rosemary and juniper are ideal to be mixed with olive oil and massage in the joint. Repeat 4-5 times a week.

Herbs for backache:

There are many different reasons for backache, such as wrong posture, muscle tension, or kidney or urinary infections. The cause of any backache must be established before any treatment can be undertaken. For example, in the case of sudden pain, lifting heavy items might have been the origin of the pain.

If suffering from backache, avoid lifting heavy weights, standing for a long period of time, and wearing high heel shoes which tilt the body off balance. Flat feet or having a slight difference between the length of your legs can also put the body off balance

Sometimes an infection in the body, like a cold or flu, can attack the back. Getting a tension reduction massage with olive, eucalyptus, and rosemary oils stimulates and relaxes muscle spasms. Sometimes backaches come from poor circulation. In that case, massage with cayenne pepper and crampbark. To soothe muscles, use lavender and chamomile. For spinal pain, use St. John's wort oil. If kidneys are weak, take an infusion of horsetail, bearberry, and Parsley.

Nutrition Reference Guide

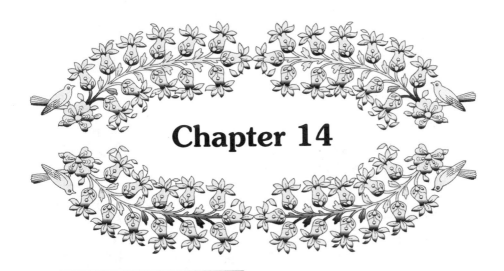

Chapter 14

Vitamins and Their Functions

itamins and minerals are nutrients that are essential to life and the health of human body. Each of the vitamins are present in varying quantities in specific foods and each is absolutely necessary for proper growth and maintenance of health.

Vitamins function with chemicals called enzymes, which are of two types, protein molecules and coenzymes. Enzymes are the foundation of the body, help in digesting foods, and are responsible for oxidation. Oxidation begins when oxygen enters the bloodstream and is trans-

ported to the cells where oxidation actually occurs. Then the wastes are removed via the lungs and urine. Without enzymes we could not breath, walk, see, feel, smell, or taste foods and the body could not break proteins into essential amino acids.

Enzymes are activators of chemical reactions, and vitamins are a fundamental part of enzymes. If you have vitamin deficiency, the enzymes for that particular vitamin will not be activated. A poorly nourished cell may actually have many enzymes without the proper (vitamin) coenzymes. Since the enzyme is low, the cell will continue functioning at a reduced rate. If proper nourishment is not received, the cell will die, affecting other organs. The signs may take weeks or months to appear. For example, particular enzymes require vitamin B6 to be activated to transmit nerve impulses to fingers. If vitamin B6 is deficient, this enzyme will not be activated and one might feel some numbness in the fingers. Vitamins are of two types: water-soluble, like vitamins B and C, and fat-soluble, like vitamins E, A, K, and D .

Antioxidant Vitamins: Vitamins A, C, and E are antioxidant or anti-free radical, protecting against nitrosamine. In polluted areas, vitamin A (beta carotene) and vitamin C lower the risk of cancer. There are many hazards that interfere with digestion and absorption of nutrients.

Beta Carotene (Vitamin A)

In the family of carotenes there are three compounds which are alpha and beta carotene and cryptoxanthene, found in corn and papaya. Beta carotene, also known as carotenide compound, is prevalent in fruits of yellow or orange color, such as peach, apricot, carrot, cantaloupe, pumpkin, banana, and sweet potatoes. Green leafy vegetables (those containing chlorophyll) are those such as spinach, turnip, and parsley. Both alpha and beta carotene are later converted during absorption into vitamin A in the liver and small intestines. Long time dosage of beta carotene, in contrast to vitamin A, has no side effect on the liver. Some research indicates that beta carotene is anti-carcinogenic. Beta carotene can be destroyed by heat, light, and air. It is susceptible to oxidation, so try to drink carrot juice right after it is squeezed. It not only helps in curing cancer, but also prevents possible susceptibility to cancer.

Spinach	8100	I.U
Papaya	1700	I.U
Parsley	8500	I.U
Beets leaves	5100	I.U
Cantaloupe	3400	I.U
Pumpkin	3700	I.U
Red bell pepper	21600	I.U
Apricot	2700	I.U
Persimmon	2700	I.U
Peach	1400	I.U
Turnip leaves	7600	I.U

The amount of daily recommended consumption for adults is between 3000-7000 I.U.

Vitamin A: Vitamin A is a fat-soluble vitamin that occurs in two forms, performed vitamin A and pro vitamin A (carotene). Performed vitamin A is concentrated only in certain tissues of animals. One of the richest sources of performed vitamin A is fish liver oil and yellow butter. Pro vitamin A (carotene) must be converted into vitamin A before it can be used. Carotene is abundant in carrot and green leafy vegetables, like spinach, dandelion, broccoli, and beet greens.

Vitamin A improves one's resistance to infection, promotes cell growth, and is essential for eyes and for treating acne and skin disorders. Vitamin A is an antioxidant, works against the development and spread of cancer, and protects cells against free radical damage that leads to cancer. Studies show that in the case of chemotherapy for breast cancer blood with high levels of vitamin A responds twice as well against toxicity of drugs than blood at a lower level. Dr. Alex Sakula (1976) announced the results of his experiments in Red Hill Hospital, England on cancer patients. He stated that in 28 patients suffering from lung cancer, the vitamin A level in their blood was less than normal. Food sources of vitamin A are butter, fish oil, cod liver oil, fish, chicken, beef liver, eggs, and dairy products. In 1982, the U.S. National Academy of Sciences established the relationship between cancer and daily diet. Dr. Bjeike (1975) reported on 8,278 cases of male smokers where 74% had lung cancer. Out of these, a third were those consuming the least amount of vitamin A. He states that smokers need greater amounts of vitamin A in their daily diet in order to prevent cancer.

The primary area of absorption and storage of vitamin A is in the upper intestinal tract, where the fat splitting enzymes and bile salts convert carotene into a useable nutrient.

Approximately 90 percent of the body's vitamin A is stored in the liver, and there is a small amount in lungs, kidneys, fat tissues, and retinas. The body will use this if enough vitamin A is not received from the diet. Adequate supply of zinc is needed to mobilize vitamin A out of its storage deposits.

The factors that interfere with the absorption of vitamin A and carotene are heavy physical activities performed four hours after consumption, excess consumption of alcohol and iron, and use of drugs and cortisone.

Since vitamin A is primarily absorbed in upper intestinal tract, the amount of absorption depends on the intake quantity, the influence of other substances present in the intestines, and the amount of vitamin stored in the body. A diet low in fat results in little flow of bile to the intestine, which can cause carotene and vitamin A loss.

Amount of vitamin A in one hundred grams of animal products

Cheese (high in fat)	1100	I.U.
Beef liver	53400	I.U.
Calf liver	32700	I.U.
Lamb liver	74500	I.U.
Chicken liver	12300	I.U.
Butter	3300	I.U.

Vitamin D

Vitamin D is a fat-soluble vitamin, and can be acquire either by ingestion or exposure to sunlight. Vitamin D aids the absorption and metabolism of calcium and phosphorus. Vitamin D is necessary for normal growth in children; without it bones and teeth do not calcify properly. In adults, it is needed to maintain stability of the nervous system, normal heart action, and normal blood clotting, as all these functions are related to the supply and utilization of calcium and phosphorus. Vitamin D is best taken with vitamin A.

Vitamin D deficiency can lead to inadequate absorption of calcium from the intestinal tract, to retention of phosphorus in the kidney, and to osteoporosis which in menopausal woman causes thinning bones. Due to the role that estrogen plays, calcium, magnesium, and other minerals have to be taken with vitamin D in order to treat these conditions and to form and maintain healthy bones by working together. Vitamin D also can combine with calcium to act as an anti-cancer agent. Lack of vitamin D can lead to high blood pressure, muscular numbness, tingling, and spasm.

Vitamin D is found in fish liver oil, fish, milk, and dairy products. There are two forms of vitamin D. Vitamin D3 is preferable since it is natural. Both vitamins D3 and D2 can be produced synthetically to form an active hormone. Studies show that overdosing on vitamin D ,the symptoms of which are nausea, loss of appetite, headache, diarrhea, fatigue, restlessness, and calcification of the soft tissues of the lungs, kidneys and bones, can even cause fatal toxicity

Vitamin E

Vitamin E is a fat soluble vitamin and an antioxidant, opposing the oxidation of vitamins A & C. Vitamin E increases the level of super oxide dismutase enzyme, which is a powerful free radical scavenger. Vitamin E is also able to prevent the oxidation of polyunsaturated fats, thus maintaining the function of organs. Vitamin E also prevents the oxidization of adrenal and pituitary hormones and promotes proper functioning of linoleic acid, an unsaturated fatty acid.

Vitamin E 1) is good for normal functioning of the nervous system, 2) reduces hot flashes and headaches during menopause, 3) relieves itching and inflammation of the vagina if applied as ointment, 4) reduces breast tenderness and other premenstrual symptoms, 5) has a dramatic effect on reproductive organs by preventing miscarriages and increasing both male and female fertility, 6) maintains cells from harmful and toxic substances, 7) promotes defenses against viruses and bacteria, and 8)eases headaches and relieves migraine attacks by preserving the oxygen in the blood for an extended period. Cosmetically, vitamin E can aid in the healing of burned tissue, prevent or dissolve scar tissues, and remove acne scars. Adequate intake of vitamin E could be helpful in counteracting premature aging and cross-linking of the skin. Studies have shown that red blood cells on people who take vitamin E supplements lived far longer than those who received no supplement.

Vitamin E is absorbed from the intestines, with bile salt and fat enters the lymph, and is transported through the blood to the liver, where a high concentration is stored. Improper absorption may cause muscular and digestive problems, such as ulcer and cancer of colon.

Daily intake of vitamin E recommended by the National Research Council is based upon the metabolic size of the body and the level of polyunsaturated fatty acids in the diet. Average daily intake is 4 IU for children, 7-12 IU for adolescents, 15 IU for adult males, 12 IU for females, which during pregnancy and lactation increases to 15 IU . The requirement increases with gains in polyunsaturated fatty acids in the diet. Air pollution also increases the need for vitamin E.

Vitamin E can be found in the oil of vegetables like corn, sunflower, wheat germ, safflower, soybean, nuts, peanuts, dark green leafy vegetables, dairy products and animal meat. Since cooking and processing cause a loss of vitamin E, choose cold pressed or unrefined oils.

Vitamin K

Vitamin K is fat soluble and the most important vitamin involved in the production of coagulation (blood clotting) factors. Vitamin K is absorbed in the upper intestinal tract with the aid of bile salt and is transported to the liver, where it is essential for some clotting factors.

Low levels of vitamin K may be related to the development of osteoporosis and have behavioral effects. The factors that destroy vitamin K are excessive use of antibiotics, ingestion of mineral oil which causes rapid excretion of vitamin K, X-ray radiation, aspirin, and air pollution. The National Research Council has estimated that the average adult daily intake of vitamin K is between 300-500 micrograms. Therapeutic doses of vitamin K are often given before and after operations to reduce blood losses.

Vitamin K can be found in liver, lean meats, egg yolk, spinach, green cabbage, tomatoes, strawberries, and whole wheat. There are three forms of vitamin K, i.e., K1 (from plants), K2(from intestinal bacteria), and K3 (synthetic).

Vitamin C (Ascorbic Acid)

Vitamin C is water soluble and known as ascorbic acid. It is normally the least stable of vitamins and is very sensitive to oxygen. Its potency can be lost through exposure to light, heat, and air which stimulate the activity of oxidative enzymes.

Vitamin C 1) helps to increase resistance to diseases, infections and cancer, 2) heals wounds and burns, 3) inactivates a variety of viruses and bacteria, 4) maintains collagen, a protein necessary for the formation of connective tissue in skin, bone, cartilage and collagen. Vitamin C can also prevent high blood pressure and hardening of the arteries which lead to heart attack and stroke, repair damaged artery walls, and prevent cholesterol deposits. Vitamin C increases the intestinal absorption of iron, may play a role in calcium metabolism, and also protects vitamins B1, B2, B5, A, E, and folic acid against oxidation. The level of vitamin C in the blood reaches to its maximum two to three hours after ingestion, then decreases by its elimination through urine and perspiration. Most of vitamin C is out of the body in three to four hours.

Vitamin C, reduces the effects of some allergies , protects the brain and spinal cord from destruction by free radicals, and helps in relieving stress. Take extra vitamin C if you are under stress, with illness, undergoing surgery, with wound or infection, using birth control pills, or smoking cigarettes, as these things deplete high levels of vitamin C from the body.

Vitamin C protects from nitrosamines. The body is exposed to nitrosamines in foods, smoke, ingestion of nitrites and nitrates, and other forms of nitrosamines. The body makes nitrosamines from foods such as vegetables, processed meats (like hot dogs, bacon, or ham), polluted air and water, and smoke. Vitamin C can block this process.

Food sources of vitamin C are fruits and vegetables like broccoli, spinach, parsley, horseradish, bell peppers, cauliflower, chives, turnips, cabbage, garlic, onions, tomatoes, guava, oranges, lemons, strawberries, kiwi fruit, papayas, watermelons, grapefruits, and gooseberries.

Vitamin C is easily destroyed when exposed to oxygen. Fruits and vegetables began to lose vitamin C as soon as cut. For example, freshly squeezed oranges quickly begin to lose their nutrient value. Since vitamin C is sensitive to heat and is lost when a large quantity of water is used during cooking, it is better to eat the vegetable raw or lightly steamed with a small amount of water.

Vitamin B Complex

The vitamins that are in this groups are B1 (thiamin), B2 (riboflavin), B3 (niacin), B6 (pyridoxine), B12 (cobalamin), B5 (pantothenic acid), folic acid, and biotin. Although all these vitamins have their own properties and biological role to play, they also have much in common. They work together and are found in the same foods. Vitamin B complex provides energy by converting carbohydrates to glucose, which is then burned to produce energy.

Vitamin B complex is necessary for normal functioning of the nervous system and may be the most important factor for the health of skin, hair, eyes, mouth, and liver. One of the important sources of vitamin B complex is intestinal bacteria. Symptoms of vitamin B complex deficiency are feeling tired, irritable, nervous, and depressed, gray hair, falling hair, baldness, acne or other skin problems, insomnia, constipation, or high cholesterol levels.

Vitamin B1 (thiamin)

Vitamin B1 is a water soluble vitamin that, with the help of a coenzyme, participates in the process of converting glucose to energy. This vitamin helps to resist diseases, decreases oxidation of lipids, and plays a major role in the metabolism of carbohydrates. Since the cells of the nervous system are extremely sensitive to carbohydrate metabolism, the brain and nerves are the first to show signs of vitamin B1 (thiamin) deficiency.

Vitamin B1 metabolism increases during pregnancy, fever, emotional stress, and overactive thyroid. Drinking lots of caffeine increases the risk of vitamin B1 deficiency. In fact, nervous symptoms are associated with thiamin deficiency, and people who drink excess tea or coffee are prone to such deficiency.

Vitamin B1 (thiamin) is rapidly absorbed in the upper and lower small intestines. It is then carried to the liver, kidneys, and heart by the circulatory system, where it may combine with manganese and proteins to become active enzymes. Thiamin is not stored in great quantity, therefore it should be supplied daily. The National Research Council recommends 0.5 milligram of thiamin per 1000 calories daily for all ages.

Sources of thiamin are blueberries, red chicory, black currants, Brussels sprouts, and red cabbage. Vitamin C has been shown to protect against thiamin (vitamin B1) destruction in some of these foods. Vitamin B deficiency diseases, like beriberi, affect the cardiovascular, gastrointestinal, and nervous systems with symptoms like insomnia, nervousness, headache, constipation, heaviness, weakness in the legs, and numbness and burning of the feet.

Foods with high content of vitamin B1(thiamin) are liver, dried beans, soybeans, peanuts, whole grains, bread, brown rice, wheat germ, egg yolk, poultry, and fish. Medium sources for this vitamin are dried fruits like prunes, nuts,and raisins, beans, broccoli, oatmeal, and Brussels sprouts. Thiamin depletes by exposure to heat or ultraviolet light. Baking meat and bread reduces the thiamin content by 15 to 25 percent, and boiling meat reduces thiamin by 50%.

Vitamin B2 (Riboflavin)

Vitamin B2 is a water soluble vitamin and occurring in foods with vitamin B1 content. Vitamin B2 functions as part of a group of enzymes involved in the breaking and utilization of carbohydrates, fats, and proteins. Vitamin B2 (riboflavin) is essential for eyes.

Vitamin B2 is absorbed through the walls of the small intestine, carried by the blood to the tissues, and excreted in urine. The recommended dietary allowance is 1.6 milligrams for adult males and 1.2 milligram for females; in pregnancy and lactation 1.5 to 1.7 milligrams is needed.

Vitamin B2 deficiency is shown by excessive sensitivity to light, inflamed eyes, and blurred vision. Vitamin B2 is needed for tissue repair and physical stresses. Riboflavin deficiency inhibits red blood cell production and causes anemia. Riboflavin works in conjunction with iron to correct iron deficiency anemia. Vitamin B2 deficiency symptoms are depression, moodiness, nervousness, and behavioral changes.

Food sources of vitamin B2 are dairy products, meat, poultry, fish, liver, kidney, beans, nuts, grains, whole grains, and vegetables like spinach, broccoli, Brussels sprouts, and asparagus.

Vitamin B3 (Niacin)

Vitamin B3 is water soluble and more stable than vitamins B1 and B2. As a coenzyme, niacin assists in the breaking and utilizing of proteins, fats, and carbohydrates. Vitamin B3 (niacin) is effective in improving circulation and reducing cholesterol and triglyceride levels in the blood. Vitamin B3 is ideal for people who have high blood cholesterol and triglycerides.

Niacin is absorbed in the intestine and is stored in the liver. The recommended dietary allowance is 16 milligrams for men, 13 milligrams for women, and 9 to 16 milligrams for children. Vitamin B3 (niacin) deficiency symptoms appear in the nervous system and are depression, weakness, and loss of memory. Food sources of vitamin B3 are beef, pork, fish, dairy products, whole wheat, eggs, and vegetables like broccoli, tomatoes, potatoes and carrots.

Vitamin B6 (Pyridoxine)

Vitamin B6 is water soluble and acts as a coenzyme in the utilization of carbohydrates, fats, amino acids and proteins. Vitamin B6 is needed for the proper growth and maintenance of almost all body functions.

A daily supply of vitamin B6 is necessary as it is excreted in the urine within 8 hours after ingestion and is not stored in the liver. Vitamin B6 is needed for turning iron into hemoglobin to produce red blood cells.

Vitamin B6 deficiency symptoms occur in the nervous system as depression, anemia, insomnia, dizziness, confusion, nervousness, a needle-like feeling in the hands and feet, seborrhea, dermatitis, and acne. If there is a low level of vitamin B6, there may be low blood glucose. It may also cause the loss of hair and water during pregnancy. The recommended dietary allowance of vitamin B6 is 2 milligram per day, which increases during pregnancy.

Food sources containing the highest amounts of vitamin B6 are eggs, fish, salmon, meat, chicken, wheat germ, peas, carrots, spinach, walnut, and sunflower seeds. Medium sources are whole grains, brown rice, banana, cantaloupe, avocado, cabbage, and beans. Heat, oxygen and light affect vitamin B6; up to 70% of it may be lost during cooking and processing.

Vitamin B12 (Cobalamin)

Vitamin B12 is water soluble and necessary for normal metabolism of proteins, fats and carbohydrates. Vitamin B12 helps in vitamin A conversion.

Vitamin B12 must be combined with calcium during absorption in the gastrointestinal tract, after which it is bound to serum protein and transported to the tissues. Highest concentrations of vitamin B12 are found in liver, kidneys, heart, brain, pancreas, and bone marrow. For better absorption, take B12 with several meals.

Vitamin B12 deficiency symptoms include a wide variety of gastrointestinal problems, nervous system dysfunction, severe physical and emotional stress, confusion, depression and moodiness, memory loss, and brain damage.

Food sources of vitamin B12 are meat (like lamb, pork, calf liver, beef, and beef kidneys,) dairy products, egg yolks, and seafood (like clams, sardines, salmon, crabs, and oyster). Vitamin B12 is not stable in the presence of heat and light which change it to oxidant, so great care is required during cooking and storage.

Vitamin B5 (Pantothenic Acid)

Pantothenic acid is part of vitamin B complex and is water soluble. It is converted to coenzymes to release energy from fats, carbohydrates and proteins, to utilize vitamins (especially vitamin B2), to synthesize cholesterol and fatty acids, to maintain the digestive tract, and to improve the body's ability to withstand stressful conditions. Vitamin B5 is found in the blood plasma, in the liquid part of lymph, and is excreted in urine. The National Research Council suggests a daily intake of 5-10 milligrams of this vitamin for adult and children.

Vitamin B5 deficiency affects the immune system, and its symptoms are headache, fatigue, insomnia, and nervousness. Food sources of pantothenic acid are eggs, potatoes, pork, beef, milk, fresh vegetables, and whole wheat. Pantothenic acid is lost when cooked, canned, frozen, or processed. For example, 50% of pantothenic acid in grains is lost during the milling process.

Biotin

Biotin is a water-soluble B complex vitamin, and as a coenzyme, is involved in the metabolism of carbohydrates. It helps in the production and oxidation of fatty acids and carbohydrates. Without biotin, fat production is impaired. Biotin is absorbed in the intestine and is synthesized by the intestinal bacteria, yet most of it is excreted in urine. Biotin is stored in the kidneys, liver, brain, and adrenal glands.

Biotin deficiency symptoms are nausea, appetite loss, numbness, depression, high blood cholesterol, hair loss and skin rash. Food sources high in biotin are chicken, lamb, pork, beef, veal, liver, soybeans, milk, cheese, saltwater fish, whole wheat flour, and rice. Biotin is stable during normal cooking and processing.

Inositol & Choline

Inositol and choline are parts of the vitamin B complex, and they promote production of lecithin, prevent fat accumulation in the liver, and remove fats from liver into the cells with the help of lecithin, therefore, inositol and choline aid the metabolism of fats and reduce blood cholesterol. Inositol and choline are essential for the health of the liver, kidneys and nerves. They play an important role in the transmission of nerve impulses.

Folic Acid

Folic acid is part of the vitamin B complex and is water-soluble. It functions as a coenzyme with vitamin B12 and vitamin C for the metabolism of proteins. Folic acid helps the formation of red blood cells and nucleic acid which are essential for growth and reproduction of cells. Folic acid is necessary for proper brain functioning, reinforces mental and emotional health, and helps in the performance of the liver.

Folic acid is absorbed in the gastrointestinal tract and is stored in the liver. Folic acid deficiency results in poor growth of hair, graying hair, forgetfulness, and mental sluggishness. As folic acid helps in the formation of red blood cells, a deficiency could lead to anemia.

The recommended dietary allowance of folic acid is 400 micrograms for adults and 800 micrograms during pregnancy. Food sources of folic acid are red meats, eggs, dairy products, grains, and green leafy vegetables.

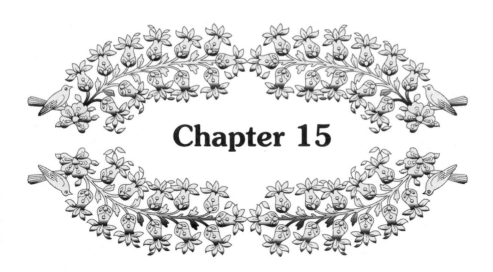

Chapter 15

Minerals and Their Function

inerals are nutrients that exist in organic and inorganic combinations. Minerals, like vitamins, act as catalysts for biological reactions, as micro-nutrients, and as coenzymes which are needed for proper composition of body fluids, bone formation, and maintenance of nerve function.

Vitamins and minerals become part of the structure of cells, enzymes, hormones, blood, muscles, and bones after being absorbed. Minerals can be stored or utilized for long periods of time. Minerals maintain the water balance needed for proper mental and physical functioning, maintain acidity/alkalinity of the blood and tissue fluids, and allow nutrients' flow in the bloodstream.

Minerals also consist of two groups: macro-minerals (like calcium, magnesium, and phosphorus, needed in large amounts) and micro-minerals (like potassium, zinc, iron, copper, chromium, and iodine, needed in smaller quantities). Minerals are stored in bones and muscle tissue.

Calcium

Calcium is a macro-mineral that helps in the formation of bones and teeth. About 99 percent of calcium is deposited in bones and teeth and one percent employed in the blood clotting process. Calcium acts with phosphorus, magnesium, and vitamins A, C, and D to 1) build and maintain bones and teeth, 2) regulate heartbeat and blood pressure, 3) prevent colon cancer, 4) regulate contraction and relaxation of the muscles and heart, and 5) absorb nutrients, especially vitamin B12. If the diet is deficient in calcium, the body will draw it from bone. If the calcium deficiency continues for a long time, eventually there is so much calcium lost from the bone that osteoporosis can occur.

Calcium absorption depends on the presence of enough vitamin D which works with the parathyroid hormone to regulate the amount of calcium in the blood. The National Research Council recommends 800 milligrams of calcium daily to maintain the necessary balance since only 20 to 30 percent may actually be absorbed.

Foods sources of calcium are dairy products (especially milk that contains lactose, a substance that may increase the absorption of calcium in the body), green leafy vegetables, seafood (like sardines, salmon, clams, oyster, and shrimp), soybeans, and soybean products, such as tofu.

Phosphorus

Phosphorus is the second macro-mineral present in every cell. It plays a major role in chemical reactions in the body. Along with calcium, it utilizes fats, proteins and carbohydrates for the growth, maintenance, and repair of cells and the production of energy. It is combined with fats in the blood that become phospholipids to break and transport fat and fatty acid. Phosphorus helps in digestion of vitamins B2 and B3 and is necessary for skeletal growth, tooth development, the functioning of kidneys, and the transfer of nerve impulses.

Seventy percent of phosphorus is absorbed from ingestion in the intestine, 88% of which is stored in the bones and teeth, along with calcium. Phosphorus deficiency symptoms are weakness, loss of appetite, and loss of calcium and bone mass. The National Research Council recommends a daily dietary intake of 800 milligrams of phosphorus for men and women, 1200 milligrams during pregnancy. If the phosphorus in the body is high, additional calcium should be taken to maintain proper balance. Food sources of phosphorus are nearly all foods, especially dairy products, meat, fish, nuts, beans and grains.

Magnesium

Magnesium is a macro-mineral situated in cells that is involved, with the help of enzymes, in the metabolism of amino acids and carbohydrates, in breaking sugar in the liver to create energy, and in the utilization of vitamins C, E, and B complex.

Along with calcium and phosphorus, sufficient magnesium is required to build strong bones, to maintain the function of the nerves, and to relax muscles. When calcium flows into muscle tissues, magnesium leaves and the muscle contracts, and when calcium leaves, magnesium replaces it and the muscle relaxes.

Magnesium deficiency may cause muscle spasms, convulsions, psychiatric problems, and depression. Studies suggest that stress may lower magnesium levels in women during premenstrual tension, and oral contraceptives have been found to lower blood magnesium as well. Since magnesium interacts with calcium, potassium, and sodium to tone the blood vessels, inadequate magnesium in the blood may cause blood vessel diseases. Vitamin D is necessary for proper utilization of magnesium.

Almost 50% of daily magnesium is absorbed in the small intestine. The rate of absorption is influenced by parathyroid hormones, the rate of water absorption, and the amount of calcium, phosphate and lactose in the body. The adrenal gland helps to regulate magnesium excretion through the kidneys.

The National Research Council recommends a daily magnesium intake of 350 milligrams for men, 300 milligrams for women and 450 milligrams during pregnancy. Food sources of magnesium are dairy products, meat, seafood, soybeans, nuts, peanuts, and whole grains like oatmeal, rice, wheat germ.

Zinc

Zinc is a micro-mineral and a component of insulin, a part of the enzyme that is needed to break down alcohol, and it helps in normal absorption and action of vitamins. Zinc is known for its role in protecting us from harmful substances. It protects the liver from damage due to certain poisons. It prevents the absorption of lead (such as lead exposure due to air pollution, car fumes, or water flow through lead plumbing), cadmium (which can be leached from galvanized pipe and exhaust fumes), and other metallic toxins. Zinc may also be protective against the harmful effects of free radicals.

Zinc is absorbed in the upper small intestine and is mostly excreted through the gastrointestinal tract, with small amount excreted through urine. Zinc deficiency symptoms are fatigue, susceptibility to infection, brittle nails, spots on the nails, lack of hair pigments, loss of appetite, and the inability to smell foods. Consumption of alcohol may flush the stored zinc out of liver and into the urine. Chronic zinc depletion can cause cancer.

The highest concentration of zinc is in the eyes and is activated by vitamin A. Zinc, taken at daily doses of at least 30 mg. with vitamin A and carrot juice, is a treatment for skin diseases, such as boils, eczema, psoriasis, and severe acne. The National Research Council recommends a daily intake of 15 milligrams of zinc for adults, increased to 30 milligrams during pregnancy and for skin disorders like acne, boils, and eczema.

Food sources of zinc are meat, poultry, seafood, liver, eggs, whole grains, nuts, and peanuts. Approximately 70% of zinc depletes from whole grains during milling process.

Iron

Iron is a micro-mineral concentrated in blood. Iron is present in many enzymes which are involve in the production of energy. About 5% of iron is found in myoglobin, an iron protein complex found in muscles, providing energy.

Iron is absorbed in the upper part of the small intestines within four hours after ingestion, then moved by blood to bone marrow. Only two to four percent of the iron in foods is used by the body. Iron is primarily stored in liver, bone, marrow, and blood. The common disease of iron deficiency is anemia (hypochromic), related to a reduction of hemoglobin in red blood cells. Other symptoms are fatigue, irritability, paleness, low energy, headache, and adverse effects on learning ability which appear after complete depletion of iron stores.

Studies indicate that iron supplementation in the case of iron deficient children improves their ability to learn. Vegetarian women, particularly during menstruation and pregnancy, are at higher risk of low iron intake and consequentially may experience severe headaches.

The National Research Council suggests a daily iron intake of 10 mg. for men and 18 mg. for women, which can be increased during pregnancy and menstruation. Food sources of iron are red meats (beef, calf, and lamb), liver, fish, poultry, eggs, milk, cereals, breads, whole grains, and vegetables like spinach, broccoli, potatoes, and fruits

Potassium

Potassium is necessary for normal growth, stimulation of nerve transmission, contraction of muscles, and hormone secretion. Potassium and sodium help maintain water balance, regulate distribution of fluids, and normalize heartbeat and nourishment of muscles.

Potassium is absorbed from the small intestine and excreted through urine and perspiration. Excessive potassium buildup may result in kidney failure. Excessive use of salt depletes potassium supplies. Potassium can be depleted by diarrhea, excessive sweating, vomiting, fever, burns, surgery, and use of diuretics, laxatives, alcohol and coffee. Potassium deficiency symptoms are nausea, vomiting, muscle weakness, muscle spasms, cramps, high blood pressure, and heart failure in extreme cases. People with high blood pressure who are using diuretics are frequently advised to eat fruits and vegetables that contain potassium like bananas, potatoes, oranges and tomatoes.

Food sources of potassium are milk, meats, poultry, fish, fruits, vegetables and whole grains. Since potassium is lost during cooking, e.g., potatoes loses up to 50% of potassium during boiling, better add a little salt substitute containing potassium chloride to boiling water to prevent the potassium from leaching out during cooking.

Selenium

Selenium is a micro-mineral which works with vitamin E in promotion of normal growth and fertility. Selenium is an antioxidant and anti-cancer mineral which preserves elasticity of tissues by delaying oxidation of polyunsaturated fatty acids, thus protecting cells against free radicals' damages. Studies indicate that selenium appears to be protective against cancer of breast, colon, lung, cervix, rectum, bladder, esophagus, pancreas, skin, liver, and prostate as well as tumors of the ovary. The same studies also indicate that smokers who die of cancer have lower selenium, vitamin A and vitamin E

levels.

Most people do not get enough selenium due to low selenium content in the soil. Since selenium preserves elasticity of tissues, deficiency may lead to premature aging, infertility, and heart diseases. In eastern Finland, which has the highest rate of heart disease cases in the world, low selenium in blood has been found to be associated with these diseases. In China, children in certain areas where the selenium of soil is low develop heart disease; this responds positively to selenium supplementation. Selenium with vitamins A & E improves skin conditions, such as acne.

Selenium is absorbed in the liver and kidneys and excreted in urine. The National Research Council recommends 50 to 200 micrograms of selenium daily.

Food sources of selenium are seafood, meat, whole grains, fruits, and vegetables. Cooking and processing deplete the selenium in the food. Vitamin C can enhance the absorption of selenium.

Copper

Copper is a trace mineral found in tissues. It helps in the absorption and use of iron and the formation of hemoglobin and red blood cells. Copper contains enzymes required for metabolism of ascorbic acid and proteins, energy production, oxidation of fatty acids, and formation of melanin (skin pigment) which converts the amino acid tyrosine to color pigments of hair and skin.

Copper is absorbed in the stomach and upper intestine. Copper deficiency symptoms are anemia, weak immunity, and bone disease. The same symptoms have been observed in infants fed only cow milk, which is very low in copper. The National Research Council recommends a daily dietary intake of 2 milligrams of copper for adults. Food sources of copper are seafood, shellfish, liver, meat, grains, nuts, cereals, and raisins.

Iodine

Iodine is a micro-mineral. Human body contains 20 to 30 milligrams of iodine, three quarters of which is in the thyroid and the rest is distributed throughout the body. Iodine is in the principal hormone produced by the thyroid gland and helps in the development and functioning of the thyroid gland.

The thyroid hormones regulate metabolism and influence physical and mental growth, the functioning of the nervous system and muscles, and circulation. Iodine is readily absorbed from gastrointestinal tract into the blood stream and then into the thyroid gland, where it is oxidized and convert to thyroxin. The National Re-

search Council suggests a daily iodine intake of 150 micrograms for men and women, 175 during pregnancy and 200 during lactation.

Iodine deficiency disease is goiter, which is a condition of thyroid gland enlargement as a result of insufficient hormone production. In some areas people suffer from goiter due to low iodine in their soil. Goiter is more commonly seen in women, especially during adolescence, pregnancy, and menopause.

Food sources of iodine are seafood and vegetables which grow near the coast. Some get their iodine from iodized salt.

Manganese

Manganese, a trace mineral, is an essential part of enzymes involved in the utilization of B vitamins and ascorbic acid. It plays a major role in the production of fats, proteins, and carbohydrates necessary for normal bone development and for functioning of the nervous system. Manganese is a component of superoxide dismutase enzyme that helps prevent aging processes, maintains sex hormone production, and helps forms thyroxin, a constituent of the thyroid gland.

Manganese is absorbed in the small intestine . Normally 4 milligrams of manganese are excreted everyday, and this amount needs to be replaced. The National Research Council recommends 2.5 to 3 milligrams daily for adults.

Manganese deficiency may affect the immune system and glucose tolerance, leading to paralysis, convulsion, blindness, deafness in infants, dizziness, ear noises, and loss of hearing.

Food sources high in manganese are nuts (especially pecans and hazelnuts), seeds, whole grains, oatmeal, cereals, seaweed, and avocado. Other fruits and vegetables contain moderate amounts, and refined grain is a poor source of manganese. Milling removes 70% of manganese.

Chromium

Chromium is the major mineral involved in insulin production and glucose regulation. Insulin is the hormone that regulates the levels of glucose in the blood. Chromium activates enzymes involved in the metabolism of glucose. Glucose is known as "blood sugar" and is the primary source of energy. Chromium depletion impairs glucose metabolism, then body relies on fat metabolism for energy.

Chromium is difficult to absorb. Only about 3 percent of dietary chromium is retained in the body. It is stored in kidneys, spleen, heart, lungs, and brain and is excreted through urine.

Even slight chromium deficiency has serious effects on body. It upsets the function of insulin and causes glucose metabolism disorders, such as diabetes and hypoglycemia. Chromium supplementation improves glucose tolerance.

There is no recommended dietary allowance for chromium, yet it is estimated between 80-100 microgram daily. Food sources of chromium are meat, especially liver, cheese, whole grains, cereals, and bread. Milling of grains depletes 80% of the chromium.

Fluorine (Fluorides)

Fluorine is a micro-mineral present as compounds called fluorides in small amounts, primarily in the teeth and skeleton. There are two types of fluorides, namely sodium fluorides, added in drinking water, and calcium fluoride. Fluorine strengthens bones and reduces decay of tooth enamel.

Food sources of fluorine are drinking water, seafood, cheese, meat, and tea. Fluorine content in plants depends on environmental conditions, such as soil. About 90% of fluorine is absorbed in the intestine, half of which is absorbed by teeth and bones and the rest excreted in the urine.

Fluorine deficiency may lead to poor teeth development and dental problems. The average diets provide 0.25 to 0.35 milligram of fluorine daily, and average adult ingests 1.0 to 1.5 milligrams.

Sodium

Sodium is an essential mineral for cell fluids, arteries, veins and capillaries. About 50% of sodium is in these fluids and vessels, and the remainder in bones. Sodium keeps the blood minerals soluble and, along with potassium, regulates the water balance and prevents deposition of minerals in the blood stream.

Sodium is readily absorbed in stomach and small intestine, then is carried by the blood to the kidneys where it is filtered and returned to the blood to maintain blood level. Excess is excreted in the urine. The level of sodium in the urine reflects dietary intake; if there is a high intake of sodium, the rate of excretion is high.

Sodium is found in all foods, mostly seafood, kelp, seaweed, poultry, and meat. Sodium deficiency can cause intestinal gas, weight loss, vomiting, muscle shrinkage, diarrhea, excessive perspiration, and fever.

The National Research Council recommends a daily sodium chloride intake of 1 gram per kilogram of water consumed. Excess sodium in the diet may cause potassium excretion.

Sulfur

Sulfur is a micro-mineral present in every cell and is called "nature's beauty mineral" as it keeps the hair glossy and smooth and the skin clear, healthy and youthful. Sulfur is prevalent in keratin, a tough protein necessary for health and maintenance of skin, nails, and hair. Sulfur works with vitamins B1, B5, and biotin as a metabolizer and with the liver to secrete bile.

Sulfur is absorbed and stored in the cells of joints, hair, skin, and nails, and any excess is excreted in urine. Sulfur deficiency causes a loss of hair and skin problems, like acne. Sources of sulfur are eggs, dairy products, fish and meat.

Drinking Water and Your Health

The average adult drinks and excretes about 2 1/2 to 3 quarts of water daily. For individuals who live in hot climates or have strong physical activities, the amount may increase to 4 quarts. Water forms a large percentage of the weight of most solid foods. For example, water content for milk is 87%, green beans 89%, and lettuce 95%. Even meat is substantially made up of water. If a diet consists of fruits and vegetables, significant water is consumed since most of them are more than 80% water.

It is probably hard to know exactly whether enough water has been ingested, thus, drink at least six to eight glasses of filtered water daily and do not rely on tea or coffee for supplementation of water. Caffeine acts as diuretic, causing loss of water from kidneys.

Though water is essential for life, yet some of its constituents can influence the quality of life. The most dangerous of these constituents are microorganisms like bacteria and viruses. Most people drink untreated water unknowingly. By chlorinating water supplies, many diseases like typhoid, intestinal worms, and skin diseases can be controlled. Other contaminates in water are toxic heavy metals and carcinogenic chemicals.

Remember that:
water is the only liquid that cleans the system; nothing can replace it.

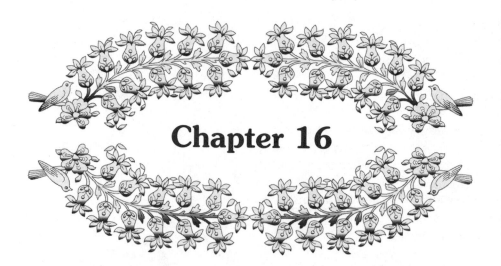

Chapter 16

What Is Nutrition?

Nutrition is the relationship between food and health of the body. Adequate supplies of all essential nutrients, like carbohydrates, proteins, minerals, vitamins, fat,, and water, are required to utilize, maintain, and balance that health.

Proper nutrition is essential for normal reproduction, resistance to infection, and the ability to repair damages.

Loss of Nutrients: Everybody needs enough vitamins and minerals to ensure good health. Most people do not eat a well balanced diet, which, according to the latest National Research Council recommendations, consists of 30% fat, 20% protein, 35% complex carbohydrates, like grains, breads, potatoes, or starchy vegetables, and 15% simple carbohydrates, like sugar, sweets, and fruits. Based on the above recommendations, average women need 2000 calories and men need 3000 calories daily.

Published reports in the United States and Europe show that most of the people, especially women, are at risk of deficiency in nutrients.

The nutrients in food content widely fluctuates depending on its growing conditions. For example, selenium is one of the most important antioxidant minerals but is depleted from many soils. There is no guarantee that the soil in which our food is being grown has adequate essential minerals. By using fertilizers, we are creating more problems. The nutritional content of factory farm animals fed on artificial diets is not the same quality. Fruits and vegetables lose their nutrients from the time they are picked. Storing and cooking cause further nutrient losses.

Vitamins deplete as food ages. For example, if a fruit contains 100% vitamin C when freshly harvested, after two months the vitamin C content may fall by 40%; loss is especially high in green vegetables. Some vegetable like potatoes, when freshly harvested in fall, may have 30 milligrams of vitamin C per 100 grams, but by spring they only have 5 milligrams per 100 gram, and by summer only one milligram per 100 grams. Orange has vitamin C, but it loses 30% of its vitamin C soon after being squeezed.

Heat, light, chemicals, and water used to process foods deplete nutrients. Freezing and canning also destroy up to 60% of the vitamin C content, 40% of vitamin B2 , and 30% of vitamin B1. Sterilization of canned foods can destroy 30% of vitamin A and 60% of vitamin B2. Cooking method also destroys 50% of vitamins, especially vitamin C. Therefore, fruits and vegetables lose large amounts of their vitamins during cooking, freezing and canning processes. Meat also loses its nutrients through cooking. For example, half of a meat's thiamin content (vitamin B1) can be lost during cooking.

Today we live and are surrounded by chemically-tainted food, water, and air.

Meats and chicken are injected with hormones and fed with antibiotics; fruits and vegetables are sprayed with pesticides; and artificial flavors or colors are added to foods. However, it has been found that certain vitamins and minerals are protective against some of these toxic substances.

Stress: If under any physical or emotional stress, one depletes stores of vitamins and minerals more rapidly. Therefore, additional vitamins must be taken.

Illness and Disease: There are many illnesses that interfere with digestion and the absorption of nutrients. For example, infections deplete vitamins and minerals, and appetite decreases during the illness. Nutrients are important for the immune system, especially at critical times. If the immune system is low, illness will deplete nutrients and lower one's resistance to infection, which in turn lowers the nutrients even more.

If taking a medication for illness, especially antibiotics, take extra vitamin C to resist the infection and fight against the bacteria or virus and take acidophilus to balance intestinal system, as antibiotics destroy both harmful bacteria and good bacteria that are beneficial for better health and absorption of nutrients. Acidophilus balances the intestinal system. Take mucopolysaccharides and mucoprotein. Mucopolysaccharides protects cells against an invasion of organisms such as bacteria, viruses, and fungi. They must be obtained from foods like crustaceans and deep sea cold water fish.

Free Radicals: In today's life, with pollution from cars, smog, chemicals dumped in water, and processed and canned foods, vitamins deplete faster from diets. It is very important to drink pure and clean water, exercise to release the pollution trapped in the lungs, and eat healthy, fresh food in order to stay healthy. Free radicals are formed by exposure to toxic chemicals in foods, water, and air, by radiation, by excessive sunlight, and by the formation of polyunsaturated fats. The body has certain defense mechanisms that keep the processes under control and they must be enhanced by certain vitamins and nutrients.

Drugs: There are many drugs that interact with nutrients, causing depletion of vitamins. Drugs like antibiotics interfere with vitamin B6 and destroy good bacteria that are existing in intestine; hormones in medications destroy water-soluble vitamins; and drugs for cholesterol limit absorption of vitamins A, E, D, and K.

Age: Many diseases, such as high blood pressure, sugar, cholesterol, and heart diseases, are associated with aging. As one ages, organs tend to function less optimally and therefore require more nutrients, especially calcium and magnesium. There are herbal remedies for prevention and treatment of such diseases; refer to the medicinal plants chapter.

Nutrition and the Immune System: The immune system is a complex of interaction between blood cells and special proteins to defend the body from harm. The immune system also has the ability to kill bacteria and viruses and to repair damaged cells before possibly growing into a cancerous tumor.

Vitamins and minerals do more than just prevent deficiencies; they are used in every process of the body. State of the art biochemistry shows that nutrient deficiency symptoms are only the last event in a long chain of reactions in the body. If enough of a specific vitamin is not received, the initial reaction occurs on the molecular level. Vitamin stores are depleted followed by depletion of the enzymes. This causes changes at a cellular level, disrupting the normal functioning of the cells which depend upon these enzymes.

Inadequate nutrition can weaken defense systems, lessen proteins and fiber, and increase fat, thus impairing immunity. Vitamins such as vitamins A, B6, B5, B12, C, E, folic acid, and minerals, such as selenium, zinc, iron, and magnesium, enhance immunity.

Defense Against Free Radicals: The body's defense system not only fights against bacteria and viruses, but it also protects us from free radicals. Free radicals are irritating and upset the processes of anti-free radical agents, such as vitamins C, E, A, beta carotene, and selenium, from repairing damaged cells. For example, 500 to 1000 mg of vitamin C a day reduces the fat peroxide level by 15%, and vitamin C and E together reduce the level by 25%. Vitamin E works with selenium as a free radical scavenger, and it protects vitamins A and C from oxidation. Enough vitamins and minerals should be taken to protect the body from free radical oxidation. For example, vegetable oils are being consumed for the ability of their polyunsaturated fatty acids to reduce cholesterol. They are high in vitamin E which is an anti-free radical agent preventing oxidation. However, the heat used for processing the vegetable oils destroys vitamin E, and therefore, extra supplement of vitamin E and selenium must be taken.

Disease Prevention: In order to be healthy, prevent diseases, and overcome pollution, emotional and physical stresses, we must take vitamins and minerals. As the actual absorption of vitamins and minerals in our diet is not 100% due to many factors, including loss of nutrients through processing and storage, supplements can be taken. However, nutritional supplements do not take the place of fresh food; one still needs a balance of carbohydrates, fats, and proteins. Taking supplements with food enhances the absorption of nutrients contained in the supplements. Although each has its own biochemical function, nutrients tend to work better together. They help each other and must be taken in proportion. Supplementation of one single nutrient may put you in risk of developing an imbalance with other nutrients.

Herbs and Nutrition: "We are what we eat" means that what you eat represents your health and physical and mental stability. Ancient Iranians believed that babies born with long foreheads would be intelligent and have extraordinary intuition. Some are. But later, as brilliant scientists and geniuses with short foreheads were observed, the belief was weakened. Today scientific knowledge of human self recognition proves that old beliefs are not entirely wrong. Being born with a long forehead means the parents must have had good health and a nutritious diet which helps in the healthy growth and development of babies. Thus, being born with long forehead indicates proper eating of a nutritious diet by parents.

Herbs, for particular ailments or as a basic regime for general well being, balance the body and promote natural energy flow. Herbs and plants play a vital role in human health.

From the ancient times, people used herbs for flavor, digestion, and their biochemical properties. Volatile oils in herbs, such as those in the mint family, marjoram, peppermint, basil, tarragon, and rosemary, can cleanse and stimulate the digestive system and increase appetite. Bitter herbs like gentian, dandelion, and centaury cleanse and detoxify the gallbladder and liver. Herbs like parsley and caraway soothe the walls of the digestive tract and reduce flatulence. And herbs like nettle help secretions which aid the pancreas to digest fats. Herbs with antiseptic properties detoxify and cleanse and are important in hot climates where contaminated food is a hazard to health. Antibacterial and preservative properties make culinary herbs and spices valuable to be used in vinegars, oils, pickles, wines, and all stored food.

Herbs not only add flavor to the diet, but they also open new horizons in eating and drinking habits. Making herbal tea and meals, due to their primary and secondary biochemical actions, will help to support health. For example, stinging nettle with burdock and yellow dock provide a delicious tea or meal to control sugar levels and purify and cleanse blood.

In modern Iranian and Mediterranean cuisine, extra herbs are used in different dishes, salads, and drinks. They also use herbs as the healer. For example, garlic is added to many diets to cleanse and purify internals and to regulate blood pressure, cholesterol and sugar. Some culinary herbs are good for mouth or gums. For example, cinnamon and watercress strengthen gums; herbs like sage are antiseptic and help in healing mouth ulcers. Herbs like mint and cloves have antiseptic and antibiotic actions. Herbs like oat calm the nervous system. Herbs like carrot and dandelion, rich in vitamin A, promote good vision and healthy bones and teeth and aid the function of the liver. Rice starch is rich in vitamin B and is used to treat diarrhea and vomiting. Watercress and parsley, sources of calcium, are good for healthy bones and teeth and healthy muscle function. Onion, rich in vitamin C and iodine, promotes growth of hair and limits cold and flu. Now that more is known about herbs and their value, they should definitely be included in the daily diet.

In Iran, hot fresh breads and feta cheese with herbs like tarragon, basil, marjoram, peppermint, watercress, and parsley are used as snacks on summer afternoons.

How to Lose Fat: Weight loss programs have been with us for years. The word weight in common language means fat. Fat is lost by burning in muscles, so you cannot melt it in saunas, steam baths or plastic wraps, rub it off with a vibrator or rolling machines, and participate in weight loss programs that recommend a processed food diet. By exact definition of needs, better ways are found and better results are achieved. Weight and fat loss may seem the same, but remember it is the fat that is intended for loss, not weight. People who concentrate on fat loss are successful.

Fat is released from storage into blood to be carried to muscles. If muscles don't burn the fat, it returns to be stored again. To succeed with a fat loss program, muscles should burn the fat. The major fault in most weight loss programs is that some of the muscle is lost, thus impeding burning of fats. Do not make this mistake! Losing muscle affects proteins, eventually decreases fat metabolism, and impairs the ability to burn fats.

You should learn and understand that your muscles are the only place where excess fat can be burned. You must not start any diet program that might impair your muscles' efficiency. Stay on a good diet. Exercising for 20 minutes a day or fast walking tones the muscles in order to burn fat. Fats regulate body temperature, and if temperature is low, fat is burned to raise it. Tone your muscles to lose more fat. People with poorly toned muscles have trouble in losing fat.

Find out how much fat loss is needed. To lose fat, remember the following:
■ Focus on fat loss rather than weight loss.
■ Muscle loss is to be avoided, as it results in decreased burning of fats.
■ Do a body fat test to know how much excess fat you need to lose.

Stand up and tighten your legs and thighs. Touch your leg. If it feels tight, your muscle is tone and you can easily lose fat, but if it feels flabby, you need to tone the muscles. Remember the age is an important factor. After the age of forty, muscles began to lose their tone.

After finding out how much fat is needed to be lost, start with muscle toning. Exercise without sweating, and take in a healthy, balanced diet and herbs to enhance metabolism of fat.

The first question is how many calories one should consume. I personally do not believe in counting calories. I know the body needs a certain amount of healthy food in order to stay healthy and in good shape. If you understand your body, listen to it, and learn what to eat in order to keep it healthy and in shape, you do not have to worry about calories. If you are a calorie counter, remember that a pound of fat has 3500 calories. If muscle metabolizes an additional 500 calories of fat per day, then usually in seven days you would burn 3500 calories or 1 pound of fat. It seems logical to eat 500 calories less everyday so that muscle will burn fat drawn from cells. Assuming that your body consumes 2000 calories a day, by taking in only 1500 calories, automatically 500 calories are drawn from fat stores. Usually athletes need and handle more calories than others. Fit people with firmer muscles have a higher percentage of body lean and a lower amount of fats. To lose fat, do as follows:

- Exercise 20 to 30 minutes everyday; do not allow sweating, as it prevents fat loss.
- Take 8 glasses of water everyday to flush sugar, salt, and fat deposits.
- Eat a healthy, fresh, nutritious diet that is low in sugar, fat, and salt, and high in fiber.
- Avoid processed foods (canned and frozen).
- Avoid refined carbohydrates.
- Meditate and relax.
- Add vegetables, like cabbage, garlic, onion, and dandelion, to your diet to burn fats.

Avoid heavy breakfasts. Instead, eat fresh fruits that contain low sugar and low fat (like plums, citrus, pears), and then do not eat until lunch. In this way body will metabolize stored fat, especially in the stomach area. Once stomach fat is reduced, it will be easier to exercise. When you eat sour fruits like citric for breakfast, not only vitamins and minerals are attained, but also these vitamins and minerals promote vitality of cells. Body metabolism gets energy from day light since sour fruits do not contain fat it helps burning the stored fat. Some herbs like blue flag, poke root and berries have the same action in the body. They increases the metabolism burn stored fat.

Drink herbal teas of chickweed and fennel, as they have slimming properties. Also include herbs that contain saponin to reduce cholesterol. Some herbs or herbal teas increase metabolism and help burn fat. Herbs such as blue flag reduce one's craving for food, and herbs such as poke root berries can be used for excess fat burning.

But first and foremost, remember to eat healthy and fresh food. Respect your body and yourself. Nothing and nobody should be more important to you than your health. Do not cheat your body under any circumstances.

"Eat healthy and live healthy forever"

Minoo's Section

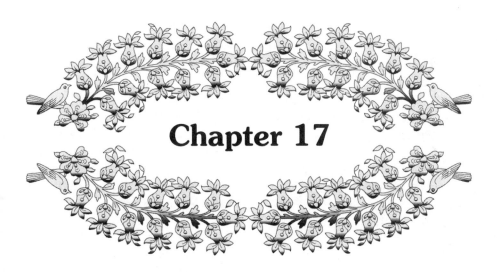

Chapter 17

Minoo's Herbal Products

Skin is a living organ. It protects your body from environmental hazard. It also reflects your inner health. Fresh radiant skin helps you to feel more beautiful. Being beautiful means living in harmony with yourself, respecting your inner balance and health, and discovering its true nature.

What could be more natural for your well-being than discovering the undoubted effect of plants and herbs? To enable you to face the world with natural beauty and radiant skin, Minoo offers a complete range of facial products to meet your personal needs.

All Minoo's facial products are formulated basically from botanical sources. The herbs that Minoo uses in her natural products are gathered from all over the world. Each product has been tested under clinically controlled conditions to ensure purity and effectiveness.

Minoo also offers an advanced training program to introduce an entirely unique application technique that allows aestheticians to reach their maximum potential.

The courses are of two to seven days duration. Training includes biochemistry, medicinal plants, aromatherapy, and acupressure massage techniques (for wrinkles, tension, headaches, and sinus drainage) besides advanced European facial techniques and skin analysis.

Minoo's advanced training course delivers the cutting edge in the distinguished difference of knowledge and professionalism. This creates the basis for an ongoing career and loyal clientele who appreciate high quality care and performance.

Minoo's facial products, facial massage techniques, and herbal remedies have helped many people with different skin disorders, wrinkles, dehydration, facial tension, low circulation, and many other physical and emotional pains.

Minoo's Herbal Facial Products:

The first step towards a healthy complexion is to ensure thorough and regular cleansing of the skin. You can use the herbal soaps, shampoos, or infusions for the body, but face and hands are so exposed to the city's grimes and fumes that they need additional deep cleansing to refresh the skin and prevent blemishes that result from pores clogging with oil.

Facial steam also helps in opening and cleaning the pores, especially in people who have oily or blemished skin. People with sensitive skin and broken capillaries should not steam very often, as steam further irritates sensitive skins. You can use facial steam of herbs that suit your skin. For example, if you have oily acne skin, steam it twice a week with fresh sage, rosemary, eucalyptus, burdock, yellow dock, pep-

permint, and parsley. In the case of dry skin, steam with lavender, chamomile, rose, and fennel.

Moisturizing the skin is the most important part of a skin regime. No matter how dry or oily your skin is, you should use a moisturizer day and night.

Minoo's Botanical Skin Care Products:

Minoo offers a complete range of skin care products for three skin types. All Minoo's botanical facial products are hydrophilic (water-based) and should be used with water and acupressure massage. Minoo's facial products are as follows:

Cleansers: Minoo's cleansers are carefully selected for Minoo's preparations. These ingredients cleanse and remove surface impurities.

Cleansers for Normal Skin: This is formulated for dehydrated skin, and skin with poor circulation. It cleanses, hydrates, and soothes the skin. Cleansing morning and evening is the key to healthy skin; this cleanser must be used morning and evening. With a few drops of water, massage it in a circular motion, wash, and follow it with Minoo's toner for deep cleansing.

Herbal ingredients of this cleanser are horsetail, rosemary, birch sap, clover blossom extract, birch leaf extract, yarrow, sage, nettle, apricot kernel oil, sweet almond oil, vegetable oil, honey, and vitamin E.

Toner for all Skin Types: This is designed for deep cleansing and controlling the pH level of skin. Toner for all skin types is formulated from herbs that have antiseptic and pH balancing properties. This toner is to be used after cleanser for removing deep impurities.

Herbal ingredients of this toner are aloe vera, comfrey, chamomile, marigold, allantoin, orange blossom, rose bud, and witch hazel.

Nourishing Cream for Dry- Normal Skin: This cream is developed to preserve the skin tissues and make the driest skins feel moist, soft, silky, and younger looking. You can team this cream with Minoo's liposome and alpha hydroxy acid, and experience the results.

This cream is to be used morning and evening on a cleansed face and neck, with few drops of water. Finger acupress it for absorption. Skin will feel toned, silky, and younger looking. Hyaluronic acid content of this cream helps hold moisture longer in the skin and attract moisture from air, holding it in the skin as well.

Herbal ingredients in this cream are parsley, fennel, honey, beta carotene, allantoin, lactic acid, hyaluronic acid, pseudo-collagen, ascorbic acid, vitamins E and A, and apricot kernel oil.

Hydro Mask for Normal-Dry Skin: This mask is developed to moisten and tone dry skin and help to increase the circulation. This mask has to be used twice a week on cleansed face and neck. It can be mixed with plain yogurt or crushed fresh fruit, like strawberry or peaches. Leave on skin for 15-20 minutes, wash, and follow with Minoo's moisturizer. Skin becomes soft, toned, smooth, and younger looking.

Herbal ingredients in this mask are parsley, fennel, honey, carotene, carrot oil, almond oil, avocado oil, vitamins E, A, and C, and lactic acid.

Cleansers for Dry-Sensitive Skin: This cleanser is developed to cleanse and soothe nervous skins that easily get red. This product should be used morning and evening, over the face and neck with few drops of water. Massage with a circular motion, wash, and follow with toner for deep cleansing.

Herbal ingredients in this cleanser are chamomile, calendula, cucumber, rosemary, comfrey, avocado oil, almond oil, safflower oil, vitamin E, A, C, and D.

Nourishing Cream for Dry-Sensitive Skin: This cream is developed to soothe and preserve skin tissues, making the driest skin tissues feel softer, smoother, moist, and toned.

The mixture is designed for sensitive skins, with all state of art ingredients to nourish, relax, and soothe the skin.

This cream contains a high percentage of hyaluronic acid, which is highly humectant, and that keeps the skin moist all the day. It is ideal to apply this cream and walk by the beach or in a foggy climate, so it can attract moisture from the air and hold it in your skin for longer period of time. This cream is to be used day and night, over cleansed face and neck with few drops of water. Finger acupress it for absorption. Skin will feel wet when using this cream.

Herbal ingredients of this cream are hyaluronic acid (humectant acid derived from beet sugar), cucumber, chamomile, calendula, comfrey, vitamin B5, vitamin A, E, and C, lactic acid, and allantoin (comfrey, beets).

Soothing Mask: This mask is designed to soothe and relax sensitive skins. You get a cooling sensation from this mask. It has the ability to reduce redness. If you have inflamed or wounded skin, apply this mask to reduce inflammation.

This mask is to be used twice a week. After cleansing, leave on for 15 minutes, wash, and follow with Minoo's moisturizer.

Herbal ingredients in this mask are chamomile, calendula, rosemary, cucumber, menthol, azulene, lavender, vitamin E, A, and C.

Cleanser for Oily Acne: This cleanser is developed for oily skins and skins with large pores, blackheads, and blemishes. It has a slight drying action that aids in the healing of skin. If suffering from acne and large pores, cleanse in the skin morning and evening. Apply this cleanser day and night over face and neck, with few drops of water. Massage in circular motion, wash, and follow with Minoo's toner.

Herbal ingredients in this cleanser are eucalyptus, peppermint, sage, rosemary, parsley, lemon oil, radish, corn oil, vegetable oil, and vitamin C .

Moisturizer for all Skin Types: This moisturizer is suitable for all skin types, especially oily skin or oily skin without moisture. This cream protects the skin from moisture loss. It has a light texture which allows fast moisture penetration in the skin.

This moisturizer has to be applied day and night on a cleansed face and neck with few drops of water, then finger acupress for one minute.

Herbal ingredients of this moisturizer are lavender, allantoin (comfrey, beet), carrot oil, hyaluronic acid, pseudo-collagen (collagen from plant), fennel, honey, and vitamins B5, E, A, C, and D.

Refreshing Mask: This mask is great for all skin types, especially oily and skin with large pores. Its cooling and refreshing effects visibly stimulate and tone the skin. Use this mask when feeling tired and fatigued or going to that special party. Apply twice a week on cleansed face and neck, leave on for 15 minutes, wash, and follow with Minoo's moisturizer.

Herbal ingredients in this mask are eucalyptus, peppermint, lemon oil, parsley, menthol, radish oil, corn oil, and vitamin C.

Acne Lotion: When the follicle becomes filled with oil, dead cells, and bacteria, it swells and ruptures. This causes debris to escape into dermis, thus, causing acne.

Minoo's acne preparation has been developed to purify and dry blemishes on the skin. It penetrates, inhibits the growth of bacteria, and retards oil production on the surface of the skin. With Minoo's acne lotion, within two to three days, acne will surface and dry. This lotion has to be used after cleansing and moisturizing of the infected area. Repeat every three to four hours.

Herbal ingredients in this acne lotion are burdock extract, tea tree oil, sage, and witch hazel.

Exfoliating Mask: As an intensive refined cleanser and revitalizing mask, this product unclogs pores, removes excess oil, and sloughs dead cellular layers. It helps to circulation and prepare the skin to receive oxygen, water, and vitamins from other Minoo's products. Skin become soft, silky, and

younger looking after the use of this mask. By using Minoo's exfoliating mask, make-up application sits better and more naturally on the skin.

This exfoliating mask is very light and gentle, and it is suitable for all skin types. If you have oily skin with large pores, use this mask once or twice a week. If you have sensitive skin, use it once or twice a month. For oily skins, steam your face with herbs, like parsley, eucalyptus, sage, or rosemary while using this mask. Place any of these herbs in a pot, add hot water, let it boil, and steam your face for 5-10 minutes while having exfoliating mask on the face. If you have sensitive skin, steam your face with lavender, chamomile or comfrey for 4 minutes with the mask on your face. If you have dry skin, steam with fennel or lavender and rose, while you have this mask on your face, for five to eight minutes. Wash and follow with Minoo's moisturizer. If not wishing to steam with herbs, use this mask in the shower or use exfoliating mask in the bathtub with windows closed to let the aroma linger for the best benefits.

Ingredients in this mask are papaya enzyme, orange, corn flour, wheat flour, oat flour, and vitamin B5 (panthenol).

Minoo's Eye Cream: The skin around the eyes is the thinnest, driest, and the most sensitive skin. To control dryness, Minoo's eye care cream will benefit individual skin types and needs. The texture is designed with all the state of art ingredients to soothe and make firm tiny wrinkles around the eyes and to help in reducing puffiness around the eyes.

Minoo's eye cream should be used both morning and evening or as soon as skin feels dehydrated, with few drops of water. Apply around the eye; finger acupress it for a minute.

Herbal ingredients in this cream are borage oil, cucumber oil, chamomile, calendula, comfrey, hyaluronic acid (sugar from beet), vitamin E, C, A, and D, vitamin B5 (panthenol), sesame oil, and almond oil.

Minoo's 7 Day Miracle Wrinkle Cream: This skin-perfecting cream is designed for all skin types. It is ideal for promoting moisture, firmness, and youthfulness in the skin. It works within a short period of time, producing visible smoothing of the skin, and prevents premature aging. Skin becomes toned, soft, and glowing.

This cream is highly concentrated, so apply it with water and use acupressure massage. It has to be applied day and night, over entire face and neck, with water and finger acupress it for a couple minutes.

Herbal ingredients in this cream are jojoba oil, parsley, fennel, chamomile, borage, royal bee jelly, hyaluronic acid (sugar from beet), vitamin C, A, E, F, D, and B5 (panthenol).

Liposome Serum as Anti-Free Radical: Free radicals are one of the major causes of skin aging. They cause up to 80% of the signs of premature aging. Liposome, as an anti-free radical, has a molecule which penetrates in the cell surface and helps to neutralize the free radicals before harming the skin. Using this product on a daily basis helps as a filter against free radicals.

Liposome anti-free radical is ideal for all skin types and ages, especially people who live in polluted areas and smokers, since carbon monoxide in tobacco reduces the oxygen in blood. Nicotine also constricts the arteries which reduces blood flow. Using liposome with acupressure massage helps in normal circulation.

Liposome should be used morning and evening on the entire face and neck after cleansing. With fingers, acupress to create a firming effect. A moisturizer has to be used with liposome.

Liposome anti free radical is derived from live active yeast (protein yeast for super oxide dismutase S.O.D.). Vitamin A, C, and E are anti free radicals or antioxidants.

Liposome Serum for Tissue & Cell Repair: Yeast derived from the live yeast cell stimulates living tissues to utilize more oxygen. Liposome T.R.F (tissue respirator factor), a cell proliferate, is able to promote wound healing, stimulate growth of connective tissues, act as an anti-inflammatory and excellent moisturizer (due to hyaluronic acid), and increase the elasticity of the skin, making it feel smoother and younger looking. The molecule in liposome T.R.F. is a very small 2 carbon atom. It penetrates within 30 to 40 seconds.

Use five drops of this serum, after morning and evening cleansing, on the entire face and neck. Finger acupress it for absorption.

Liposome tissue and cell repair is made from live active yeast protein for wound healing and contains hyaluronic acid and vitamin E.

Glycol Multi Fruit Acid Cream (Alpha Hydroxy Acid):

This particular alpha hydroxy acid cream has been developed from a variety of fruit acids to normalize the acid mantel on the skin, where the extraordinary transformation starts. Fruit acid gently dissolves layers of lifeless cells that dull your skin's appearance. It will return skin's brightness, clarity, smoothness, and tone. With Minoo's AHA treatment you will get maximum fruit acid efficiency, without risk of irritation.

This fruit acid is great for all skin types, problems, and conditions. It can act as a moisturizer on oily skins. This cream has to be used morning and evening on the entire face and neck, with few drops of water. Finger acupress it for couple of minutes for absorption, and follow with Minoo's moisturizer.

Herbal ingredients in this cream are lemon, orange, bilberry, sugar cane, allantoin (comfrey), pseudo-collagen, and aloe vera extract.

Pigmentation Cream:

This cream will slow excess production of melanin, help to lighten brown spots caused by the sun, hormonal disorder, or acne scars, and fight against uneven skin pigmentation. Skin will become even and glow.

This cream has to be used over cleansed and moisturized skin every day and night. Night is the ideal time; massage it in for absorption. Results appear in four to six weeks, if used daily.

Sunburns:

This is inflammation of the skin caused by exposure to ultraviolet rays. Usually, fair skins damage more and faster than darker skins, as fair skin has little protective pigments. Damage to fair skin causes redness, discomfort, broken capillaries or sensitivities, and wrinkles. Damage to darker skin starts with redness and further oily pigments are increased.

More serious sunburns cause swelling of skin and tissues that leads to blister peel. It is known that sunbathing can cause skin cancer. Modern sunscreen products are only effective superficially. Sun also causes wrinkles and skin to turn leathery due to damage by free radicals from sun.

If you have a fair skin, you are more at risk of skin damage. Therefore you should avoid direct rays of the sun. If you have to be in the sun for a few minutes, wear a hat and sunglasses, apply sun screens that contain vitamin E, aloe vera and comfrey to soothe and protect skin, apply heavy moisturizers that contain hyaluronic acid, and drink plenty of water to prevent dehydration.

If sunburned, a soothing and healing lotion containing lavender and comfrey, like Minoo's hand and body lotion, can be applied. Lavender, chamomile, and comfrey soothe, moisturize and relax sunburned skin. If you do not have Minoo's hand and body lotion, mix 1/2 cup of natural plain yogurt and 5 drops of lavender oil and apply on the skin. While still tacky, cover the area with cotton. For example, if shoulders are burned, after application wear an old T-shirt. Repeat the application. You can also apply raw grated potatoes to affected area and repeat the application everyday until complete healing. Minoo's Liposome (T.R.F.) is very healing and reduces inflammation and discomfort of the skin.

Minoo's Sunscreen: If you like to have a healthy and young complexion,

avoid the sun as much as possible. Long exposure can be very unsafe for the health of your skin.

Minoo has prepared sun protection for all skin types. Remember not to stay in the sun for a long time, even if you have protection on your skin, because nothing is guaranteed for 100% protection, especially if you have a fair complexion. Fair complexion means less pigments for protection, and usually fair skin is thinner.

Sunscreen moisturizer is a long lasting moisture-enhancer with antioxidant for ultimate anti-aging protection, as well as blocking skin damage from ultraviolet rays. This non-greasy protection is formulated from herbs like aloe vera, comfrey, evening primrose, panthenol, cucumber and vitamin E to soothe, moisturize and prevent skin burning.

It needs to be used during the daytime under make-up, especially if your skin is exposed to sun, and if your skin is peeling, use it day and night for protection.

Hand and Body Lotion: As we grow older, skin loses its oil and moisture because the body does not produce the skin-lubricating sebum oil from its sebaceous glands nor retain water in the quantities that it did when younger. Therefore, we ought to take more care of our skin by drinking more water and by using heavy moisturizer and acupressure to protect against dehydration and wrinkles.

Minoo's hand and body cream is intensive care, protecting the skin from dehydration and cracking in wintertime. The cream has to be used all over the body after each shower, and on hands after each hand washing, especially washings done with soap.

Minoo's hand and body lotion is prepared from soothing and moisturizing essential oils of herbs, like olive, chamomile, comfrey, lavender, wheat germ, soy bean, jojoba, avocado, rose, and orange.

How to Give Yourself a Facial:
There are many different ways to keep a healthy complexion forever. Consider your skin like a saving account... the more you deposit, the more interest is received. The more attention that you pay to your skin by taking good care of it, the more you will be proud of it when you are older. Never is too late; start from today! Respect your skin, and take better care of it.

As I mentioned in former chapters, the keys to a healthy complexion are:
▪ Healthy and balanced diet.
▪ Drinking enough water.
▪ Getting enough sleep and exercise.
▪ Avoiding sun, dry heat and air.
▪ Cleansing morning and evening to remove make-up and impurities from your skin.
▪ Protecting the skin from harsh environmental influences (free radicals).

▪ Avoiding emotional stresses.
▪ Giving acupressure massage and facial exercise every night for a few minutes.

▪ Getting facials on a regular basis, or getting a mini-facial once a week in order to keep your pores clean and help in receiving oxygen and vitamins.

With Minoo's facial products and facial massage techniques, your problem is solved no matter whether you have an acne problem or a most sensitive, dehydrated skin. With any skin type and condition that you have, never forget to keep it clean and nourished.

Once a week, after you cleanse your skin with Minoo's cleanser and toner, apply exfoliating mask and steam your skin with herbs for few minutes, then extract your impurities and blackheads by wrapping a clean cloth around your index finger and actually try to remove them. If you let blackheads and impurities sit on your skin, the result would be clogged pores, and oxygen would be prevented from getting to the skin, thereby causing acne and further damages. After extraction of impurities, apply five drops of Liposome on your face and neck and deep acupress with middle and ring finger for at least one minute. Liposome penetrates the skin very quickly. Then apply Glycol multi fruit acid cream on the entire face and neck. If you do not wish to used fruit acid, apply the moisturizer that suits your skin, then deep acupress with water for 2 minutes.

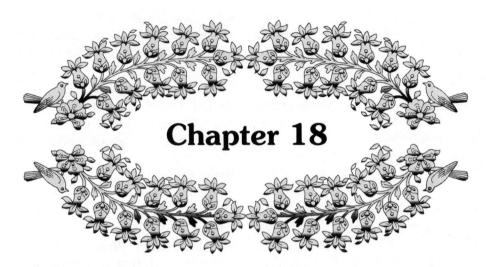

Chapter 18

Minoo's Massage Techniques

inoo has developed unique application mas sage technique for professional aestheticians, her acupressure massage focus on facial muscle oxygenation, wrinkle reduction, tension and headache reduction.

Anti-Aging Acupressure Massage With Moisyurizer:

Place two thumbs between the brows, and place middle and ring fingers in the outer corner of eyes. Apply pressure, deep and gentle. With the back of middle and ring fingers, start from the outer corner of the eyes. Press, and move to the inner corner. With second, middle, and ring fingers, press around the eyes, and keep moving to the mouth area. Give pressure to the line around the eyes, lips, and forehead with thumb, second ring and middle fingers, and finally piano tap. Repeat this 3-5 times.

After acupressure anti-aging massage, apply the mask that suites you on the entire face and neck. Leave on for 15 minutes, wash with warm water, follow with cool water, and apply moisturizer. Finger acupress eye cream around the eyes with few drops of water for absorption.

Facial and Relaxation Massage for Aesthetician:

This is a massage technique developed by Minoo for professional aestheticians.

This unique application can create a loyal clientele who appreciate real European facials and professionalism.

This relaxation and tension reduction massage starts after deep pore cleansing and oxygenation, one step before the final mask. It takes 15-18 minutes, depending on physical and emotional conditions. For example, if client suffering from headache, headache reduction massage is recommended, or if suffering from sinus pressure, sinus drainage massage is suitable. General tension and acupressure massages are as follows:

Back Tension Reduction Massage:

- Place both hands on the back of your client, close to brow line.

- Massage upwards in circular motion.

- Go through each cervical and give acupressure massage.

- If you feel any tension or tightness, hold your middle and ring fingers and release the tension by giving deep acupressure massage.

- Come up and end your massage at the base of the neck, where muscles are situated.

- Place both thumbs on both sides of shoulders, usually tension is around the shoulder and neck, press deep for few

seconds.

- Massage deep in circular motion to loosen the tension. Repeat 5-7 times depending on tension or tightness.

Shoulder Tension Reduction Massage:

- Rest both thumbs on the shoulders.

- With 2nd, 3rd, 4th, and 5th fingers circle massage both shoulders clockwise.

- Repeat 3-5 times.

Decollet Tension Reduction Massage:

- Strike from breast bone up to shoulders alternately with right and left hands.

- Repeat 3-5 times

Neck Tension Reduction Massage:

- Slide the 3rd and 4th fingers of both hands gently down the neck.

- Exert light pressure with 2nd, 3rd, 4th, and 5th fingers on the head, turning muscles upward behind ears.

- With light pressure, slip under jaws, gently forward with 3rd and 4th fingers.

-Repeat 3-5 times.

Neckline Tension Reduction Massage:

-Rest both hands on shoulders.

-Strike with pressure towards neckline.

-Lightly press with middle finger and with pressure of fingertips. Slip gently down the trapezius muscle towards shoulders.

-Repeat it 3 times.

Chin Tension Reduction Massage:

-Make circular movements alternately with 3rd and 4th fingers of both hands from under the center of the chin.

-Rotate the right hand counterclockwise and the left hand clockwise.

-Steadily rest the thumbs on the chin.

-Repeat 3-5 times.

Laughing Lines Tension Reduction Massage:

-Place the 2nd and 3rd fingers of both hands in the center of chin.

-Move fingertips upward along mouth-nose line to the root of nose.

-With the 2nd, 3rd, 4th and 5th fin-gers, glide under cheekbones, slowly up to ears.

-Repeat 3 times.

Lips Tension Reduction Massage:

-Place the 3rd finger of the left hand flat over the center of upper lip.

-Place 3rd finger of right hand on the center of lower lip.

- Circulate fingertips of both hands around the mouth.

-Repeat 3-5 times.

-Place middle and ring fingers of both hands on the upper lip.

-Press deep horizontally and vertically.

-Repeat 3 times.

Temple Crossing Movements:

-Rest both hands gently on temples.

-Slide them down the cheeks to chin, then cross under chin, and return in opposite direction up the cheeks to the forehead.

-Cross both hands in the middle in or-der to start the same procedure.

-Repeat 5 times.

Temple and Side Massage:

- Place the ring and middle fingers on both sides of the face.

- Massage deep, stop, and acupress it when at temples.

- Place the ring and middle fingers of both hands on temples.

- Press gently and move toward the inner corners of both eyes.

- Repeat 3 times.

Eye Tension Reduction Massage:

- With the 2nd and 3rd fingers of the left hand, spread the skin on outside corner of the eyes.

- Glide, with circular movements, the 3rd finger of right hand from inner corner of the eyes to nerve endings.

- With light pressure, slowly return the skin under eyebrows to its starting position.

- Repeat 3 times on each eye.

- Place ring and middle finger of each hand on outer corner of the eyes.

- Move with pressure and go around the eyes, and do brow lifting.

Tension Reduction Massage of Lines on Forehead:

- Place the 2nd, 3rd, and 4th fingertips of the right hand at the root of rose.

- Then spread fingers slightly over right side of forehead and move upward to hairline with light pressure.

- Do the same with left hand over the left side of forehead.

- Repeat 5 times.

- Strike the 3rd and 4th fingers of both hands, with light pressure, from the root of nose upward over forehead.

- Repeat 5 times.

- Place thumbs of both hands between the eyebrows.

- Place the middle and ring fingers of both hands at the outer corner of the eyes.

- Gently acupress the middle and ring fingers to the inner corners of the eyes.

- Move the thumbs towards the outer corner of the eyes.

- Place 2nd, 3rd and 4th fingers of both hands over the forehead horizontally.

- Acupress deep across.

-Repeat 3 times.

- Then, with the same finger, deep acupress vertically towards the hairlines.

-Repeat 3- 5 times.

Temple/ Forehead Tension Reduction Massage:

-Place the 3rd and 4th fingers of both hands at the root of nose.

-Make 3 circular movements in the direction of temples.

-There rest them flat with light pressure.

-Repeat 5 times.

Eyebrows Tension Reduction Massage:

-Place thumbs above and inside the corners of eyebrows (parallel).

-Lift eyebrows gently between thumbs.

-Glide the 3rd fingers on sides.

-Lightly press the 3rd fingertips at the outer corners of the eyes.

-Glide around the eye, over nose bridge, to the inner corner of the eyebrows.

-Repeat 5 times.

Final Relaxation Massage:

-With slight pressure, rest both hands on the temples.

-With horizontal soft movements of both hands, strike alternately over the forehead, from one temple to the other.

-There, rest the fingers for a while, with light pressure.

-Lightly press with the middle fingers and move slowly down to the neck, dıcolletı over the shoulders, back to the neck, jaws, chins, and from the corner of mouth up to sides of nose bridge, from nose to the nerve endings of the eyes.

-With both hands, slowly return over eyebrows to the forehead.

Final Calming Movements:

-Cross the 2nd, 3rd, 4th, and 5th fingers of both hands on top of each other.

-Place them on the chins (rest the 5th fingers on the chin-neck line, the 2nd fingers under the lower lip).

-Return sideways to the outer corners of the mouth.

-Then tuck the thumbs under laughing lines and strike with insides of both hands upward to the root of nose and forehead.

-Then turn hands, and with the 3rd and 4th fingers, gently strike the forehead downward over the temples along the outer cheekbones.

-Then place the hands around the chin.

-Repeat 3 times.

Compression:

-Place palms of both hands on sides of the face.

-Place the thumbs above the eyebrows, and the other fingers should touch the lower jawbone. Increase the pressure slowly and loosen again.

-Repeat 3 times.

Acupressure Anti-Aging Massage:

-Place both thumbs between the brows and the middle and ring fingers in the outer corner of the eyes.

-Start from the outer corner of the eyes, press the back of middle and ring fingers deep and gentle.

-Move the 2nd middle and ring fingers to the inner corner.

-Press around the eyes and keep moving to the mouth.

-Press the line around the eyes, lips, and forehead with the thumbs and the 2nd, middle, and ring fingers.

-Place both ring fingers' nails on the outer corner of the eyes.

-Press and move to the inner corner of the eyes with acupressure massage.

-Place both palms on the outer corner of the eyes, and press deep.

-Move towards the mouth, knuckle the finger and acupress around the mouth and chins.

-Move upward to the temples and forehead and rest with acupressure.

-Rest the muscle of both the thumbs on the outer corner of the eyes.

-With light pressure, move downward to the lips and chins, and upward to the temples and forehead.

-Finally piano tap, rest both your hands on the forehead's sides, gently pull with the fingers, and end it at the ears.

Headache Reduction Massage:

Tension headaches usually start from the neck.

-Concentrate on the neck, especially base of the neck (the center of headache).

-First, acupress massage the shoulder with both thumbs for a minute.

-Then, with the 2nd, 3rd, 4th, and 5th fingers of both hands, go through neck cervical; massage, and end it at the base of neck.

-Repeat 5-7 times

-Place the ring and middle fingers of the left hand on the base of neck.

-Then, place the middle and ring finger of the right hand between the brows.

-Finally, place the thumb of right hand on the skull.

-Press all three places at the same time and with the same pressure (very deep pressure).

-Press and hold for 10 seconds.

-Repeat 7-10 times, depending on the severity of headache.

-Place the middle and ring fingers of both hands on the base of neck, and thumbs on the temples.

-Press hard, but be gentle on the temples.

-Repeat 5-7 times, and each time for 10 seconds.

-With both thumbs and index fingers, pull the ear, massage and press.

-Ear massaging is very relaxing and releases the tension and pain.

-Repeat this 2-3 times on each ear for 5 seconds.

-With both hands' thumbs and index fingers, lift the brows and massage.

-Repeat 2-3 times.

-Place the 2nd, 3rd, 4th, and 5th fingers of both hands on the forehead, press it hard, and keep moving towards the hairlines.

-Place middle and ring fingers of both hands on the temples, and acupress massage deep in the circular motion for one minute.

-Place the 2nd, 3rd, 4th, and 5th fingers of both hands on dıcolletı, and press to release lactic acid deposits. Massage with both hands' fingers in circular motion.

Sinus Drainage Massage :

-Turn on the steamer, and put in a few drops of pure eucalyptus oil or fresh eucalyptus leaves.

-Steam for a few minutes for inhalation.

-While inhaling, give sinus drainage massage.

-Place the middle and ring fingers of both hands on the sinus area.

-Starting from below the eyes, deep acupress, and keep moving downward to the mouth.

-Place the ring and middle fingers of both hands between the brows.

-Press hard, and keep moving upward to the forehead. End it at the hair-lines.

-Lift the eyebrows with the thumbs and index fingers.

-Massage and acupress.

-Repeat this massage 4-5 times

-Excess mucus will be released through the nasal passages.

-It is recommended to eat lots of raw onion and inhale eucalyptus.

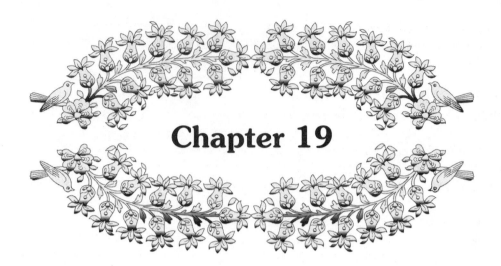

Chapter 19

Herbal Food Recipes

In previous chapters we analyzed the herbs, their biochemical constituents, and energetic, therapeutic, cosmetic, and medicinal values. As we know, there are many herbs and plants that are used for their nutritional properties, flavor and color. Many people use herbs to flavor or garnish their meals, but, main meals can be made with herbs too. Since early times, raw wild herbs and vegetables have been collected and dishes prepared to be eaten, especially by people in Iran and Mediterranean countries. The earliest surviving salad recipe includes quanti-

ties of plants and fresh herbs.

These mixtures are often nutritious, as each leaf, bud, flower, and seed provides different minerals and vitamins. Most Iranian housewives have some knowledge of the medicinal values of herbs and make their salads according to the needs of the household, attempting to balance cool plants, such as cucumber, endive, and lettuce, with warming aromatic herbs, such as tarragon, parsley, dill weed, dried or pickled herbs, small weeds, and herbs that survive throughout the winter.

Many of the herbal salads must be eaten early in the year, while they are still fresh and before becoming bitter and harsh. Some herbs, like dandelion leaves, need to be blanched in boiling water for few minutes to reduce their bitterness.

It is often necessary to eat herbs or

vegetables when fresh, since most herbs and vegetables deplete their vitamins and minerals with heat and cooking.

Spring salad herbs include leaves of borage, watercress, yarrow, sorrel, dandelion, corn, and lime leaves. To flavor spring salads, use fennel, lovage, caraway, and chervil.

The following recipes, from Iran, and Mediterranean countries, show the way which you too can use herbs for your dinner recipes, like soups, salads, stews, poultry, seafood, desserts, a variety of dishes with rice, etc. The recipes in this section serve four people.

Persian Noodle Soups (Aasheh Rashteh):

This very traditional soup is highly nutritious and contains a variety of cereals and herbs. This is also a great meal for vegetarians. Soy and other beans in this soup substitute for meat.

3 cups of combined soy, black, garbonza, and large kidney beans.
1/2 cup of lentils
4 bundles of each: parsley, spinach, cilantro, and chive.
1 cup of chopped onion
1 package of Japanese noodles
5 cloves of garlic, minced
2 cups of cream cheese and yogurt, blended together
A pinch of salt, pepper, and turmeric

for garnishing and taste.
1 tablespoon of dried mint

Cook soy, black, garbonza, and kidney beans. Cooking will take at least three hours. Chop spinach, parsley, cilantro, and chive. Wash and cook them in a separate big pot with at least 6 cups of water. As you are cooking the herbs, add lentils, as lentils cook faster than the rest of the beans. Add noodles. Sauté the onion, add turmeric to sauté, and pour it in the pot to cook with noodles and herbs. Cook for at least 20 minutes, then add all the cooked beans to the herbs and noodles. Lower the flame, and let the soup settle for at least 30 minutes more.

Once soup is ready, in a separate frying pan, sauté garlic just for one minute. Add the dried mint to it for garnishing. Serve the soup in a casserole dish. Garnish the top with cream, sauté of garlic, and mint. This soup serves at least 8 people.

Turnip Soup:

This soup is great for colds, coughs, sore throats, and sinus infection.

1 cup of chopped onion
1 cup of chopped turnip
1 cup of chopped carrots
1 cup of chopped potatoes
1 cup of chopped broccoli and cabbage
1/2 cup of oatmeal
3 cups of fresh chicken broth

5 cloves of garlic
1/2 cup of fresh lemon juice
1 tablespoon of chopped rosemary
Salt and a pinch of ginger.

Boil the chopped vegetables and oatmeal in chicken broth for 30 minutes. Add salt and pepper, ginger, and lemon juice.

Whole Grain Soup (Aasheh Jou):

3 cups of combination of whole barley, wheat, burger, oat, and brown rice.
2 cups of combination of soybeans, black beans, garbonza beans.
4 cups of chopped parsley, cilantro, spinach, and chives.
1 large onion, chopped
1/2 cup of olive oil
3 cloves of garlic, minced
2 cups of yogurt with cream cheese, mixed
Garlic and salt.
1 teaspoon of turmeric
Salt and pepper.

In a big pot, wash all the grains and beans, except oat. Add enough water to cover all the ingredients. Let it boil for at least 3 hours or until all the grains are tender. Then add chopped herbs and let it cook. In a frying pan, sauté onion with olive oil. Add turmeric, the onion, and barley flakes with the rest of ingredients to the pot, and let it boil on a low temperature for at least 20 minutes. Serve this soup either with

the blended cream and yogurt or lemon juice.

Herbal Summer Soup (Aabdough):

This summer herbs soup is very refreshing and great when the weather is very warm and you do not feel like eating a hot cooked meal. This recipe serves at least 4 people.

1 cup of chopped cucumber
3 cups of plain yogurt
3 cups of minced herbs, oregano, marjoram, thyme, basil, mint, tarragon, watercress, dill weed, and chives
1 cup of chopped onion and garlic
1/2 cup of chopped walnut
2 cups of ice cube
2 pieta breads, chopped (you can use crunchy, dried bread)
1 tablespoon salt
1 teaspoon fresh or black pepper.
2 cups of water

Mix all the ingredients in a big bowl. Add ice and water, and leave it for few minutes. Serve it. This is a delicious, satisfying, and refreshing summer soup. You can also add raisins to this soup.

Herbal Rice (Saabzi Poulo):

This rice can be served either with chicken, fish, or herb soufflé.

3 cups of basmati rice, wash and soak in water for a few hours

4 cups herbs, minced: parsley, cilantro, leeks, chives, mints, and dill weed
1/2 cup of rosemary and fenugreek (you can use dried fenugreek)
5 cloves of garlic, minced
1 cup of olive oil
3 tablespoons salt
1/2 teaspoon saffron.

In a big pot, boil the rice until half tender. Rinse the rice in a colander. Pour one cup of olive oil in the same pot. After the rice is rinsed, pour one layer of rice in the pot and one layer of chopped herbs and garlic. Continue to the top. After all the rice and herbs are combined in the pot, put the pot on a stove with high temperature for few minutes. Once steams appear, turn the flame down, and let it cook for at least 45 minutes. Serve this rice with fish or chicken.

Wash a whole chicken, empty the interior, and stuff it with chopped garlic and rosemary. Sprinkle saffron all over the chicken and add 1/2 cup of water and some lemon juice. Let it bake for at least an hour. Serve it with herb rice.

If you like to serve this rice with fish, clean and empty the interior and stuff it with rosemary and lemon peel. Sprinkle saffron all over the fish with some lemon juice. Let it bake for at least an hour. Serve it with herbal rice

Herbal Soufflé (Koukou):

This soufflé can be served either with herbal rice or as a sandwich with bread.

1 cup of each herb, finely minced: parsley, cilantro, leeks, chives, mint, spinach
1 cup combination of fenugreek, dill weed, and rosemary(If you can't find fresh fenugreek, use 1 tablespoon dried)
5 eggs
5 cloves of garlic
1 tablespoon of all purpose flour
1/2 teaspoon of baking soda.
1 cup of olive oil
1/2 teaspoon of black pepper
1/2 teaspoon of turmeric
1 teaspoon of salt.
a pinch of saffron

You can either bake or fry the soufflé, whichever way you prefer. To fry the soufflé, pour olive oil in the frying pan and preheat it. In a big bowl, mix all the herbs, garlic, salt, pepper, saffron, turmeric, flour, and baking soda. Add the eggs, and beat it for at least 5 minutes. Pour the ingredients in the preheated frying pan and let it fry slowly. Lower the flame and let it fry. Once the bottom part is fried, turn it over to the other side to cook. Once other side is cooked too, cut it like a cake. Serve with rice or bread.

Fenugreek Stew (Ghormeh Saabzi):

This soup is an aromatic and delicious traditional soup in Iran. This stew can be made either with lamb, beef, or chicken breast. This recipes serves at least 4 people.

3 cups of basmati rice
2 pounds of chopped leaned beef or chicken breast.
1 large onion, chopped
4 cups of well-minced parsley, chives, and fenugreek
1 cup of kidney beans
1 cup of olive oil
1 teaspoon of black pepper
1/2 teaspoon of turmeric
1/2 teaspoon of saffron.
1 tablespoon salt
1/2 cup of dried lemon or fresh lemon juice.

In a large pan, sauté onion and meat. Add salt, pepper, turmeric, and 2 cups of water. Wash the kidney beans. Mix them with meat and onion, sauté, and let it cook.

In a separate frying pan, fry the herbs with olive oil on low flame until brown. Empty the fried herbs in the pot and let it cook with the rest of ingredients on low flame for at least 3 to 4 hours. Add dried lemon or fresh lemon juice 30 minutes before serving.

The rice has to be soaked at least few hours before cooking. Empty the washed and soaked rice in a large pot with few cups of water. Half cook, rinse, and pour it back in the pot with some olive oil. Let it cook on low temperature. Once the rice is done, serve it with stew.

Meat Ball With Herbs (Koufteh):

Meat ball with herbs can be made as large as you like. This is a great meal for parties, and you can also make a sandwich with it. You can either bake or boil it. This meatball can be stuffed or not. The recipe below is for stuffed meat ball, and if you do not care for this, avoid stuffing.

1 cup of rice
1 cup of split beans
2 cups of well-minced tarragon, parsley, marjoram, and mint
1 large onion, chopped
2 pounds of ground leaned beef, veal, or chicken breast
5 cloves of garlic
1 cup of olive oil
1 tablespoon of salt
1/2 teaspoon of black pepper
1 egg
1/2 teaspoon of saffron
Ingredients for stuffing:
1/2 cup of ground walnut
1/2 cup of bilberry
1/2 cup of chopped fried onion
1/2 cup of plums, pitted
2 boiled eggs

Wash the rice and split beans. Boil

them with one cup of water for 10 minutes. Put them in the food processor with the herbs, garlic, salt and pepper; blend them until mixed well together. Place this in a bowl, add ground meat and egg, and start massaging them with your hand until well mixed. Make a big ball with these ingredients. If you wish to stuff them, make a hole in the middle of the meat, put the stuffing in the middle and close it. If you wish to boil it, prepare sauté of one large onion with olive oil, add turmeric and 5 cups of water. Place the meat ball in the pot with fried onion and water, and let it cook for at least 3 hours. When serving, slice it to the desired size.

If you wish to bake it, , pour 3 cups of water in a deep and large casserole dish. Add fried onion and saffron, cover, and bake it for at least 2 to 3 hours. You can garnish it with ground tomatoes, minced parsley, and basil.

Sweet Nut Rice (Shirin Poulo):

This rice is served with chicken.

2 pounds of chicken breast
4 cups of basmati rice, washed and soaked in 5 cups of water
1 cup of almonds
1 cup of raisins
1/2 cup of orange peel (soaked in water for 2 hours)
1/2 cup of pistachios
1 cup of olive oil

1/2 teaspoon of saffron
1/2 cup of sugar

In a large frying pan, pour olive oil and sauté raisins, pistachios, almonds, and orange peel for few minutes. Add 1 cup of water and 1/2 cup of sugar, and let it boil for only 2 minutes.

Boil the soaked basmati rice until half tender, and rinse it. Pour the rice back in the pot, add 1 cup of water and 1/2 cup of olive oil, and let cook slowly for 30 to 40 minutes.

Wash the chicken breast and cut it to small pieces. Add 1 cup of water, salt, and saffron, and bake it for 30 minutes.

After the rice is cooked, serve the rice in a tray, one layer of rice and one layer of fried ingredients (almond, pistachio, raisin and etc.), and prepared chicken breast. Continue to fill the tray with rice, chicken, and other ingredients. Serve it with salad.

Bilberry Rice (Zareshk Poulo):

This rice is served with chicken breast. This rice and sweet rice are formal dishes and can be served at weddings and formal parties.

1 cup of bilberry, cleaned and washed
1 cup of almond, chopped and cleaned.

1 tablespoon of saffron, soaked in 1/2 cup of hot water
3 tablespoons of sugar
2 pounds of chicken breast, cleaned and cut
4 cups of basmati rice, soaked in water and salt
1 cup of olive oil.

In a large frying pan, sauté bilberry, almonds, and sugar with 1/2 cup of olive oil. Add sugar and 1/2 cup of water, and let it boil for 2 minutes.

In a pot, pour 6 cups of water, rice, and salt. Boil until half tender. Rinse the rice and put back in the pot with 1/2 cup of olive oil and 1/2 cup of water. Cook on low temperature.

Chicken breast can be baked or boiled. For baking, add 1/2 cup of water and a pinch of saffron, and let it bake for 30 to 40 minutes.

When serving in a big dish, try putting one layer of rice and sprinkle the saffron, then one layer of bilberry, and almond. Put the chicken around it.

Stuffed Cabbage Leaves or Grape Leaves (Doulmeh kalam):

This recipe can be served with bread. You can make it either with cabbage leaves or grape leaves or both.

1 pound of large cabbage leaves or grape leaves.

2 cups of rice and split beans.
2 cups of finely chopped tarragon, parsley, chives, and mint
1/2 cup of finely chopped onion
5 cloves of garlic, finely minced.
5 large fresh tomatoes, blended well so that it looks like a sauce.
1 pound minced beef or minced chicken breast.
1/2 tablespoon of salt, black pepper, and turmeric
1 cup of olive oil
1/2 cup of water.

Use the large cabbage leaves. Steam for 2 minutes until a little tender.

Cook rice and split beans until tender. Cook the chicken breast or beef, and mix all the minced herbs, meat, rice, beans, onion, garlic, salt, pepper, and turmeric.

In 2 cabbage leaves put 2 tablespoons of ingredients and wrap. Place in casserole dish and keep stuffing the cabbage leaves until cooked.

Pour blended tomatoes over the stuffed cabbages, with oil and 1/2 cup of water, and let it bake for at least one hour. Serve it with some fresh lemon for better taste.

Stuffed Tomatoes and Bell Pepper (Dolmeh):

This recipe can be served with bread.

2 cups of rice and split beans

3 cups of minced parsley, tarragon, marjoram, mint, and chives
1 large onion, minced
5 cloves of garlic, minced
1 pound of minced chicken breast
2 cups of tomato sauce
5 large bell pepper
4 large tomatoes
1 cup of olive oil
1 cup of water
1 tablespoon black or fresh pepper
1/2 teaspoon of turmeric and 1 tablespoon of salt

In a pot, cook rice and split beans until tender. In a large frying pan, sauté minced chicken breast with all the herbs, onion, and garlic. Add salt, pepper, and turmeric. Add cooked rice and split beans to the herbs.

Empty the tomatoes and bell peppers, and stuff them with the prepared ingredients. Place the stuffed tomatoes and bell pepper in a casserole dish and sprinkle the tomato sauce over them with 1/2 cup of water and 1/2 cup of olive oil. Bake for 1 hour, and serve it with fresh lemon for even better taste.

Herbal Salads

Spring salads have usually been a good source of nutrition, and herbs can be added to the salads for extra flavor and beautiful colors. You can use a variety of herbs for their nutrition, flavor, color, and aroma.

For example, dandelion is nutritious and an excellent source of vitamin A, iron and other minerals. It has cleansing and stimulating effects on liver and gallbladder. Watercress and fennel are healing, and nasturtiums can be used for their colors as well as flavor. Cucumber, mint, lemon balm, and marjoram are soothing and refreshing, and if you have kidney problems, lovage and celery can be added to your salads.

Following recipe shows you how to make your fresh herbal salads. There is also a recipe for dressing.

All Herbs Salads With Dressing:

3 oz of chopped dandelion leaves
2 oz of chopped watercress
2 oz of chopped spinach
2 oz of chopped green onion
1 cup of chopped parsley
1 small romaine lettuce
1 cup of nasturtium flowers for garnishing and flavoring

Dressing Recipe:

3 cloves of garlic, minced or ground
1 teaspoon of ground black pepper
1 teaspoon of salt
1 tablespoon of fresh minced marjoram
2 fresh lemons, squeezed
1 cup of organic yellow mustard
1 tablespoon of olive oil

In a big salad bowl, mix all the herbs

and garnish with nasturtiums flowers. Mix all the salad dressing ingredients in a jar and shake well. Serve with hot fresh bread.

All Herbs Salads Without Dressing:

This herbal salad is very refreshing and satisfying. In summer or spring, you should have it with fresh pieta bread and feta cheese. It is actually a good snack for summer afternoons. Recipe is for 2 to 3 people.

1 cup of chopped fresh basil
1 cup of chopped fresh mint
1 cup of chopped fresh tarragon
1 cup of chopped fresh parsley and cilantro
1 cup of chopped fresh marjoram
1 cup of chopped fresh oregano and dill weed
1 cup of chopped fresh watercress
1 cup of sliced radishes and green onion
1 cup of chopped fresh chives
16 oz of fresh low fat feta cheese
6 fresh warm pieta breads

Wash all the herbs before chopping. In a big bowl or big basket ,mix all the herbs, and add feta cheese. Serve it with bread.

All Veggies and Herbs Salads:

This salad can be served either with bread or the main meal. It serves 4 to 6 people.

1 head of lettuce
3 pickling cucumbers
1 cup of cherry tomatoes, fresh
4 stalks of celery
1 stalk of broccoli
3 fresh carrots, shredded
1 horseradish, chopped
1 cup of chopped red cabbage
1 large red onion, chopped
1/2 cup of chopped cilantro
1 large bell pepper, chopped
1 cup of chopped dandelion
1 cup of sprout beans
1 cup of alfalfa
1 cup of chopped mushroom
1 cup of chopped parsley and dill weed
4 cloves of garlic, minced
1/2 cup of olive oil
Salt and black pepper
Fresh lemon juice or vinegar

In a big bowl, mix all the vegetables and herbs. Add olive oil, salt, pepper, and lemon juice.

Green Onion Salad:

This salad can be served as a meal or snack, and it can be served with bread or a meal.

1 bundle of green onions, chopped
2 large potatoes, steamed and chopped
1 clove of garlic, ground
2 cups of celery and endive, minced
2 tablespoons of low fat mayonnaise

2 fresh lemons, squeezed
1 teaspoon black pepper
1/2 teaspoon of salt
1 tablespoon of minced dill week
1 tablespoon of olive oil.

In a big salad bowl, mix all the ingredients. Let it sit for 15 minutes. This is a good snack or meal and can be served with fresh wheat bread.

Iranian Tomato Salad:

This is a traditional Iranian salad that is served with meals. It can also be served with bread as a snack.

2 large fresh tomatoes, chopped in small pieces
3 large English cucumber, chopped in small pieces
1 large red onion, chopped
3 hot chili peppers, minced
1 teaspoon of fresh dill weed
1 clove of garlic, minced.

Dressing

1 fresh egg white
1/2 cup of olive oil
1/2 cup of vinegar
Pinch of black pepper

In a bowl, beat the egg whites for at least 10 minutes manually, or two minutes with electric mixer, until creamy. Add olive oil, vinegar and pepper while beating. This dressing is very delicious and is served with other salads too.

In a big bowl, mix all the vegetables and add the dressing, Serve with meal.

Pasta Salad:

This salad is like a meal; you can serve it by itself or with bread.

2 cups of shell pasta
1 cup of minced chicken breast or bacon
1/2 cup of minced onion
1/2 cup of celery, minced
1/2 cup of minced parsley and garlic
1 cup of olive oil
2 tablespoons of Dijon mustard
1/2 cup of mayonnaise (organic low fat)
1/2 teaspoon of caraway
Black pepper and salt
3 fresh lemons

Cook the pasta until tender. In a frying pan, sauté chicken breast with olive oil and garlic. Mix all the ingredients, and add the mayonnaise and mustard. Squeeze the lemons and mix the salad. Serve with bread or by itself.

Vegetables and Herbs Omelet:

This recipe is a mixture of herbs, vegetables, and proteins. It is highly nutritious and is a great meal as well as snack. The recipe is good for 2 to 3 people.

6 large organic eggs.

1 large tomato, chopped
1 bell pepper, chopped
1 cup of sliced mushrooms
1 thinly sliced leek
4 thinly sliced scallions
1 cup of chopped fresh herbs like tarragon, marjoram, dill leaves and parsley
1 cup of chopped cauliflower and
broccoli
1 cup of chopped dandelion and
spinach.
1 tablespoon of minced chili pepper
and 1 teaspoon salt.
1/2 cup of virgin olive oil
1/2 cup of grated cheddar cheese.

Beat the eggs, and mix the rest of the
ingredients. Bake for 30 minutes at
350(F in a nonstick dish. Uncover the
last 5 minutes to brown the top. Before serving, sprinkle the cheese, and
serve it with bread.

Appendix

Herbal Teas

Herbal tea for menstrual cramps

Primary herbs: borage, cramp bark, peppermint, motherwort 1 tablespoon each

Secondary herbs: ginger root, valerian, chamomile 1 teaspoon each

Place the herbs in boiling water (for each tablespoon add sixteen ounces of boiling water). Simmer for twenty minutes. Strain, add honey, and drink hot. Use three to four cups daily as needed.

Herbal tea for constipation

Primary herbs: dandelion, centaury, gentian, agrimony 1 tablespoon each

Secondary herbs: senna, peach leaves, parsley 1 teaspoon each

Place the herbs in boiling water and simmer for fifteen minutes. Strain and drink one cup before bedtime for catharsis, blood cleansing, and purification.

Herbal tea for colds and coughs

Primary herbs: coltsfoot, licorice, hyssop, blood root, barberry 1 tablespoon each

Secondary herbs: lavender, ginger root, sage 1 teaspoon each

Place the herbs in boiling water and simmer for twenty minutes. Strain, add honey and fresh lemon juice to taste. Drink while hot. Take three to four cups a day as needed to relieve cold and flu.

Herbal tea for tension headache

Primary herbs: valerian, vervain, rosemary 1 tablespoon each

Secondary herbs: chamomile, hops, skullcap 1 teaspoon each

Place the herbs in boiling water. Simmer for twenty minutes. Strain, add honey, and drink hot. Take three to four cups daily.

Tension headaches are usually located at the base of the head just above the nape of the neck. Apply acupressure massage to the muscles above the nape at the base where the pain is centered. Also massage the skull and temples for ten to fifteen minutes.

Herbal tea for migraine headache

Primary herbs: feverfew leaves, rosemary, hops 1 tablespoon each

Secondary herbs: skullcap, borage, valerian, chamomile 1 teaspoon each

Fresh feverfew leaves work best for this formula. First, grind the leaves to release their flavor and medicinal properties. Place the herbs in boiling water, and simmer for at least twenty minutes. Strain, and drink with natural honey or brown sugar. Fresh fever-

few leaves can be eaten with fresh wheat bread to relieve migraine headaches

Herbal tea for high blood pressure

Primary herbs: hawthorn, yarrow 1 tablespoon each

Secondary herbs: skullcap, borage, valerian 1 teaspoon each

Place the herbs in boiling water and simmer for twenty minutes. Strain, add fresh lemon juice, and drink two cups as needed. Garlic also helps in treating high blood pressure. Daily one should either add two cloves of garlic to salad or eat one clove with bread for detoxification and keeping the blood pressure low.

Fruit tea for high blood pressure

Primary fruit: bilberry, sixteen ounces

Wash the bilberries, and soak in one-half gallon of water for several hours. Boil ten minutes, and strain. Drink cold. As an option, add a pinch of salt. Bilberry juice lowers the blood pressure immediately, cleanses and purifies the blood.

Herbal tea for cleansing the liver and gallbladder

Primary herbs: dandelion, centaury, gentian 1 tablespoon each

Secondary herbs: rosemary, peppermint, agrimony 1 teaspoon each

Place the herbs in boiling water, and simmer for at least twenty minutes. Strain, and drink two to three cups per day to cleanse aforementioned organs. Repeat once a week, especially in cases of heavy, greasy diet.

Herbal tea for kidney and bladder stones

Primary herbs: Agrimony, goldenrod, white birch 1 tablespoon each

Secondary herbs: Marshmallow root, parsley, horsetail 1 tablespoon each

Place the herbs in boiling water, and simmer for twenty minutes. Strain, and drink three to four cups a day. Drink fresh radish juice and plenty of drinking water.

Herbal tea for urinary infection

Primary herbs: Gravel root, goldenrod 1 tablespoon each

Secondary herbs: Horsetail, parsley 1 teaspoon each

Place the herbs in boiling water, and simmer for at least twenty minutes. Strain, and drink three to four cups daily. Cranberry juice, along with plenty of drinking water, is also effective in cases of urinary infections.

Herbal tea for the nervous system

Primary herbs: Skullcap, vervain, melissa 1 tablespoon each

Secondary herbs: Chamomile, passionflower, cowslip 1 teaspoon each

Place the herbs in boiling water, and simmer for at least twenty minutes. Strain, and drink hot; three to four cups daily as needed. Natural honey can be added to the tea.

Herbal tea for skin disorder

Primary herbs: Burdock root, yellow dock, blue flag 1 tablespoon each

Secondary herbs: Nettle, licorice, skullcap, chickweed 1 teaspoon each

Place the herbs in boiling water, and simmer for twenty minutes. Strain and drink three to four cups daily. Eight glasses of pure drinking water must be added to the diet.

Herbal tea for insomnia

Primary herbs: Skullcap, valerian 1 tablespoon each

Secondary herbs: Mugwort, passionflower, cowslip 1 teaspoon each

Place the herbs in boiling water, and simmer for twenty minutes. Strain, and drink one to two cups two hours before bedtime.

Glossary

Every field or profession has its technical vocabulary. Therefore it is to be expected that a number of words used by botanical pharmacology may not ring a bell in the ears of the average person. Following are some of the most important technical words pertaining to the present book.

Alcohol: A large group of compounds often found in volatile oils or in plants that contain volatile oils. An alcohol are characterized chemically by the presence of the -OH (hydroxyl) group.

Alkaloids: Chemical compounds that contain nitrogen (N2). Plants that contain alkaloids have various physical effects, including alleviating pain, reducing blood pressure, and causing spasms. Many of these compounds are very poisonous.

Alternative: Medicines, often prescribed in the form of tea, whose effect on the body is gradual, not immediately noticeable.

Antiperiodics: Substances which can allay or prevent the return of periodical symptoms, such as fever.

Antipyretic: Helps the body to lower fever. Antipyretics are found in herbs such as aloe vera, elder flower, peppermint, angelica, and pennyroyal.

Antispasmodic: Herbs containing antispasmodic help to prevent spasms or cramps such as painful menstruation, intestinal cramping, or muscle shock. Herbs in this category are black haw, cramp bark, back cohosh, chamomile, valerian, and skullcap.

Antiseptic: Any plant or chemical product that causes destruction of micro-organisms or bacteria to prevent infection or diseases.

Aromatic: A plant, drug, or medicine with a spicy scent and pungent taste. Examples: ginger, sweet flag, lavender, rosemary, rose, clove, cinnamon, and angelica. Aromatics tend to stimulate the digestive system.

Astringent: A substance that causes dehydration, tightening, or shrinking of tissue and is used to stop bleeding, close skin pores, and tighten muscle. This class of substances is found in plants such as agrimony, sage, oak bark, burdock, ginger, raspberry leaves and willow bark.

Bitter principle: Bitter principle represents a grouping of chemicals that have an exceedingly bitter taste. The bitter principles have been shown to have therapeutic effects. They stimulate the secretion of all the digestive juices and also stimulate the activity of liver and gallbladder, helping toxin elimination. They are found in herbs like gentian, dandelion, centaury, and wormwood.

Carbohydrates: Nutritional substances in plants, including sugars, starches, and polysaccharides, that combine with other substances to produce pectin and mucilage, which soothe and protect.

Cardiotonic: Herbs that have cardiac tonic effects, like hawthorn, and motherwort.

Cathartics: Substances and herbs that strongly evacuate the colon and relieve constipation. Cathartics stimulate secretions of the intestines, often with drastic physical results.

Decoction: Preparation of herbal tea made by woody, waxy, or root parts of herbs in water. They usually contain no volatile oil. Boiling may destroy the properties of the plant. A decoction without an added preservative, such as alcohol, should not be kept for long, but should be freshly prepared, especially in hot weather.

Demulcents: Herbs or medicines which are soothing to the intestinal tract, usually of an oily or mucilaginous nature. Examples: olive oil and glycerin, although they are quite different substances.

Diuretics: Herbs or medicines tending to increase the production and discharge of urine. We find diuretic properties in many herbs. They do no harm to the body; probably do good. Found in herbs like dandelion, juniper, bayberry, parsley, and yarrow.

Emetics: Chemical agents which cause vomiting. Many plants have emetics properties; some more than others. Almost everyone knows that it is not herbs alone which induce vomiting; taste, motion, and smell as well as emotional upsets will do the same.

Emollients: Materials which soothe the skin rather than internal membranes. They are moisturizers which soften, soothe, or protect the skin especially against dehydration, and they are found in herbs like comfrey, Irish moss, chickweed, and slippery elm.

Expectorant: Herbs or remedies that help the body expel excessive secretion of phlegm which accumulates in the lungs. This is accomplished by coughing, sneezing, and spitting. Many plants are valuable for this purpose.

Flatulence: Gas in the stomach or bowels. From the beginning of time herbs have been used to treat flatulence. Common examples are mint, sweet flag, and marjoram.

Flavonoid glycosides: Products of a common group of yellow plants, they have a wide variety of actions such as diuretic, circulatory stimulant, anti-inflammatory, and antispasmodic.

Glycosides: These plant chemicals are of two types: (1) those that have a strong effect on the heart, known as cardioactive glycosides (they are derived from plants like foxglove) and (2) bitter glycosides known as purgative which are blood purifying and detoxifying (they are derived from plants like gentian, dandelion, and centaury).

Infusion: Preparation method for herbal tea that consists of steeping the herbs in water by pouring boiling water over them. Usually the green parts of the herb are used (flower, leaves, and stem), and volatile oil is isolated by the method. Infusion is a simple and quick way of extracting the medicinal principle from fresh or dried plants.

Lignin: A chemical contained in plants that helps penetration of nutrients through layers of tissue and absorption of the nutrients through the body.

Mucilage: Gel-like substance with molecules made up of polysaccharides (chains of sugar units). When they soak up water, a sticky jelly is produced. Mucilage content in plants indicates they have a soothing and anti-inflammatory effect when applied on the skin, usually in cosmetics. Mucilage also protects against irritation and inflammation in the mucous membranes of the throat, lungs, kidneys, stomach, and urinary system. Found in herbs like slippery elm.

Phenol: Many plants contain this chemical compound, often combined with sugar to form glycoside that is antiseptic and reduces inflammation when taken internally. An example is salicylic acid, the natural forerunner of aspirin. Salicylic acid is found in many plants such as wintergreen and white willow. Herbs that contain phenol are antiseptic, including clove, thyme, marjoram, and bayberry.

Plant acids: These are organic acids found throughout the plant, for example, citric acid in lemon or salicylic acid in strawberry.

Purgative: Cathartics that stimulate the action of the intestines, often with drastic physical manifestations.

Saponins: Act as natural cleansers. The plants containing these chemical compounds act like a soap when mixed with water. Saponins help dissolve fat and decrease cholesterol levels. There are two kind of saponin, triterpenoid and steroid. Steroid saponins have a direct effect on hormonal activity. They are found in herbs like licorice. Triterpenoid saponins have a strong expectorant effect, and they also help in the absorption of nutrients. They are found in herbs like cowslip root.

Sedative: Any herb that reduces nervous tension and aids relaxation.

Tannins: Plants containing chemical compounds like tannins usually react with protein to produce a leather-like coating; they promote healing and numbing; they reduce inflammation and irritation. Tannins contract tissues of the body, drawing them together and improving the resistance to infection.

Tinctures: Infusion describes a solution of organic material in water, but tincture refers to a solution in alcohol. Many plants have their properties locked up in oil, resin, or wax which is not soluble in water. Where the plant material is in the form of sugars, salts, or gums, warm or cold infusions will dissolve the medicinal substance. You can make tinctures with plants that contain oil. Use only medicinal grade alcohol with the plants. Let the mixture stand for two to three weeks, strain, and take two to three tablespoons a day as needed.

Volatile oils: Plants contain these chemical compounds which are natural alcohol; they usually act as antiseptic and antibacterial agents; they have a strong aroma and taste. Volatile oils are a mixture of 50% alcohol and 50% hydrocarbon, and they often enhance the moisture-retaining properties of a plant's leaves.

Waxes: Combinations of an alcohol and a fatty acid.

Yin Yang: The female and male principles of polarity in Chinese remedies.

Index